D1349046

Intra-operative Diagnosis of CNS Tumours

INTRA-OPERATIVE DIAGNOSIS OF CNS TUMOURS

Tim H. Moss MB ChB PhD FRCPath

Consultant Neuropathologist, Frenchay Hospital, and Honorary Senior Clinical Lecturer in
Neuropathology, Bristol University, Bristol, UK

James A.R. Nicoll BSc MB ChB MD MRCPath

Senior Lecturer in Neuropathology, University of Glasgow, and Honorary Consultant in
Neuropathology, Institute of Neurological Sciences, Southern General Hospital NHS Trust,
Glasgow, UK

James W. Ironside BMSc MB ChB FRCPath

Senior Lecturer in Pathology, University of Edinburgh, and Honorary Consultant in
Neuropathology, Western General Hospital, Edinburgh, UK

ARNOLD
A Member of the Hodder Headline Group
LONDON • SYDNEY • AUCKLAND
Copublished in the USA by Oxford University Press, Inc. New York

First published in Great Britain 1997
Arnold, a member of the Hodder Headline Group,
338 Euston Road, London NW1 3BH

Co-published in the United States of America by
Oxford University Press, Inc.,
198 Madison Avenue, New York, NY10016
Oxford is a registered trademark of Oxford University Press

British Library Cataloguing in Publication Data
A catalogue record for this book is available from the British Library

Library of Congress Cataloging-in-Publication Data
A catalog record for this book is available from the Library of Congress

ISBN 0 340 67737 6

Publisher: Georgina Bentliff
Production Editor: James Rabson
Production Controller: Sarah Kett
Cover designer: Terry Griffiths
Composition by Scribe Design, Gillingham, Kent
Colour reproductions by DP Graphics, Holt, Wiltshire
Printed and bound by Bath Press Colour Books, Glasgow

CONTENTS

Despite the considerable advances in tumour imaging and localizing techniques seen in the last decade, neurosurgeons continue to have good reason to seek intraoperative advice from pathologists, perhaps more so than their general surgical colleagues. Lesions requiring a diagnostic biopsy which are deeply seated in the central nervous system often cannot be sampled under direct vision, and the need to cause minimal disturbance to adjacent areas of eloquent brain places additional restrictions on a surgeon seeking diagnostic tissue for paraffin histology. Even when a large craniotomy is performed, surgeons planning to remove or debulk intrinsic tumours with diffusely infiltrating margins will often be influenced in the extent of their procedure by intra-operative confirmation of the histological type or malignant grade of the lesion. As in any surgical discipline, there will also inevitably be occasions when pre-operative investigation fails to suggest a likely diagnosis for an intracranial lesion, and the nature of the surgery must be guided almost entirely by the pathologist's intra-operative advice.

Owing to the generally soft texture of central nervous tissue and many of its neoplasms, the neuropathologist is not restricted to cryostat sectioning for giving intra-operative advice, but also has the option of using the smear cytology technique. Frozen sections have been the mainstay for rapid diagnosis of central nervous system tumours in the past, and are still used routinely in some neuropathology laboratories today, but smear cytology has become increasingly accepted as an alternative approach. The earliest advocates were Eisenhardt and Cushing in the late 1920s,[1] and the currently used wet film method was brought in by Dorothy Russell a few years later.[2] More recently, intra-operative smears have been popularized by the neuropathology department at the Institute of Neurological Sciences in Glasgow, who acquired considerable practical experience of the technique in the early 1970s.[3,4]

Although smear preparations have contributed enormously to the intra-operative diagnosis of central nervous system tumours, it should be emphasized that the technique is by no means always possible or infallible, and there remain instances when frozen sections need to be used, either in preference to smears or occasionally in conjunction with them. Some tumours occurring within the central nervous system are simply too tough to smear satisfactorily, whilst in other situations the diagnosis does not become apparent without the architectural features of the lesion, which may be lacking in smear preparations. This book concentrates on the use of smear cytology in intra-operative diagnosis, but draws attention to the possible need for frozen sectioning wherever this is felt to be important. Chapter 18 in particular deals with the best approach to central

nervous system lesions which are not usually soft enough to make satisfactory smear preparations.

Intra-operative diagnosis relies heavily on knowledge of the clinical circumstances and can almost never be undertaken satisfactorily if smears or frozen sections are interpreted in isolation. Details of the patient, the radiological features of the lesion and the surgeon's observations all need to be taken into account when drawing up a shortlist of possible differential diagnoses, and will help to maximize the information yielded by the microscopic findings. Sometimes simply knowing the precise site of a tumour can enable a confident diagnosis to be made when the appearance of a smear or frozen section cannot be regarded as entirely specific for a particular tumour. The signal characteristics of the lesion on radiological scans or even just the age of the patient can also be equally important in this respect, and ideally the pathologist should be able to discuss all these details directly with the surgeon before attempting to come to any firm conclusion. This guide emphasizes the significance of clinical information in each of the sections describing individual tumour types, paying particular attention to the way that diagnostic possibilities suggested by the intra-operative pathology can be refined by details such as the patient's age, the location of the tumour and its gross appearance at surgery. In addition, Chapter 6 is devoted entirely to this topic, giving checklists and a general overview of the possible differential diagnoses relating to varying clinical circumstances.

Our intention has been to provide a practical work of reference rather than just an atlas of micrographs, but the examination of smears and frozen sections is obviously a highly visual exercise and the text has been heavily illustrated. Help is more likely to be needed when the classical features of a lesion are not apparent and care has been taken to include difficult and atypical cases alongside those showing the more expected appearance of each tumour type. The figures are all in full colour because even with a fundamentally monochrome stain like toluidine blue, illustration in black and white often fails to convey the tinctorial subtleties which are so important when seen down the microscope. Staining practice for central nervous system smears varies between different institutions, but haematoxylin-eosin and toluidine blue are by far the most commonly used stains, and most pathologists tend to base their experience almost exclusively on one or the other in routine practice. Smears from the same tumour can appear surprisingly different down the microscope depending on which stain is used, and so representative fields illustrating both haematoxylin-eosin and toluidine blue staining have been included in each chapter, sometimes in direct parallel to each other. For frozen sections, haematoxylin-eosin is almost inevitably the stain of choice and has been used throughout.

The information contained in this book is aimed primarily at neuropathologists, since it is they who usually have to provide intra-operative advice during neurosurgical operations. It is designed to be used not only by those in training, but as a practical bench reference for pathologists at all levels of experience. The process of giving intra-operative advice during neurosurgical procedures remains a continuous learning process throughout the course of a professional career, and possible differential diagnoses are less likely to be overlooked in the heat of the moment if a suitable source of reference is always readily to hand. Even for experienced individuals, it is also reassuring to be able to check the cytological features of lesions which are displaying an atypical appearance in smear preparations, or those which are only rarely encountered in routine practice. In addition to neuropathologists, there are general histopathologists who are sometimes called upon to provide intra-operative advice for neurosurgeons, and this book may perhaps encourage them to consider smear cytology as an alternative to frozen sections on these occasions. Finally, we would recommend it to the neurosurgeons themselves, who need to understand the strengths and limitations of intra-operative smear cytology and how they can help to optimize the information it yields. The surgeon not only plays an important part in the selection of the tissue sample for smearing or sectioning, but must also decide when to seek diagnostic advice in the first place, and consider how information about the nature of the lesion being operated on might alter the immediate surgical management of the patient. In the end, good intra-operative diagnostic practice is a matter of close co-operation and mutual understanding between surgeon and pathologist, who both need to be equally aware of what it involves and what can be achieved.

ACKNOWLEDGEMENTS

We would like to thank Ms B.A. Mackenzie and Mrs M. Hughes for secretarial assistance and the MLSO staff in each of our laboratories for their invaluable technical support throughout this project. We are also indebted to our neurosurgical colleagues in Bristol, Glasgow and Edinburgh, with whom we work to provide a diagnostic service, both during and after surgery.

References

1. Eisenhardt L, Cushing H. Diagnosis of intracranial tumours by supravital technique. *Am J Pathol* 1930; **6**: 541–52.
2. Russell D S, Krayenbuhl H, Cairns H. The wet film technique in the histological diagnosis of intracranial tumours: A rapid method. *J Pathol Bacteriol* 1937; **45**: 501–505.
3. Marshall L F, Adams H, Doyle D, Graham D I. The histological accuracy of the smear technique for neurosurgical biopsies. *J Neurosurg* 1973; **39**: 83–8.
4. Berkeley B B, Adams J H, Doyle D, Graham D I, Harper C G. The smear technique in the diagnosis of neurosurgical biopsies. *N Z Med J* 1978; **87**: 12–15.

The Role of Intra-operative Diagnosis in Neurosurgical Practice

1.1. Indications for the Use of Rapid Diagnostic Techniques

The main indications for seeking intra-operative advice on central nervous system tumours can be summarized as follows:

1. **Where knowledge of the precise nature of a tumour will affect the surgeon's intra-operative management during a definitive surgical procedure.** This often involves guiding a decision on how radical an excision should be attempted, either because the malignant grade of the lesion is relevant to this, or perhaps because the operative findings are not those expected from the clinical and radiological features.
2. **Where the object of the surgical procedure is to obtain biopsy material for a definitive paraffin section diagnosis.** This is often in the context of a freehand or guided needle biopsy, and careful division of each sample is needed to ensure that the smears or frozen sections give a result which will also be represented in the paraffin sections. The intra-operative result safeguards the surgeon against being in the wrong location, or inadvertently sampling purely necrotic or reactive tissue associated with the lesion. The main point of the exercise lies in achieving a definitive histological diagnosis rather than altering immediate surgical management. It is therefore worth noting that the smear or frozen section in these circumstances does not necessarily have to give a precise diagnosis in its own right, merely the information that the tissue sampled is likely to prove diagnostic in paraffin sections.
3. **Where a radical excision is being performed on a tumour of known diagnosis and the surgeon needs help in defining the margins of the lesion with adjacent brain tissue.** The diagnosis may have been confirmed by a previous biopsy or by a sample taken earlier in the same procedure. This is usually most relevant to infiltrating gliomas, where the margins of solid tumour with more diffusely involved brain are not obvious macroscopically, or where the surgical activity is close to eloquent areas of central nervous tissue which are still clinically functional.

The pre-operative diagnosis of central nervous system tumours has become increasingly refined over recent years due to the introduction of sophisticated imaging techniques, most notably computerized tomography and magnetic resonance. In many cases, the availability of techniques like these means that the surgeon has a very good idea of the likely nature of an intracranial or spinal mass lesion before operating and can plan the operative procedure with some confidence. If the likely diagnosis is available pre-operatively in this way, and assuming that the findings at operation are typical and the lesion is in need of radical resection, then there may be little call to seek diagnostic advice at all during surgery. Examples might include uncomplicated pituitary adenomas or meningiomas which have been readily identified by pre-operative imaging and prove straight forward to resect. To request an intra-operative smear or frozen section in such cases is not likely to be of any value to the surgeon and may simply waste the pathologist's time. It must be remembered, however, that even sophisticated pre-operative investigations can prove misleading, and if the appearances at operation are not those expected for the presumptive diagnosis, the situation changes entirely. A surgeon embarked on a procedure appropriate for one type of tumour but confronted by the macroscopic features of something quite unexpected is perhaps more in need of urgent help from the pathologist than at any other time.

A different situation arises when pre-operative investigation fails to give a clear indication of the likely nature of the lesion and a decision is made to perform a biopsy as initial procedure, specifically to obtain a tissue diagnosis. If the tumour is being biopsied under direct vision through a small craniotomy and the surgeon does not wish to proceed any further, then intra-operative advice may again be unnecessary, always assuming that the abnormal tissue is easily identifiable macroscopically. However, in many instances there is good cause to check that the biopsied tissue is likely to prove diagnostic after processing for paraffin histology. This is especially the case when deep lesions are being sampled 'blindly' or using image-guided or stereotactic needle techniques. So long as each sample obtained is divided in a representative way, a smear or frozen section of one portion of the biopsied tissue may save the embarrassment of a wasted procedure and the risk to the patient that a repeat operation involves. In our experience, this use of intra-operative advice is sometimes misunderstood, especially by more junior surgical staff, and the pathologist arrives at the operating theatre door with the news that the tissue sample submitted is non-diagnostic only to find the patient already in the recovery room. Reassurances that 'plenty more' has been sampled for paraffin histology frequently prove fruitless in these circumstances, since all the samples are usually taken in close proximity to each other, and if one is necrotic or simply reactive in nature, they all turn out to be. Another problem arises when the sample submitted intra-operatively shows diagnostic tumour material, but because part of it was not held back for formalin fixation, and differently located samples used for this, the paraffin sections again fail to give a definitive diagnosis. Finally, when only tiny amounts of tissue can be biopsied for technical reasons, these pitfalls must be set against the risk of wasting valuable diagnostic material by attempting to make intra-operative smears or frozen sections at all. This can sometimes jeopardize the definitive paraffin histology diagnosis in circumstances where the intra-operative result was not going to alter the immediate surgical management. Situations where this dilemma might need to be addressed include ventriculoscopic biopsies being performed through a burr hole, and biopsies from eloquent areas such as the brainstem or cord in patients with minimal or no clinical deficit.

When considering the role of smear preparations, it is worth remembering that use of the technique need not be confined to the intra-operative period. In situations where the diagnosis is not known at the time of surgery but will not alter the immediate surgical management, a 'cold' smear, i.e. one that is fixed but not stained or examined immediately, can provide a useful interim security measure in the period before definitive histology results are available. This is most useful where a mass lesion needs emergency decompression regardless of its nature, and no pathologist is available to give intra-operative advice. Should the patient's condition deteriorate post-operatively and the diagnosis thus become urgently needed to guide decisions on further management, the smear can be stained and examined in advance of the paraffin sections. An example might be where post-operative haemorrhage follows debulking of an astrocytic tumour of unknown malignancy, and further intervention is only considered justified if the lesion is of low grade. A related situation occurs when a smear or frozen section was not made at all, or failed to give a decisive result, but an early diagnosis again becomes necessary to aid decisions on immediate post-operative management. In such circumstances it may be worth having an enclosed tissue processor with an emergency short processing schedule. If some of the biopsy tissue is earmarked for this immediately after it becomes apparent that the intra-operative preparations are unsatisfactory, then preliminary paraffin sections can sometimes be examined within only a few hours of surgery and a clinical dilemma averted.

1.2. THE SMEAR TECHNIQUE: ADVANTAGES AND LIMITATIONS

Smear cytology has become increasingly popular in the last few decades as an alternative to frozen sections for the rapid diagnosis of central nervous system tumours. The soft texture of most of these lesions lends itself particularly well to the smear technique, which has many practical advantages over cryostat sectioning, and is used in preference in many contemporary neuropathology laboratories. The technique is not infallible, however, and its limitations need to be clearly understood so that it can be employed effectively, and where appropriate in conjunction with intra-operative frozen sections.

The main advantages of smear cytology for intra-operative diagnosis are as follows:

1. **Speed.** Results are available much more quickly than with the cryostat. This can save valuable time when repeated intra-operative samples are needed, for example to guide the surgeon to the correct location, or to give information on the margins of infiltrating tumour.
2. **Ease of preparation.** Creating and staining smear preparations are easy skills to acquire and results can be of consistently high quality even in relatively inexperienced hands. If so desired, the surgeons can smear the tissue themselves, thus ensuring that the areas of interest down the operating microscope are the ones that are examined by the pathologist. For out-of-hours cases, most pathologists can quickly learn to prepare and stain the smears without the need to call in a laboratory scientist.
3. **Technical simplicity.** No specialized equipment is needed and smears can be prepared and stained easily in a small area using only an extraction hood/cabinet. If the main pathology laboratory is some distance away, this makes it easy to set up a diagnostic 'out station' within the operating suite, to facilitate more direct communication with the surgeon at the time of surgery.
4. **Cytological preservation.** As with other cytological techniques, smears give a very high quality of cytological information in comparison with that available from cryostat sections. Nuclear detail in particular forms a very important role in the interpretation of smear preparations.
5. **Small sample size.** Large areas of smeared tissue can be examined from a very small sample, thus maximizing the information available when there are technical limitations on the size of the biopsy. This is especially important when stereotactic or ventriculoscopic procedures are being used.

Important limitations of the technique include:

1. It relies on the tissue or lesion being soft enough to smear out satisfactorily. This is most often the case for central nervous lesions, but by no means always

so. Even intrinsic tumours can become too tough to smear if they have undergone desmoplasia, and some types of glial tumour, including subependymomas, can make very poor smears simply because they are naturally very dense, fibrillary lesions. In general, systemic tissues make poor smears and tumours arising from non-CNS elements need assessing on an individual basis. Some meningiomas and nerve sheath tumours, for example, are ideal candidates for smear preparations, whilst others produce impenetrably thick results unsuitable for diagnostic purposes. Where smears are attempted on tissues which are really too tough, excess pressure may be needed to get a thin enough film and this frequently results in mechanical smear artefacts which again make the end result unsatisfactory (see Chapter 4). It is worth noting that calcification in a tumour does not necessarily exclude the smear technique, as may be the case with frozen sections. On the contrary, calcospherites in a glial tumour or psammoma bodies in a meningioma may provide useful diagnostic clues in the smear.

2. The currently available experience of interpreting smear preparations is very largely confined to lesions of central nervous tissue and its immediate coverings, with a few notable exceptions such as Schwannomas, lymphomas and some intracerebral metastases. Even where systemic tumours *are* soft enough to attempt smear cytology, the microscopic features may be confusing to interpret for most pathologists, beyond perhaps an estimation of likely malignancy. In consequence, it is probably better to plan a frozen section from the outset for lesions such as extradural tumours of the skull base and spine.

3. Whilst smear preparations give excellent cytological detail, much of the familiar histological architecture of tumours is not apparent. Examples include typical vascular patterns, tumour cell palisades and most types of rosette, including those of ependymomas and primitive neuroectodermal tumours. There are again notable exceptions, such as the whorls of meningiomas, but many of the visual cues which pathologists rely on in paraffin and frozen sections are absent in smears. In their place, a different set of features are 'artefactually' produced by the mechanics of the smearing process, for example the perivascular papillary formations of astrocytic tumours, and with suitable experience these can become equally helpful.

4. Like any other sampling procedure, the effectiveness of the smear technique relies on accurate localization by the surgeon. Many glioblastomas, for example, have entirely necrotic centres and a wide surrounding area of diffusely infiltrated brain or cord. Tissue inadvertently sampled from such areas can easily produce non-diagnostic or even misleading results. The smaller fragments of tissue used to make smear preparations probably make them more vulnerable in this respect than frozen sections, although with smears it is easier and quicker to

compensate by examining material from several different locations in the area of abnormality. In addition, the use of stereotactic and computer guidance techniques in neurosurgery has greatly improved the accuracy of sampling for intra-operative smear preparations in recent years.

1.3. ROLE OF INTRA-OPERATIVE CRYOSTAT SECTIONS

Even in laboratories dedicated to the use of smear cytology, cryostat sectioning continues to play an important role in the rapid diagnosis of CNS tumours. In practice, however, the frequency with which it is employed is very much a matter of personal preference. Some pathologists will only resort to the cryostat if the tissue sampled is so tough that it cannot be smeared at all, or the results are too thick to be useful. This means that the need to perform frozen sections can be avoided in a high proportion of intra-operative requests, but has the disadvantage of prolonging the time taken to reach a conclusion should the smears prove unsatisfactory in the event. In other laboratories, smear preparations and cryostat sections are routinely undertaken in parallel on all intra-operative requests. Such a protocol avoids creating further delay if the smear preparations turn out to be inconclusive, and also provides the pathologist with the diagnostic advantages of both techniques on all cases. It could well be argued that such a 'belt and braces' policy represents the gold standard for the intra-operative diagnosis of CNS tumours, but given the high proportion of cases in which smear cytology alone provides adequate information, many would regard the extra time, trouble and expense of this approach as unwarranted, especially for out-of-hours requests. A middle course can be adopted by relying on smear preparations in the first instance, but only after taking into account the individual details of each case. It is often possible to tell in advance whether biopsy tissue is unlikely to smear satisfactorily, as for example with orbital, skull base or extradural spinal lesions, and thus arrange to cut frozen sections from the outset in such cases.

Whatever approach is adopted, it still needs to be recognized that the increased work and delay of cutting frozen sections will prove necessary in some circumstances, if only because the cytological information does not enable sufficiently detailed diagnostic comment to be made, and the pathologist is hoping for further clues. Despite taking into account all the available clinical and radiological data, the information available from some smear preparations may not be sufficiently specific to satisfy a particular surgical dilemma, and this is clearly not something which can be predicted in advance. Regardless of individual policy, therefore, we feel that it is advisable for the pathologist to maintain the option of examining frozen sections in any intra-operative request, even if this is only kept in reserve as a back-up procedure.

To summarize, the *minimum* indications for the use of intra-operative frozen sections follow on directly from the limitations of the smear technique outlined in the previous section, and can be broadly grouped into the following two categories:

1. **The tissue is unsuitable for smearing.** This can sometimes be predicted in advance, or the surgeon may be confronted by an unexpectedly tough lesion at operation. Occasionally it may appear possible to create a smear using rather more pressure than normal, but after staining it is either found to be too thick or the cytological detail is obscured by crush artefact. In addition to tumours with a tough texture, a number of other types of lesion are intrinsically unsuited to the smear technique for differing reasons. These include many forms of cysts, especially those with an epithelial lining, vascular malformations and primary lipoid tumours, where the adipocytic cells tend to fracture on smearing. These and related problems are discussed in more detail in Chapter 18.

2. **The smear is technically adequate, but fails to give the pathologist sufficient diagnostic information.** This may simply be due to a lack of personal experience on the part of the pathologist, or perhaps because of a genuinely atypical or inconclusive cytological appearance. The need to cut frozen sections in such a situation will be at least partly dependant on the reasons for seeking intra-operative advice in the first place. For example, when the procedure is being performed purely to obtain material that will be diagnostic in paraffin sections, intra-operative comment can usually be limited to confirmation that viable tumour is present. In contrast, a surgeon embarked on a major debulking procedure is likely to press for as precise a diagnosis as possible if the findings are not those expected, or if the surgery proves unusually problematic. There is, of course, no guarantee that cryostat sections will be of any more practical help than the smear in these circumstances, but it is nevertheless always an option worth exploring and in our experience further diagnostic comment is very often possible.

1.4. ACCURACY OF INTRA-OPERATIVE DIAGNOSIS

Even where there is time to apply routine techniques, surgical pathology cannot be regarded as an exact science, and the pathologist's final report may sometimes have to be a matter of opinion rather than a single, unarguable conclusion. By comparison with paraffin section histology, the comment possible from urgent intra-operative smear cytology is more often likely to fall short of a single, confident diagnosis which can be easily audited against the final outcome. Despite its speed and simplicity, the technique clearly lacks many of the advantages that a histological section can confer, and for this reason should always be regarded as an interim measure pending more definitive information. To a certain extent, the same is true of intra-operative frozen sections. Extra information may sometimes become available down the microscope, but urgent cryostat histology still deprives the pathologist of many of the advantages of routine paraffin methods, including special stains and immunocytochemistry. Moreover, the pathologist's assessment of an intra-operative request stems not just from interpretation of the cytology or cryostat histology down the microscope, but relies heavily on a subjective appraisal of the clinical and radiological details in each individual case. All these observations need to be born in mind when attempting to judge the diagnostic accuracy of rapid intra-operative preparations. It should also be remembered that it is possible to provide useful information without knowing the precise diagnosis, and from the surgeon's point of view, *successful* intra-operative comment does not necessarily have to be diagnostic or even totally conclusive.

Having said all this, our personal experience of using smear cytology in the diagnosis of central nervous system tumours has been very encouraging, and there have been very few occasions where the intra-operative conclusion has proved to be totally incorrect or misleading once the result of paraffin histology is available. It should be emphasized that this recommendation assumes that cryostat sections can also be examined if the smears prove unsatisfactory or difficult to interpret. Struggling with cytology alone in these circumstances will inevitably increase the risk of seriously misleading the surgeon. For this reason, any formal audit of intra-operative diagnosis in neurosurgery should ideally assess the outcome when the two techniques are used in collaboration, but there are unfortunately no published studies of this type. A single, rather old review of 412 intra-operative frozen section examinations performed without smear cytology has reported only a 76% concordance with the paraffin section result when the criterion used was the definitive histological type of the tumour[1]. However, this figure rose to 90% when assessment of malignancy was compared, and the authors concluded that the technique could be used with almost complete assurance to distinguish non-neoplastic tissues from true tumours and primary glial lesions from metastatic ones. It was therefore emphasized that the results must be interpreted in the light of what the surgeon needs to know at the time of surgery, rather than as an absolute comparison with the paraffin section result. The largest series examining the diagnostic accuracy of intra-operative smear preparations comes from the Institute of Neurological Sciences in Glasgow, where smear cytology alone led to a correct diagnosis in 94% of 609 surgical cases.[2] The effect of the intra-operative result on the surgeon was again emphasized, and it was noted that in only 1.8% of the series could the pathologist's report have adversely affected the immediate management of the patient.

It is probably reasonable to conclude that smear cytology is a useful, safe and reliable technique for giving intra-operative advice, so long as its limitations are clearly understood. The routine use of frozen sections in isolation is unlikely to prove any more reliable, and the best results of all will almost certainly come from judicious use of the two approaches in conjunction with each other. Neither technique can be really effective without full knowledge of the clinical circumstances, both to guide interpretation down the microscope and to help understanding of how much the surgeon needs to know at the time of operating. If intra-operative diagnosis is regarded as a purely interim measure, then the pathologist's comment can be tailored to the amount of information available and the reason for seeking advice in the first place. In this way, it is nearly always possible to avoid giving misleading advice, even where the smears are technically difficult or have an inconclusive microscopic appearance.

References

1. Groves R, Hesselvik M The diagnostic accuracy of the frozen section examination in neurosurgery. *Acta Neurol Scand* 1966; **42**: 268–74.
2. Hume Adams J, Graham D I, Doyle D *Brain biopsy. The smear technique for neurosurgical biopsies.* Chapman & Hall, London, 1981.

TWO
PREPARATION AND STAINING OF SMEARS

2.1. LOGISTICS

A pre-requisite for the provision of a service for rapid intra-operative diagnosis is good communications between the operating room and the laboratory. This is essential both for rapid transport of the specimens and communication of results and ideally is achieved by close proximity of the laboratory to the operating theatre. However, the situation is clearly dictated by local geography and if the main laboratory is located at some distance in the same hospital, or on a different site altogether, it may be appropriate to have a satellite laboratory in the operating suite. The pathologist is called to the satellite laboratory when an intra-operative diagnosis is required. The minimum equipment it needs to contain includes a ventilated safety cabinet for handling the tissue and a microscope. If the facility also provides for examination of frozen sections then a cryostat is required with possible duplication of expensive equipment in the main laboratory. A further advantage of the pathologist working in close proximity to the operating room is the ability to view the relevant scans. In any case, direct dialogue between the pathologist and the surgeon is recommended to allow discussion of the clinical history, the radiographic and operative findings and the pathological features in order to achieve a specific diagnosis or to narrow the differential diagnosis (see Chapter 5). This is particularly important when the pathological findings are equivocal or non-diagnostic and further specimens may need to be sent by the surgeon.

In some centres in which smear preparations are the method of choice for rapid intra-operative diagnosis the arrangement is for the neurosurgeon to select the tissue to be smeared and to make the smear preparations in the operating room, from where they are transported to the laboratory in fixative. However in many centres fresh tissue is sent from the neurosurgical theatre to the laboratory; there are a number of advantages to this arrangement and we regard it as preferable. If fresh tissue is received in the laboratory samples can be selected from multiple areas of a specimen for smearing. If a first set of smears is non-diagnostic then it is possible to return to the specimen to make further smear preparations. If it is felt that frozen sections may be helpful, then these can be prepared without having to request more tissue from the operating theatre specifically for this purpose. Tissue may be selected for fixation in glutaraldehyde for subsequent electron microscopy if it is thought that this may aid in the diagnostic process. Samples may be sent for microbiological analysis if the results of smears suggest that the lesion may represent an infective process. Tissue can be frozen readily and stored for subsequent genetic or histochemical analysis.

If fresh tissue is sent from the operating theatre to the laboratory it should be carried in a tightly closed container within a polythene bag and transported rapidly so that it does not dry out and the diagnosis is not delayed. The specimen should be labelled with patient identification data and accompanied by a request form on which is written corresponding patient identification data and relevant clinical information including the site of the lesion and a brief history. The laboratory must be prepared to receive the specimen, either by being in a perpetual state of readiness during operating hours or by having advance warning for each individual specimen. On arrival in the laboratory the specimen is logged into the departmental information system.

2.2. SELECTION OF TISSUE

It is essential to respect the potential safety hazards of fresh central nervous tissue. The tissue which has been removed from the patient may be potentially infective: consider, for example, HIV, hepatitis B, tuberculosis, herpes simplex virus and Creutzfeldt Jakob disease. Central nervous tissue may contain as yet unknown infective agents responsible, for example, for dementia or oncogenesis. Fresh tissue should be handled entirely within an appropriate ventilated safety cabinet subjected to regular maintenance inspections. The specimen should be handled whilst wearing disposable gloves, on a disposable surface and preferably with disposable instruments.

The size of the specimen may dictate how it is handled. With small specimens there is little scope for choosing which areas to sample. This is especially so for stereotactic biopsies or small biopsies from brainstem or spinal cord lesions when the question is often whether or not to smear at all (see Chapter 1). If tissue is limited only smears should be made because frozen sections consume more tissue. With larger resection specimens selection of the area to sample is more important. With experience, on macroscopic examination of the specimen there is usually little difficulty in identifying normal grey and white matter. Areas of solid tumour, or other pathology, are identified by alterations in colour and texture. Intrinsic tumours are often grey or brown in colour and firmer than brain tissue. Central nervous tissue which is diffusely infiltrated by glial tumour may look macroscopically normal but feel abnormally tough or rubbery in texture. Necrosis, identified by its very soft pus-like consistency, and areas of haemorrhage are often found in high grade tumours. These areas are best avoided for the purposes of intra-operative diagnosis as viable tissue is required to classify the tumour. Larger specimens allow the possibility of making frozen sections in addition to, or instead of smears; it is then the choice of the pathologist to use one or other method, or both. If sufficient tissue is available frozen sections have the advantage of sampling a greater cross-sectional area. On the other hand several smear preparations may be made from different parts of a large specimen. Frozen sections alone are prepared if the tissue is too tough to smear satisfactorily. If the material is largely calcified, soft areas are sought; if no suitable areas of tissue are found then imprint preparations may be made (see Chapter 18).

2.3. MAKING SMEAR PREPARATIONS

When the tissue samples have been inspected and an area of interest selected, a 1–2 mm cube of tissue is dissected with a scalpel and placed at one end of a clean slide, previously labelled with the patient's name and the laboratory number. A second glass slide is used to lightly compress the tissue and is then slid rapidly along to make a smear of the tissue. The pressure required to make satisfactory smears depends to a large extent on the consistency of the tissue. If the tissue is pressed too firmly then crush artefact is introduced. If too little pressure is applied the smears may be too thick for satisfactory interpretation. With experience and persistence even quite tough tissue, such as that from a fibrous meningioma, can be smeared satisfactorily. Chapter 18 suggests how to deal with lesions which may be difficult to smear. A remarkable amount of useful information can be obtained while smearing the tissue. For example, with experience it is usually possible to gain a good idea as to whether the tissue smeared is relatively normal central nervous tissue or tumour or other abnormal tissue. Special mention is made of pituitary lesions: adenomas are usually significantly softer to smear than pituitary gland. This provides useful additional information when attempting the difficult task of distinguishing intra-operatively between anterior pituitary gland and adenoma.

When the smears have been made the remaining tissue should be returned to the specimen pot and the lid replaced to prevent it drying out. It may make sense to leave the residual tissue unfixed for the time being in case further smears or frozen sections are subsequently

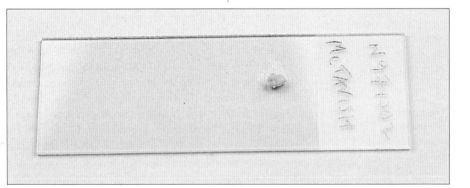

Figure 2.1
To make a smear preparation a 1–2 mm diameter piece of tissue is placed at one end of the slide

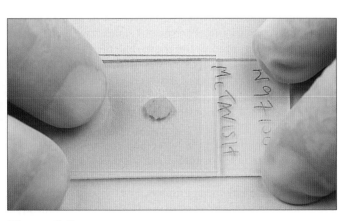

Figure 2.2
The tissue is compressed lightly with a second slide

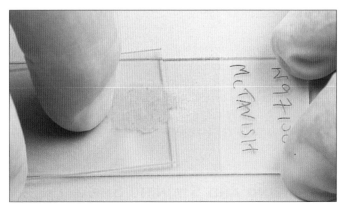

Figure 2.3
The second slide is drawn rapidly along to smear the tissue. The index finger of the right hand is controlling the pressure exerted on the tissue. The pressure is modulated according to the toughness of the tissue to make a satisfactory smear.

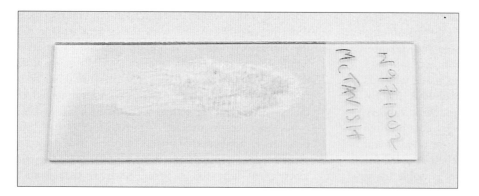

Figure 2.4
The completed smear which is immersed into fixative and stained without delay

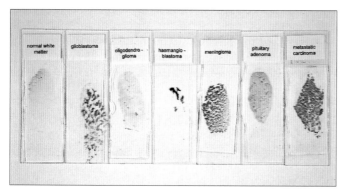

Figure 2.5
The smear preparation has been stained with toluidine blue and coverslipped and is ready for examination under the microscope

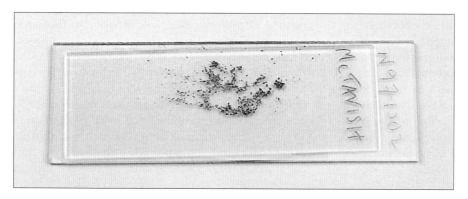

Figure 2.6
Different types of tumours smear with very different patterns which can be appreciated when the preparations are made. Oligodendrogliomas and pituitary adenomas smear uniformly, with little cohesion between the cells, in a similar fashion to brain tissue. In contrast, glioblastomas, metastatic carcinomas and most meningiomas tend to form clumps of cells which are visible to the naked eye. Tough tumours, such as the haemangioblastoma illustrated here, smear poorly.

required. For example if the tissue is too tough to have smeared well, or if examination of the smear preparations suggests that information about the tumour architecture may be diagnostically helpful (e.g. in a suspected ependymoma), the specimen can be re-examined and further samples taken.

2.4. FIXING AND STAINING SMEAR PREPARATIONS

When the smear preparations have been made they should be immersed in fixative immediately before they dry out. For tough tissue which has smeared poorly a short period of air drying of up to a minute may be found to benefit adhesion of the tissue to the slide during the subsequent staining procedure. Different departments vary somewhat in their preferred fixative. Many departments use 95% alcohol (industrial methylated spirit). Some find that the addition of small quantities of either acetone or acetic acid is beneficial, particularly if the smears are to be stained with haematoxylin and eosin. Others have a preference for fixation in a mixture of 50% ether and 50% alcohol. It should be noted however that this mixture has a potential risk of explosion if stored in an operating theatre where diathermy is used. In the absence of a long standing favourite fixative it is probably appropriate to adopt a policy of trial and error, starting with one of the standard choices, to find a fixative which suits local circumstances and the choice of staining method.

A number of staining methods may be used including toluidine blue, haematoxylin and eosin, methylene blue and Papanicalaou. The various stains have their relative advantages and disadvantages but the preference of an individual pathologist relates largely to the stain with which most familiarity has been gained. Our preference is to stain with toluidine blue or haematoxylin and eosin and a method for staining with each of these is shown in Table 2.1. Staining with toluidine blue has an advantage in being a faster and more simple method. Toluidine blue has additional advantages for smears of glial tumours as it highlights cytoplasmic processes by staining them metachromatically. On the other hand, haematoxylin and eosin has advantages in certain situations, for example it can help in the difficult process of distinguishing pituitary adenoma from anterior pituitary gland by showing variation in the staining intensity of cytoplasm in the latter. Some laboratories prefer to run both stains in parallel to obtain the

Table 2.1

Staining methods for smear preparations

Toluidine blue
1. Rinse slides briefly in water
2. Stain with 1% aqueous toluidine blue for 30–60 seconds
3. Rinse slides briefly in water
4. Dehydrate rapidly through a graded series of alcohol (e.g. 95%, 99%, 99%)
5. Clear in xylene or alternative clearing agent (e.g. Histoclear)
6. Mount using a suitable synthetic mounting medium

Haematoxylin and eosin
1. Rinse slides briefly in water
2. Stain in haematoxylin (e.g. Harris's haematoxylin or Mayer's haemalum) for 60 seconds
3. Rinse slides briefly in water
4. Differentiate in acid alcohol (e.g. 1% hydrochloric acid in 70% alcohol) for a few seconds
5. Rinse slides briefly in water
6. Blue in Scott's tap water substitute for a few seconds
7. Rinse slides briefly in water
8. Counterstain with 0.5% eosin for 30 seconds
9. Rinse slides briefly in water
10. Dehydrate rapidly through a graded series of alcohol (e.g. 95%, 99%, 99%)
11. Clear in xylene or alternative clearing agent (e.g. Histoclear)
12. Mount using a suitable synthetic mounting medium

benefits of both methods. In the final analysis it is a question of using a method, or methods of choice, in a consistent manner to maximize experience.

While staining the preparations it is important that they are handled gently so as not to dislodge the smeared tissue. This happens relatively rarely but may do so if the tissue has been tough and smeared poorly, forming thick clumps upon the slide. After staining the smears are dehydrated, cleared and mounted. Stained smear preparations can be under the microscope being examined as little as 5 minutes after the specimen has arrived in the laboratory. After a diagnosis has been made and reported to the operating theatre the remainder of the specimen should be fixed in formalin and processed for paraffin histology.

2.5. FROZEN SECTIONS

Methods of preparing frozen sections vary considerably from department to department and no specific method is prescribed here. As a general principle it is important that the tissue is frozen rapidly so as to avoid ice crystal artefact. The variety of methods used for freezing the tissue include direct immersion in liquid nitrogen, immersion in isopentane chilled with liquid nitrogen, surrounding by dry ice and spraying with an instant freeze aerosol. Sections are cut on the cryostat and our preference is subsequently to fix the sections either in 95% alcohol or 10–20% formalin. Briefly microwaving the cryostat sections improves the morphological detail. Our preference is to stain the sections with a rapid haematoxylin and eosin method, similar to that shown in Table 2.1 for smear preparations. Of other stains which may be used for cryostat sections, van Gieson can be performed rapidly and may help if there is uncertainty over the distinction between neuropil or glial fibres and collagen.

When a diagnosis has been made the tissue is thawed, fixed in formalin and processed to paraffin wax. Keeping it as a separately identified specimen allows subsequent comparison of the paraffin and frozen sections from the same piece of tissue.

THREE

INTERPRETATION OF SMEAR CYTOLOGY

Before attempting to use the smear technique for intra-operative tumour diagnosis, it is important to become familiar with the cytological features of normal nervous tissues, and to be able to distinguish tumour from reactive and other non-neoplastic states. The quickest way to study smears of normal tissue is to create a set of preparations from identified areas of a reasonably fresh autopsy brain specimen, and we would certainly commend this practice to any who are new to the technique. Different brain tissues show widely varying appearances when smeared, and assessment of features such as cellularity and texture of neuropil clearly relies on an awareness of what is normal in any given structure. It also follows that the site of a biopsy needs to be taken into account when deciding whether or not pathological alterations are present in an intra-operative smear preparation. For the inexperienced, it is even possible to confuse normal tissue with tumour, as for example when cerebellar granule neurones are misconstrued as lymphoma, or inadvertently incorporated normal choroid plexus is wrongly interpreted as a papilloma.

Florid reactive changes are perhaps more likely to cause difficulty in the interpretation of smears, and are almost inevitably present in the brain tissue surrounding a neoplastic lesion. An unwary pathologist may sometimes be persuaded that such changes are diagnostic, when in reality the biopsy procedure has only sampled the reactive margins of a tumour. The problem is compounded if the adjacent reactive tissue is diffusely infiltrated by tumour cells, as around many gliomas. It also has to be remembered that the lesion being biopsied may not be a neoplasm at all, but an unsuspected primary reactive process such as a maturing infarct or an abscess. Smears of these can again be mistaken for glial tumours on cursory examination, especially if alternative diagnoses are not considered at the time. We would not want to convey the impression that the smear technique is at all misleading in suitably experienced hands, simply that it is wise to have a good grounding in the cytological appearances of normal and reactive tissues. It is also vital to keep asking the question 'is this definitely tumour?' when confronted with smears of abnormal tissue thought to have been sampled from a neoplastic lesion.

3.1. APPEARANCE OF NORMAL NERVOUS TISSUES WHEN SMEARED

Cerebral cortex

Smears of cortical tissue inevitably show abundant neurones, which lack the uniform orientation seen in histological sections. They also vary widely in appearance depending on the area sampled. Biopsies from most sites contain neurones of pyramidal type, with prominent clumps of Nissl substance and triangular or elongate cell bodies forming dendritic branches. The size of these pyramidal cells will depend on the cortical laminae from which the specimen was taken, but they can range up to the proportions of giant Betz cells if the primary motor cortex is involved. In most cortical smears there is also a prominent population of small, compact neurones which lack obvious perinuclear cytoplasm. Like pyramidal cells, these have typical, rounded nuclei, with pale chromatin and prominent nucleoli. Larger cortical neurones of any type may contain cytoplasmic lipofuscin granules, which are brown if haematoxylin eosin staining is used but have a distinctive turquoise colour in toluidine blue preparations. In addition to neurones, smears of normal cerebral cortex also contain a rather sparse mixture of resident glial cells with varied nuclear morphology and no discernible perinuclear cytoplasm. Oligodendroglial nuclei are small, hyperchromatic and rounded, whilst those of microglia are dark but more elongate. Fibrous astrocyte nuclei have an irregular ovoid shape with pale, speckled chromatin. The neuropil of normal cerebral cortex appears as a fine, felt-like background in smear preparations, which is eosinophilic or pale blue depending on whether haematoxylin eosin or toluidine blue staining is used. If the tissue is very thinly smeared, the background neuropil is likely to be very faint and difficult to discern. Thin-walled capillary blood vessels are usually quite a prominent feature of cortical smears, and are often arranged in a delicately branching meshwork.

Deep cerebral grey matter

Smear preparations from normal basal ganglia share many cytological features with those of cerebral cortex, but usually show more pronounced neuronal heterogeneity. Large stellate or globose neurones are often a prominent feature, particularly if the biopsy involves structures such as the globus pallidus. Smaller neurones tend to be compact rather than pyramidal in shape, but there may be a combination of the two, again depending on the precise site being sampled. Lipofuscin granules are likely to be more abundant than in cortical smears, especially where there are abundant neurones of large size. The smeared background neuropil of deep grey matter structures often has a coarser texture, similar to that seen in smears from white matter. Calcospherites may also be present, particularly in specimens from older patients.

White matter

The background neuropil of smeared white matter is typically coarser and more fibrillar in texture than that of grey matter, and is often more strongly stained because of the greater proportion of myelinated fibres present. Unlike reactive tissue, it does not normally show metachromasia with toluidine blue staining. A varied mixture of oligodendroglial, microglial and astrocytic nuclei are visible, but are usually difficult to identify individually. They are more abundant than in cortical smears of similar thickness, especially the small, dot-like nuclei of oligodendrocytes. In contrast to their reactive counterparts, normal glial cell nuclei are quite small and do not have discernible perinuclear cytoplasm. White matter smears tend to be less vascular than those of grey matter, with vessels that are less prominently branched and of more variable calibre.

Cerebellar cortex

Biopsies of cerebellar lesions not infrequently include cortical tissue, which has a very distinctive appearance in smear preparations. Granule layer neurones are usually the most conspicuous feature, forming loose clusters of small, rounded, dark nuclei without discernible cytoplasm. These are interspersed with areas of smooth neuropil from the molecular layer, which contains sparse astrocytic and oligodendroglial nuclei. In addition, large Purkinje neurones are often present, either embedded in the areas of molecular neuropil or mixed in with granule neurone nuclei. Purkinje cells can appear quite polymorphic in smear preparations and do not always show the expected unipolar morphology. When a tumour is suspected clinically and cerebellar smears are non-diagnostic, less experienced observers need to be careful not to mistake the normal granule cells for a small round cell tumour such as lymphoma or medulloblastoma. Closer inspection will reveal that the granule cell nuclei are, in fact, far too small and uniform to be confused with tumour cells.

Brainstem and spinal cord

The appearance of smears containing brainstem or cord tissue will obviously depend on the particular site of the biopsy, but in general terms there is most likely to be a mixture of white matter features and neurones of variable morphology. Smears of the brainstem often resemble those from cerebral basal ganglia, whilst those from the cord may show purely white matter features of long tract tissue, or contain a variable population of pyramidal or compact neurones.

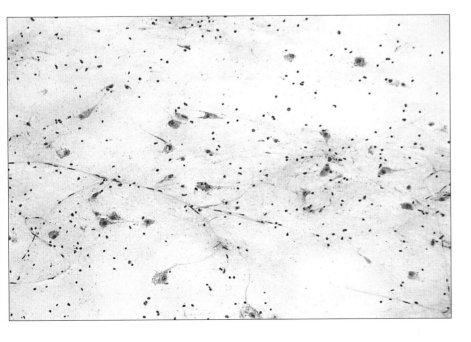

Figure 3.1
Normal cerebral cortex. The smear contains numerous pyramidal neurones, with large nuclei and characteristically triangular cell bodies. The neuropil has a smooth texture and condenses around delicate capillary blood vessels. Dot-like glial nuclei are also visible in the background. Smear preparation, toluidine blue, ×110.

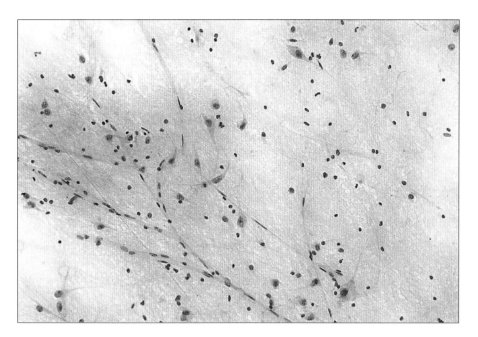

Figure 3.2
Normal cerebral cortex. The appearance of this smear is similar to that shown in Fig. 3.1, but the background neuropil is more intensely stained, emphasizing its felt-like texture. The neurones vary in size and are triangular, rounded or stellate in shape. There is again a prominent meshwork of branching capillary vessels. Smear preparation, haematoxylin eosin, ×175.

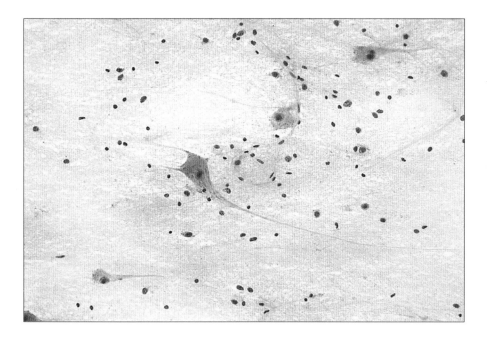

Figure 3.3
Normal motor cortex. Some small round neurones are present, but this smear is dominated by giant Betz motor neurones. Their large size enables a clear appreciation of neuronal cytology. Clumped Nissl substance gives the cell bodies a characteristic tigroid appearance. The nuclei are large, round and pale with a single prominent nucleolus. The tiny, dark nuclei in the background represent the resting glial cell population of normal cortical tissue. Smear preparation, haematoxylin eosin, ×175.

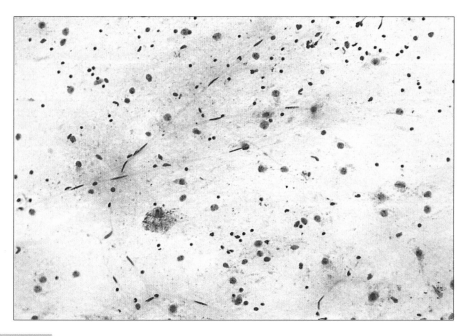

Figure 3.4
Normal putamen. The prominent, branching capillaries and fine neuropil are similar to those of cortical tissue. Instead of being mainly pyramidal, however, the neurones seen here are nearly all small and compact with rather indistinct cytoplasm. They are recognizable largely by their pale round nuclei. In addition, there is a single, much larger neurone which is globose in shape and has a cytological appearance typical of deep grey matter origin. Smear preparation, toluidine blue, ×220.

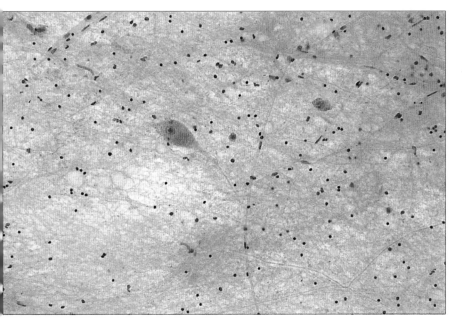

Figure 3.5
Normal globus pallidus. The neuropil here has a slightly coarser appearance, more like that of white matter. Delicate capillaries are again present and there is a prominent background population of oligodendroglia with tiny, very dark nuclei. The two large neurones are of different shape and size, and their cell bodies contain golden brown lipofuscin. This has a grey-green colour when toluidine blue staining is used. Smear preparation, haematoxylin eosin, ×175.

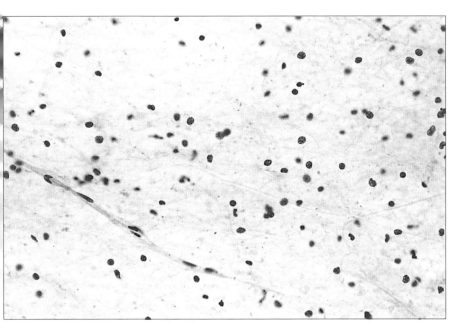

Figure 3.6
Normal white matter. There is a varied population of small glial nuclei which are mostly rather darkly stained. These cells are not separately identifiable but will include resting astrocytes, oligodendroglia and sometimes microglia. By comparison with cortical tissue, the glial nuclei of white matter are usually more abundant and the background neuropil rather coarser in texture. Smear preparation, toluidine blue, ×350.

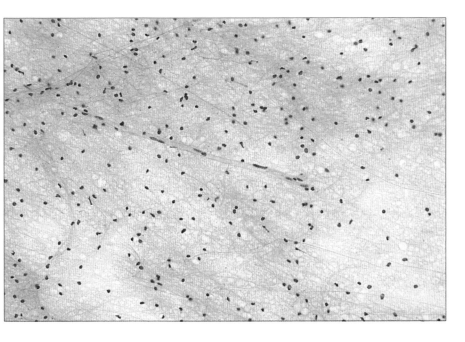

Figure 3.7
Normal white matter. At lower magnification, the glial cell nuclei of white matter give the smear a 'pepper and salt' appearance. The majority are likely to be oligodendroglial nuclei, which are very small, round and darkly stained. Blood vessels are usually much less prominent than in grey matter and more likely to be of larger calibre. Note the uniform appearance of the background neuropil, in contrast to that of reactive tissue (compare Figs 3.14, 3.16). Smear preparation, haematoxylin eosin, ×175.

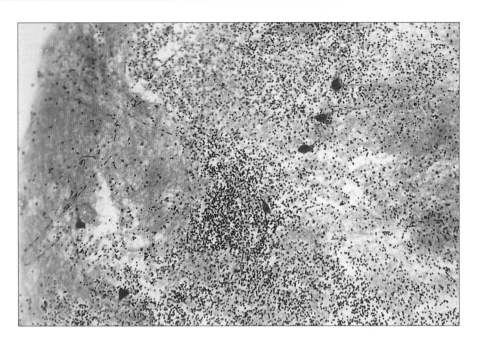

Figure 3.8

Normal cerebellar cortex. Even quite deep biopsies taken from the cerebellum are likely to include some cortical tissue, which has a varied and distinctive cytological appearance. Areas of smooth, rather bland neuropil from the molecular layer alternate with cellular granule layer tissue. It is important for less experienced observers not to mistake the latter for infiltrating small round cell tumour. Even at low magnification the situation should be obvious if large Purkinjie neurones are also present, as in this example. Smear preparation, toluidine blue, ×110.

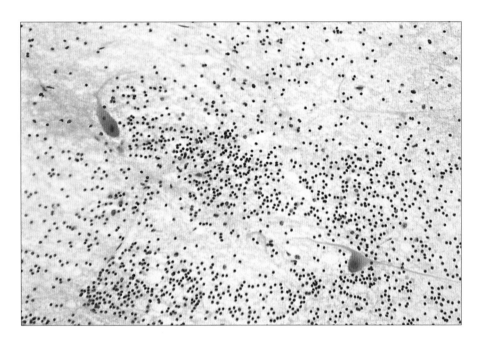

Figure 3.9

Normal cerebellar cortex. The features are similar to those of Fig. 3.8. The nuclei of granule layer neurones are very small, darkly stained and monotonous. No surrounding cytoplasm is discernible. They tend to be grouped loosely into separate clusters, rather than being evenly distributed across the smear. Typical Purkinje neurones are again seen in this field, with very prominent axonal and dendritic processes. Smear preparation, haematoxylin eosin, ×175.

3.2. MISCELLANEOUS ELEMENTS WHICH MAY BE ENCOUNTERED IN ROUTINE SMEAR PREPARATIONS

Choroid plexus tissue is occasionally introduced into smear preparations during attempted biopsies of para- or intraventricular lesions. The appearances can be virtually indistinguishable from those of benign choroid plexus papillomas, leading to potential confusion if the biopsy has missed the real tumour. Fragments of normal choroid plexus are tough and more thickly smeared compared to most papillomas, and show more numerous and prominent fibrovascular cores within the papillary fronds. It should be noted, however, that the epithelial layer often appears to be more than one cell layer in thickness, due to an artefact of the smearing process (see Chapter 9 and Figure 9.1). **Normal ependymal lining** may also appear in smears from deep paraventricular biopsies, and is usually dispersed amongst the white matter neuropil in the form of fragmented, epithelial-like sheets. The ependymal cells have uniform, rounded nuclei and compact but rather ill-defined perinuclear cytoplasm. **Arachnoidal cells** are sometimes incorporated into smears made from more superficial biopsies, or those where intact leptomeninges have been punctured by the biopsy needle. The cells again have very uniform cytological features, but their nuclei are more ovoid than those of ependymal cells and they show a predictable tendency to form spherical nests or whorls. **Rosenthal fibres** are a feature of low grade astrocytomas, especially those of pilocytic type (see Chapter 6). However, they may also be encountered in smears of any chronically gliotic tissue and do

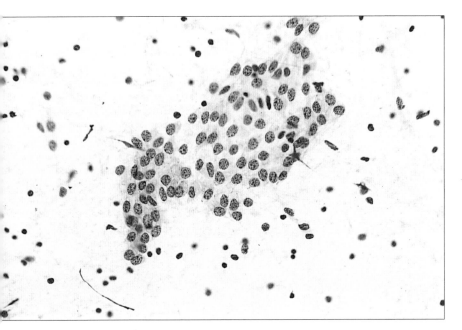

Figure 3.10

Normal ependyma. Fragments of ventricular lining may be inadvertently incorporated into smears made from deep paraventricular biopsies. Unless an observer is familiar with their cytological appearance, they can sometimes be mistaken for tumour in a non-diagnostic specimen. The smearing process usually breaks normal ependymal epithelium into sheet-like fragments, which become dispersed in the adjacent white matter. The cells are very uniform, with rounded nuclei and a uniform chromatin pattern. Their cytoplasm is discreet, but with slightly ill-defined margins. Smear preparation, toluidine blue, ×350.

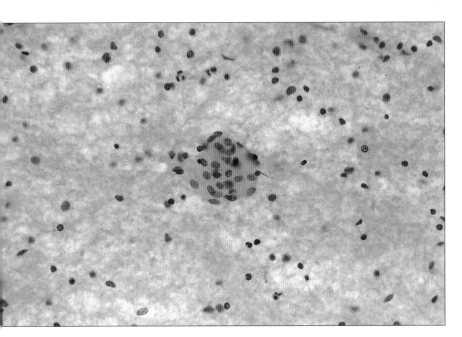

Figure 3.11

Normal arachnoidal tissue. Fragments of leptomeninges can find their way into biopsies which are superficial, or those where a biopsy needle has been advanced down through the pial surface without completely dividing the meningial membrane. Such pieces of meningial tissue are usually too bulky and tough to smear properly, but occasionally small arachnoidal nests or whorls may be encountered, as demonstrated here. Smear preparation, haematoxylin eosin, ×350.

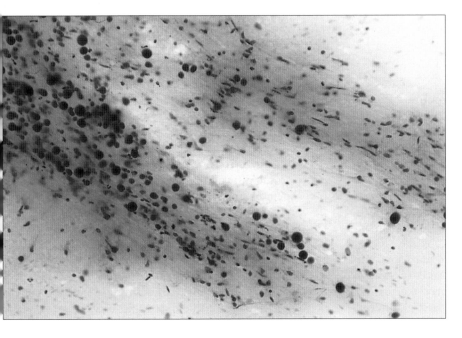

Figure 3.12

Corpora amylacea. In toluidine blue stained preparations, these appear as very dark, homogeneous, blue-coloured blobs of varying size. They are dark grey when haematoxylin eosin staining is used and may show concentric lamination. Corpora amylacea are most likely to be encountered in biopsies from the spinal cord or deep midline parts of the cerebrum, but they can also occur in any area where there is degeneration or gliotic scarring. Smear preparation, toluidine blue, ×175.

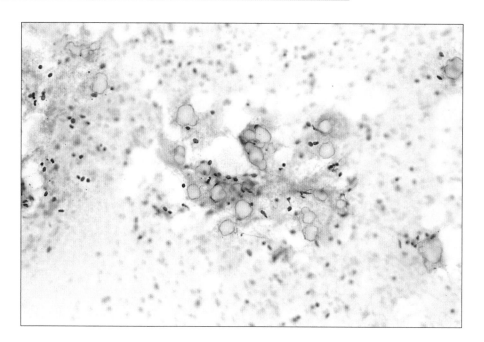

Figure 3.13
Calcospherites. In addition to the psammoma bodies of meningiomas, small calcified bodies may be found in any glial tumour, especially oligodendrogliomas. They also occur in areas of old glial scarring and in some normal deep grey matter structures with ageing. The ones shown here were from a biopsy of a calcified dysembryoplastic neuroepithelial tumour, although the intra-operative smear was not diagnostic. As often occurs, these calcospherites have repelled the stain and appear as irregular, translucent bodies with a slightly refractile quality. Smear preparation, toluidine blue, ×220.

not necessarily indicate the presence of tumour. Closely related **granular bodies** are rounded rather than elongate and tapering in shape. Both stain brightly turquoise or purplish with toluidine blue but are eosinophilic if haematoxylin eosin staining is used. **Corpora amylacea** are most often seen in smears taken from deep cerebral structures or spinal cord white matter, and may be very numerous. They have an intense, dark turquoise colour if toluidine blue staining is used but are basophilic in haematoxylin eosin preparations, sometimes with a discernible concentric architecture. **Calcification** is most often tumour-related, as in meningiomas and some low grade glial tumours, but calcospherites may also appear in smears of non-neoplastic tissue. They are more likely to be encountered in biopsies from older individuals, especially if there is cerebrovascular disease or deep grey matter structures are biopsied. Those that contain iron pigment will be an extremely dark brown or greenish colour depending on the stain used. The remainder tend to repel the stain, appearing as irregular, translucent bodies with a slightly refractile quality.

3.3. REACTIVE CHANGES

Central nervous tissue responds in a relatively stereotyped way to a wide variety of insults, and the resulting reactive changes are readily appreciated in smear preparations. These cytological alterations vary in degree of severity and chronicity, but it is important to remember that they are non-specific, and by themselves give no indication of the underlying pathological cause. They may be observed as a result of diffuse insults such as ischaemia, or because the tissue sampled is adjacent to a focal lesion which has been missed by the biopsy. Such a lesion may well be a neoplasm of some sort, but unless there is good cytological evidence of diffuse tumour infiltration (see below), it may equally be something entirely benign, such as an infarct or abscess.

As a further note of warning, florid reactive cytological changes can themselves be misinterpreted as glial neoplasm by an inexperienced observer, and familiarity with the range of reactive appearances that may be encountered in smear preparations is essential to prevent this.

The most distinctive cytological feature of acutely reactive brain is the presence of hypertrophied astrocytes. These tend to be widely scattered throughout the smear, without tendency to cling to blood vessels, and are best appreciated at relatively low magnifications, where the depth of field is greater. Their nuclei are larger than those of resting astrocytes, with paler chromatin and often a prominent nucleolus. This may sometimes cause confusion with compact neurones. However, most examples have a prominent blush of perinuclear cytoplasm, sometimes eccentric to the nucleus, which tapers in a stellate fashion to form radiating fibrillar processes. In extreme cases, the hypertrophied astrocytes may have two or even three nuclei and show quite marked pleomorphism, but they can usually still be identified as reactive cells by the distinctive stellate appearance of their perinuclear cytoplasm. Reactive brain tissue also contains an increased number of microglial cells undergoing reactive change. Sometimes they will appear as 'rod cells', with elongate dark nuclei and indistinct cytoplasm, but in more severe reaction there may be fully mature phagocytes. These have central dot-like nuclei and a discreet halo of clear or foamy cytoplasm, although the latter is often very pale and difficult to see except at high magnification. It should be noted that reactive glia are undergoing active proliferation, and occasional mitotic figures should be expected, especially if the changes are florid. As a result of this proliferation, smear preparations of reactive brain tissue are hypercellular compared to normal grey or white matter, although the impression of hypercellularity in smears always needs to take into account the thickness of the tissue film in the area being examined.

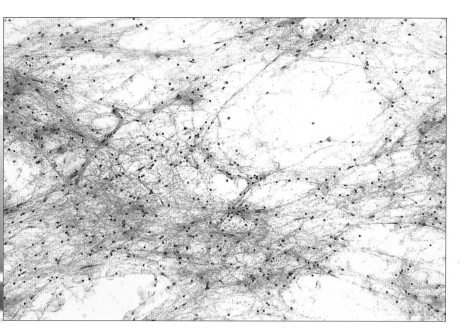

Figure 3.14
Gliotic white matter. The most striking change at this magnification is the coarse and irregular fibrillar change of the neuropil. Compare the appearance with that of the normal white matter neuropil seen in Fig. 3.7. A similar change occurs in some low grade astrocytic tumours but these are usually much more cellular than the tissue here. Smear preparation, haematoxylin eosin, ×110.

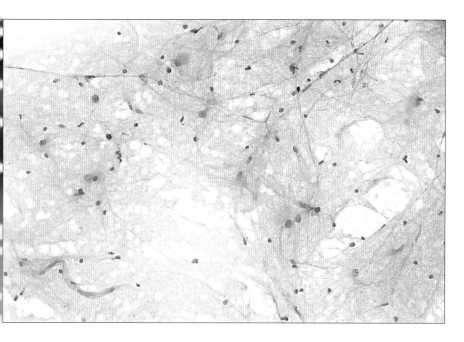

Figure 3.15
Acutely reactive brain. The neuropil here has a rather wet look, with vacuolar spaces caused by oedema. There are also some abnormally coarse fibrillar strands. Numerous hypertrophied astrocytes are present, with stellate flares of perinuclear cytoplasm. Smear preparation, haematoxylin eosin, ×220.

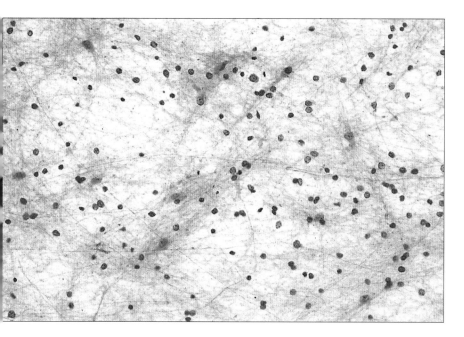

Figure 3.16
Reactive white matter. The neuropil is coarsely fibrillar by comparison to normal white matter (compare Fig. 3.6). The reactive astrocytes have hypertrophied nuclei and a characteristic stellate appearance, with radiating fibrillar processes. Smaller nuclei in the background belong to other glial cell types and there is an overall impression of increased cellularity. Smear preparation, toluidine blue, ×220.

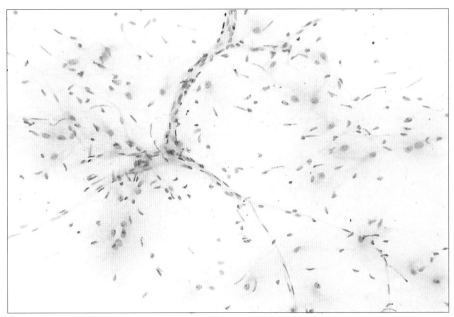

Figure 3.17
Acutely reactive brain. The smear is hypercellular, with a mixture of hypertrophied astrocytes and other glial cells with variably shaped nuclei. The large astrocytes have a typical stellate appearance with flares of radiating cytoplasmic processes. Amongst the remaining cells, those with elongate, rod-like nuclei represent activated microglia. The blood vessels present are hypercellular and prominently branched as a result of reactive proliferation. Smear preparation, haematoxylin eosin, ×175.

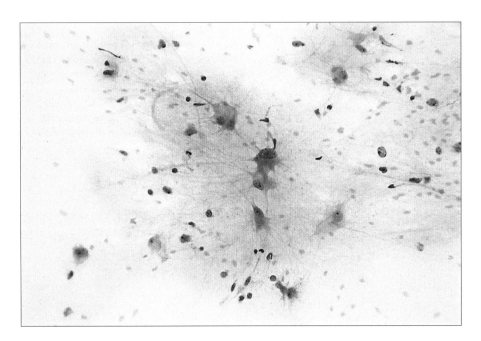

Figure 3.18
Chronic reactive change. Hypertrophied astrocytes can become quite pleomorphic in chronic reactive states and may show a wide range of cytological atypia, including multinucleation. Although sometimes more bizarre than neoplastic cells, they tend to retain their characteristic stellate appearance and are rarely numerous enough in a smear to be mistaken for tumour. The biopsy illustrated here was taken from an area of delayed radiation change. Smear preparation, toluidine blue, ×220.

The background neuropil is also altered in acute reactive states, tending to have a more coarsely fibrillar texture than normal, and may sometimes show slight metachromasia if toluidine blue staining is used. Capillary blood vessels frequently show quite marked proliferative changes, appearing larger and more prominently branched than normal. In addition, there may be endothelial cell hyperplasia, with plumper nuclei and thickened, hypercellular vessel walls. These changes can simulate the vascular alterations seen in malignant glial tumours, although reactive tissue rarely shows such pronounced 'glomeruloid' vascular budding.

3.4. DIFFUSE INFILTRATION BY GLIAL TUMOUR

Most intrinsic tumours of central nervous tissue have a tendency to diffusely infiltrate the surrounding brain or cord, regardless of their grade of malignancy. The process may extend a considerable distance from the main tumour mass, and some types can have no clearly defined, solid central area at all. Such behaviour can pose considerable problems for intra-operative diagnosis. Despite the use of sophisticated imaging and localising techniques, it is all too easy to end up with a biopsy of diffusely infiltrated tissue rather than diagnostic tumour. With low grade gliomas in particular, it is not always possible to tell from radiological scans which areas of abnormal signal represent solid tumour, and which indicate brain diffusely infiltrated by tumour cells. This obviously becomes easier if there is focal contrast enhancement, indicating higher grade and presumably solid tumour. Highly malignant gliomas, however, often have only a narrow rim of viable solid tumour separating a necrotic centre from the surrounding infiltrated brain. In such cases the pathologist is not infrequently presented with smears which are either

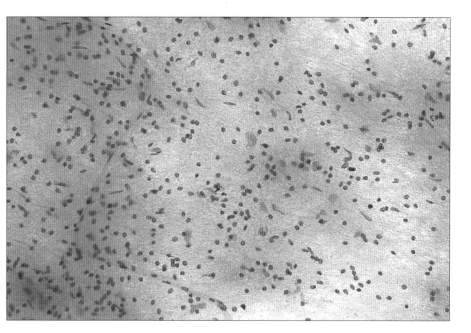

Figure 3.19
Diffusely infiltrated white matter. The smear is markedly hypercellular (compare Fig. 3.7), but typical reactive astrocytes are not an obvious feature. Instead, the excess nuclei give the impression of a rather monotonous, 'cloned' population, suggesting predominance of a single glial cell type. The infiltrating tumour in this case was a low grade astrocytoma and there are no specific cytological features of neoplasia, even at higher magnification. Smear preparation, haematoxylin eosin, ×175.

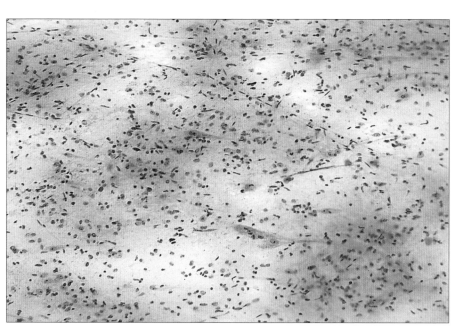

Figure 3.20
Grey matter infiltrated by low grade astrocytoma. Large neurones are easy to identify in this smear and there are some reactive changes, perhaps more easily appreciated at higher magnification. In addition, however, there is an increased cellularity which seems out of proportion to these changes, with a population of medium-sized glial cell nuclei which cannot be specifically identified. Compare with the normal grey matter in Fig. 3.1 and the purely reactive changes seen in Figs 3.16 and 3.17. Smear preparation, toluidine blue, ×110

entirely necrotic (see below) or just diffusely hypercellular. It is important to remember that if the intra-operative smears show only hypercellular, diffusely infiltrated brain, then the material for paraffin sections is likely to be similar, resulting in an ungradable or even non-diagnostic final biopsy result. On the other hand, intra-operative evidence of diffuse tumour infiltration may be a useful positive finding in some circumstances, for example if the surgeon is using smears to check the margins of an excision cavity.

Smear preparations of tissue diffusely infiltrated by glial tumour inevitably show non-specific reactive changes like those described above, together with residual normal elements of the infiltrated brain, including neurones if grey matter is involved. The tissue film nearly always appears significantly hypercellular, usually to a degree which seems out of proportion to the reactive changes present. In particular, there is likely to be an obvious population of glial cell nuclei which lack the cytological features of either reactive astrocytes or activated microglia. These excess nuclei frequently give a monotonous or 'cloned' impression, suggesting predominance of a single cell type rather than the varied mixture of cells seen in purely reactive brain tissue. At higher magnification, obvious cytological atypia or frequent mitotic figures may help confirm the impression of diffusely infiltrating glioma, always bearing in mind the range of such abnormalities which can be encountered in purely reactive circumstances. Blood vessels often show quite marked tumour-related hyperplasia in the diffusely infiltrating margins of high grade gliomas, and if there is very florid, glomeruloid proliferation in a smear, this in itself may suggest more than simple reactive change.

Having said all this, there are inevitably going to be some instances where it is not possible to be certain whether a reactive, hypercellular smear preparation represents brain diffusely infiltrated by glial tumour or not. More smears can be requested, or the surgeon asked to review the precise location of the biopsy site relative to the radiological abnormality, but such tactics are not always successful. Frozen sections may be useful in some cases, but in the absence of unarguable cytological atypia, it can still be difficult to decide whether the hypercellular tissue represents diffuse tumour infiltration or just reactive change. In our experience, it is important for the pathologist not to be pushed into making an intra-operative diagnosis of diffuse glioma in such circumstances, regardless of clinical pressure to do so. At the very least this might lead to a non-diagnostic result from paraffin sections and thus a wasted surgical procedure. At worst lies the possibility that tumour is not present at all, and the surgeon has biopsied purely reactive tissue adjacent to a non-neoplastic lesion such as an abscess.

3.5. NON-NEOPLASTIC LESIONS THAT MAY BE ASSOCIATED WITH REACTIVE CHANGE

Abscess and cerebritis

Cerebral abscesses and acute focal cerebritis may sometimes be difficult to distinguish radiologically and clinically from nervous system tumours. In particular, scans of bacterial abscesses at a certain stage of evolution show ring enhancement, mass effect and surrounding oedema which can be very like the image produced by malignant glial tumours with a necrotic centre. For the pathologist, material biopsied from the brain adjacent to either lesion is likely to show very similar reactive changes in smear preparations, making intra-operative diagnosis difficult unless the central parts of the lesion are accurately sampled. Even then, degenerate pus aspirated from the centre of an abscess can sometimes be mistaken for necrotic tumour debris from the middle of a glioblastoma. Perhaps most important of all is the need to distinguish between smears sampled from the viable rim of a glioma and those showing the florid proliferative changes of tissue taken from the wall of an immature bacterial abscess. Less experienced observers have been known to confuse the two appearances, and making the correct diagnosis in these circumstances has clear management implications applicable to the time of surgery.

Smear preparations from the wall of an abscess are usually hypercellular with very florid reactive changes, but these features may not be immediately apparent because much of the tissue tends to be tough and thickly smeared. There is typically very pronounced vascular proliferation, and the reactive elements often adhere to vessels in thick papillary clumps not unlike those seen in smears of some gliomas. At higher magnification, however, typical reactive astrocytes rather than tumour cells will be identified at the margins of these masses of tissue, intermingled with a variable population of macrophages and inflammatory cells. The latter

tend to smear out individually away from the thicker clumps of tissue and will be a variable mixture of polymorphs and mononuclear cells depending on the type and age of the abscess. If polymorphs are very numerous, then a diagnosis of acute infection is relatively straightforward, but where the infiltrate is more predominantly lymphocytic, it needs to be remembered that perivascular lymphocyte cuffing can also be seen in tissue from glial tumours and other, non-neoplastic lesions such as infarcts. With more chronic abscesses, including tuberculous lesions, inflammatory cells may be limited to a sparse lymphocytic infiltrate, and the cytology dominated by thickly smeared masses of epithelioid macrophages with small round nuclei and rather poorly defined perinuclear cytoplasm. Such preparations can be very difficult to interpret, and frozen sections are advisable wherever the tissue is too tough to smear properly or it is not possible to make a confident distinction between an inflammatory process and glial tumour using smear cytology.

Infarction

Cerebral infarcts at a particular stage of evolution can exhibit striking radiological enhancement and mass effect, and sometimes they may be mistaken clinically for a glial tumour. Judging by our experience, most pathologists can expect to receive the occasional intra-operative smear from a maturing infarct accompanied by a confident clinical diagnosis of glioma. As with infection, there are clear implications for immediate management, and it is only too easy for the pathologist to fall into the trap of concurring with the clinical diagnosis unless the possibility of a non-neoplastic lesion is constantly kept in mind.

The cytological appearance of infarcted nervous tissue will obviously depend on the age of the lesion, but those most likely to be confused with glial tumour are infarcts in the acute proliferative phase. Smears from such lesions are typically very cellular with florid reactive features and abundant evidence of vascular and glial cell proliferation. Mitoses are frequently encountered, and there are usually abundant capillary vessels showing prominent branching and endothelial cell proliferation. Cytological detail is often difficult to resolve in thickly smeared areas, and the combination of hypercellular tissue and proliferated vessels may give an initial impression of glial tumour to the inexperienced observer. Where the tissue is more thinly smeared, typical reactive astrocytes are usually easily identified, set in a coarsely fibrillar background. The most distinctive feature of acute infarction is the presence of swollen foamy macrophages with abundant clear cytoplasm. These are again most easily observed away from thicker clumps of tissue, where they tend to smear out into thin sheets. Their clear cytoplasm is not easily apparent at low magnifications, leaving the impression of numerous, small dot-like nuclei scattered across the smear. Depending on the age of the infarct, elongate fibroblastic cells and rod-shaped nuclei of activated microglia may also be identified, and the overall effect is that of a varied mixture of cellular elements rather than the monomorphic population more typically associated with glioma smears.

Demyelination

The most likely demyelinating lesions to be biopsied for diagnostic purposes are probably acute plaques in patients not previously known to have multiple sclerosis. Smears from these will show floridly reactive features and are often impossible to distinguish from early infarction or non-specifically reactive tissue. As with infarcted tissue, hypertrophied astrocytes and a variable population of foamy macrophages is to be expected, depending on the age of the lesion. Lymphocytic infiltration may also be a prominent feature in some cases and the diagnosis of an inflammatory lesion or lymphoma may be considered, especially if there is pronounced perivascular cuffing.

The same comments are largely true for smears made from lesions of progressive multifocal leucoencephalopathy, although here the degree of pleomorphism in the reactive astrocytes is more likely to misleadingly suggest a glial neoplasm. Transformed oligodendrocyte nuclei can occasionally be identified, especially if haematoxylin eosin staining is used, but this cannot be relied upon. In both cases, intra-operative suspicion of demyelinating disease will rely heavily on clinical and radiological features, and even then the pathologist can often do no more than confirm that abnormal tissue has been sampled for paraffin section diagnosis.

Vascular malformations

Vascular malformations occasionally present atypically as mass lesions, usually because of chronic haemorrhage or infarction in the surrounding brain. Such lesions may

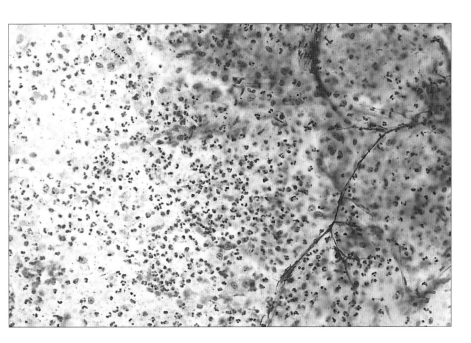

Figure 3.21
Acute bacterial abscess. The smear consists of abundant, partly necrotic polymorphs intermingled with thicker clumps of macrophages and reactive glia. Infection should always be considered when polymorphs are very numerous, as they are relatively inconspicuous in infarcted brain or necrotic glioma tissue. As the abscess matures, polymorphs become less prominent and smears are more likely to show a mixture of tough connective tissue elements and reactive brain. Smear preparation, toluidine blue, ×175.

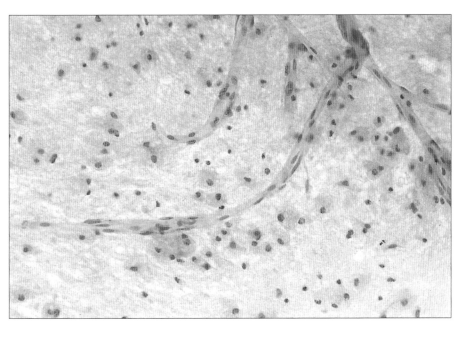

Figure 3.22
Acute infarction. In the earlier stages of infarction reactive changes predominate, including hypercellularity and florid proliferation of blood vessels. In addition, there is already likely to be a background population of globose macrophages, like those seen here. Mitotic figures may be encountered, and there is a risk of mistaking the tissue for glial tumour if a high magnification lens is not used to specifically identify the types of cell present. Smear preparation, haematoxylin eosin, ×220.

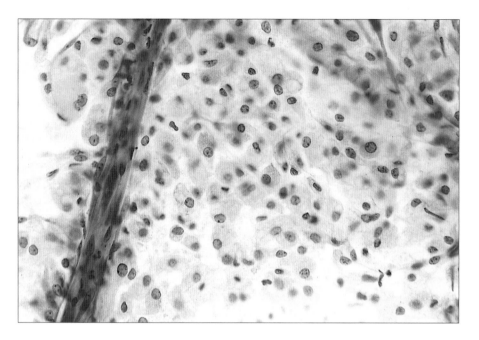

Figure 3.23
Maturing infarct. In established cerebral infarcts, smears typically show sheets of lipid-laden macrophages with abundant foamy cytoplasm and uniform, small, rounded nuclei. The macrophages are intersected by a meshwork of proliferated blood vessels and are most easily seen when they smear out into a monolayer, away from thicker clumps of tissue. Smear preparation, toluidine blue, ×350.

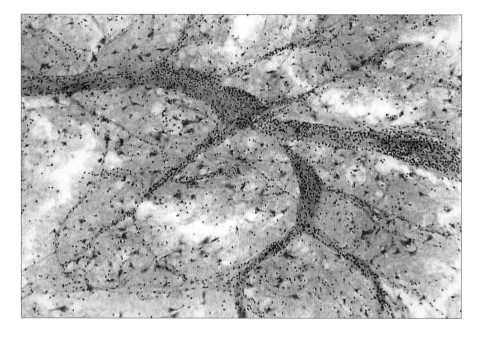

Figure 3.24
Arteriovenous malformation. Vascular malformations may be clinically mistaken for tumour if they present as a mass lesion due to maturing infarction or haemorrhage. In this case, the abnormal area was biopsied and intra-operative smears contained these large and strikingly hyperplastic blood vessels. In distinction from malignant glial tumours, the background tissue showed only reactive changes. When abundant old blood pigment is present, this is also a useful feature. Smear preparation, toluidine blue, ×110.

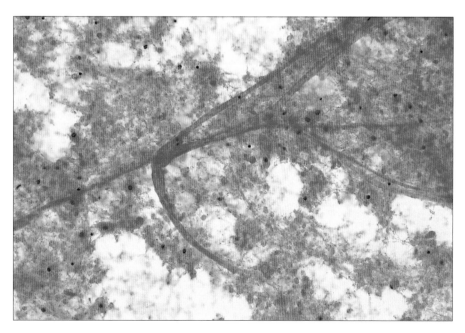

Figure 3.25
Necrotic glioblastoma tissue. The outlines of branching tumour vessels are clearly seen, with entirely necrotic tumour tissue clinging to them in a vaguely papillary fashion. The tissue has an floccular, almost amorphous appearance, although at higher magnifications the ghost outlines of some cells are visible. Nuclear staining is only visible in a small number of scattered macrophages. As in infarcted brain tissue, polymorphs are usually scarce or absent in smears of necrotic gliomas. Smear preparation, haematoxylin eosin, ×175.

be biopsied on the assumption that they represent tumour, and diagnostic advice sought intra-operatively when no obvious tumour tissue is found. The most likely culprit is a diffuse arteriovenous malformation, and smear preparations from the abnormal area will usually show abundant, hyperplastic blood vessels intermingled with reactive or infarcted brain tissue. It is clearly important not to be mislead by the abnormal vessels and mistake the appearances for infiltrating or necrotic glial tumour with unusually prominent vascular proliferation. At higher magnification only the cytological features of reaction or infarction will be identified in the background, often intermingled with abundant old blood pigment. If the vascular elements have made the tissue too tough to smear properly, then frozen sections will be needed to confirm the diagnosis. It is worth noting that although arterialized veins can appear very abnormal in smear preparations, they will not show the glomeruloid budding associated with proliferated vessels in malignant glial tumours.

3.6. TUMOUR NECROSIS

Recognizing small areas of necrosis in glioma smears is obviously important for assessment of tumour grade, but occasionally the pathologist is confronted by entirely necrotic tissue sampled from the centre of glioblastomas or metastases. It is well to remember that totally necrotic intra-operative preparations cannot be considered entirely diagnostic, and unless some viable tumour tissue is seen in the smears, material saved for paraffin sections is likely to prove equally unsatisfactory. The cytological features of necrosis will obviously vary with the type of tumour concerned and the age of the necrotic change, but in general there is a distinct pallor of the tissue, with loss of nuclear staining and blurring of other cytological detail. If a toluidine blue stain is used, the necrotic tumour tends to assume a uniform pale turquoise colour, whereas in haematoxylin eosin stained preparations it is faintly eosinophilic. Scattered polymorphs may be present, but these are never numerous. In contrast to infarcted brain, reactive astrocytes and macrophages are not usually seen. Scattered pyknotic tumour cell nuclei are often still apparent, and the ghost outlines of dead cells may be visible at high magnification. In malignant glial tumours, the necrotic fibrillar background assumes an amorphous, greasy appearance and may be faintly metachromatic if toluidine blue staining is used. Ghost blood vessels are often prominent, and as in viable glioma smears, necrotic tumour tissue may continue to cling to these in a loosely papillary fashion.

FOUR

ARTEFACTS

A number of appearances may be encountered in smear preparations and frozen sections which are artefacts. These artefacts may be caused by events in the neurosurgical operating theatre or while the specimen is in transit to the laboratory. Alternatively the artefacts may be introduced in the laboratory while the smears or frozen sections are being made or stained. The account which follows is not intended to be an exhaustive catalogue of such changes, but merely to be a reminder that these changes can occur. An awareness of artefacts allows modification of the process of acquiring, smearing or sectioning and staining the tissue to ensure that they occur infrequently. In addition, an awareness of the different appearances of the various artefacts should prevent them from being misleading in the attempt to achieve a diagnosis.

4.1. BEFORE THE TISSUE REACHES THE LABORATORY

Artefacts introduced in the neurosurgical operating theatre include those due to thermal damage, whether by diathermy or laser coagulation, and crush injury due to physical trauma from instruments. Not surprisingly such artefacts occur most commonly in highly vascular lesions in which haemostasis may be difficult to achieve and in tough lesions which may be physically difficult to remove. Both forms of tissue damage can completely transform the appearances of cells in ways which are familiar from paraffin histology. Extraneous material may be introduced in the operating theatre and this may give rise to confusion. For example, both bone dust and glove powder may be confused with calcospherites or psammoma bodies. Awareness of the characteristic concentric laminations in a psammoma body is helpful (see Chapter 14). Occasionally haemostatic sponge may be present in the specimen sent for an intra-operative diagnosis and it may be mistaken for spicules of calcification or may do no more than distract from the diagnostic process.

If the tissue is allowed to dry out it becomes completely useless for making either smears or frozen sections. Not surprisingly this occurs most frequently with very small pieces of tissue which have a high surface area to volume ratio. Very small pieces of tissue, such as stereotactic biopsies, tend to be the most precious in the sense that no more material may be available. Drying out of the specimen can be prevented by the addition of a few drops of saline to the specimen pot in the operating theatre, ensuring that the lid of the specimen pot is tightly closed and that the specimen is transported to the laboratory without delay.

4.2. SMEAR PREPARATIONS

Artefacts may be introduced in the laboratory when the smears are made, although with experience their occurrence is minimized. If too much pressure is applied to the tissue sandwiched between the slides then the cells become streaked. When this occurs the cells may become spindle-shaped with elongated nuclei and appear to have cell processes so that they can look remarkably like the cells of a pilocytic astrocytoma. This is readily recognized as an artefact because the cells are orientated in parallel in line with the direction in which the tissue is smeared, in contrast to the randomly orientated cells in an astrocytic tumour. Crush or streaking artefact occurs most commonly either in lesions which are very soft, in which exertion of modest pressure has damaged the tissue, or in very tough lesions on which considerable pressure was exerted in order to get the tissue to smear at all. Experience allows appropriate modulation of the pressure required to smear tissues of very different consistencies.

Tough lesions, even when smeared optimally, often produce thick clumps of cells on the slide. When these are stained and viewed under the microscope the lesion may appear densely cellular as a consequence of the thickness. Examples of lesions in which this may occur and may be misleading include subependymoma and pilocytic astrocytoma. These are generally rather sparsely cellular tumours in sections, but as they are tough, they often appear relatively hypercellular in smears. Uncertainties in this situation can be resolved by resorting to frozen sections.

Shrinkage and crumpling of the nuclei may occur if the smears are allowed to dry after they have been made and before they are placed in fixative. Occasionally only the most superficial layer of cells in the smear has dried and the appearances may mislead one into thinking that mitoses are present in a benign tumour.

The staining methods employed with smear preparations are simple and artefacts are rarely introduced. If the smears are inadequately stained or inadequately cleared, which is particularly likely to occur in the centre of tissue clumps in thick smears, then the staining may not be intense enough to allow interpretation

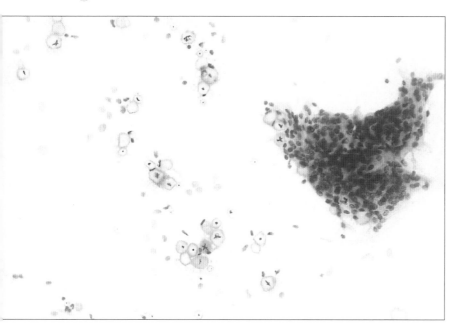

Figure 4.1
Glove powder. Glove powder is an example of extraneous material which may arrive from the neurosurgical theatre with the specimen. It has been intentionally introduced into this smear of a meningioma devoid of psammoma bodies for the purpose of this illustration. The particles of glove powder are generally smaller than psammoma bodies and lack concentric laminations. For comparison psammoma bodies are illustrated in Figs 14.8 and 14.9. Smear preparation, toluidine blue, ×700.

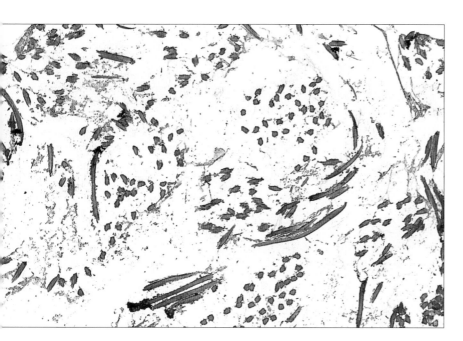

Figure 4.2
Haemostatic sponge. This material may also accompany a specimen arriving from the neurosurgical theatre, particularly from operations in which haemostasis has been difficult. It could be mistaken for spicules of calcification in either smear preparations or frozen sections. Frozen section, haematoxylin eosin, ×90.

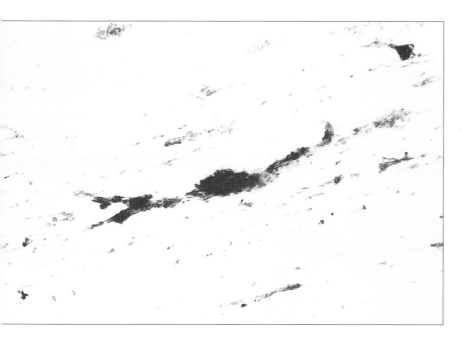

Figure 4.3
Drying artefact. If tissue has been allowed to dry before smear preparations are made then they are uninterpretable as illustrated here. Smear preparation, toluidine blue, ×350.

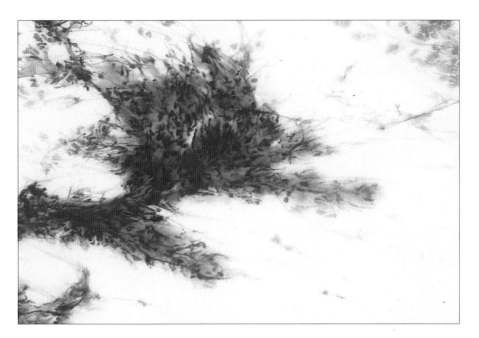

Figure 4.4
Crush artefact. If excessive pressure is applied when making the smear the appearance of the tissue can be dramatically altered. This may occur when attempting to make smears from tough lesions as illustrated here. This is a smear of a haemangiopericytoma which at low power now appears to have a fibrillar architecture and resembles an astrocytic tumour (see Figs 14.18 and 6.13 for comparison). Smear preparation, toluidine blue, ×350.

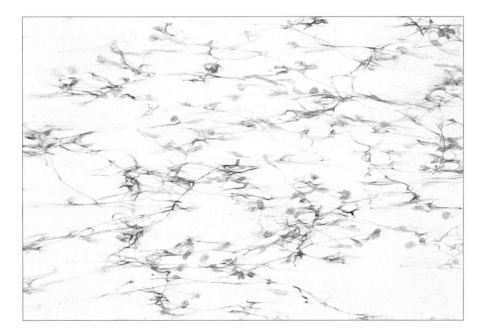

Figure 4.5
Crush artefact. Crush artefact may also occur when only moderate pressure is applied while smearing a very soft lesion. Illustrated here is a central neurocytoma the cells of which are now streaked and somewhat resemble those of a pilocytic astrocytoma (see Figs 10.13 and 6.28 for comparison). Smear preparation, toluidine blue, ×700.

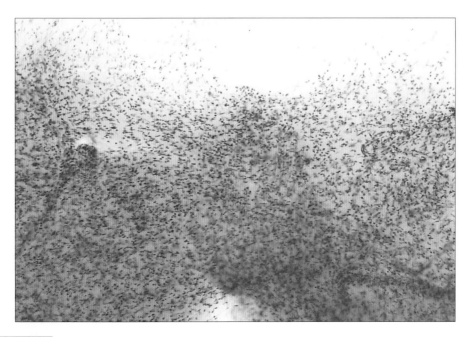

Figure 4.6
Smears of tough lesions. Illustrated here is a smear preparation made from an optic nerve pilocytic astrocytoma. Due to the tough consistency of the tissue it has smeared into thick clumps which may be interpreted as suggesting the tumour to be densely cellular. Sections of the same piece of tissue are shown below (Fig. 4.7) for comparison. Smear preparation, toluidine blue, ×350.

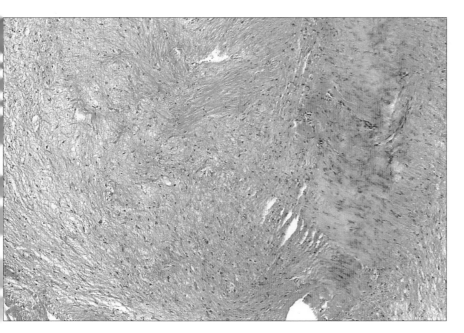

Figure 4.7
Illustrated here is a section of the optic nerve pilocytic astrocytoma shown at the same magnification in a smear in the figure above (Fig. 4.6). Despite the potentially misleading appearance of the smears, in sections the lesion is of very low cellularity. Paraffin section, haematoxylin eosin, ×350.

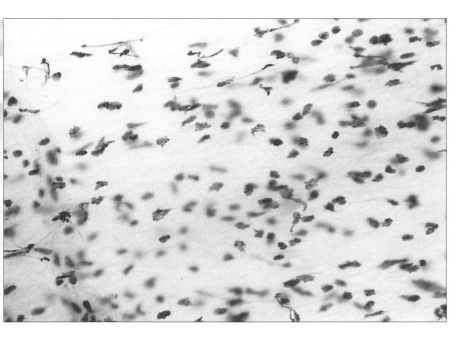

Figure 4.8
Drying artefact. If after the smears are made they are allowed to dry in air before immersion in fixative the superficial layer of cells may become altered in appearance. The nuclei may shrink and crumple, as illustrated here in a low grade astrocytoma, and be mistaken for mitotic figures. Subsequent paraffin sections of this tumour contained no mitoses. Smear preparation, toluidine blue, ×1400.

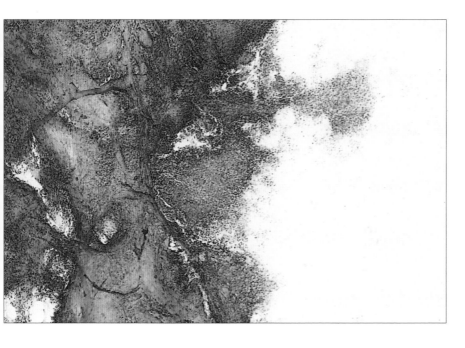

Figure 4.9
Staining artefact. Inadequate staining occurs particularly in the centre of thick clumps of tissue as illustrated here. This rarely causes a problem as the thinner layers of cells at the margins of the clumps are likely to be adequately stained. Smear preparation, toluidine blue, ×90.

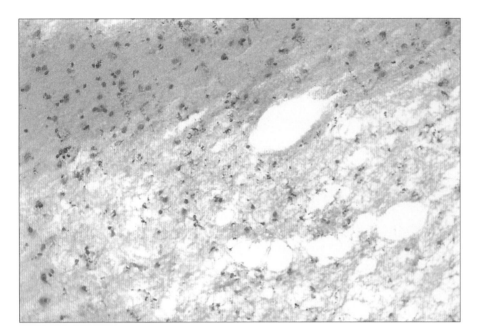

Figure 4.10
Ice crystal artefact. The illustration is of normal cerebral cortical tissue which was frozen slowly deliberately to introduce ice crystal artefact. The neuropil at the top and left is relatively well preserved in contrast to that below and to the right which is disrupted and contains vacuoles. In addition, the cellular and nuclear morphology is severely disrupted. Frozen section, haematoxylin eosin, ×700.

of the cytology. However, even in smears where this is a prominent artefact there are usually well stained cells around the margins of the tissue clumps and smeared between them which allow accurate interpretation of the smear.

4.3. FROZEN SECTIONS

Artefacts specific to frozen sections include ice artefact due to slow freezing of the tissue which allows ice crystals to form. Ice artefact can severely distort the morphology of cells and introduce vacuoles into the tissue section rendering it useless for diagnostic purposes. This form of artefact is avoided by adopting a method for rapid freezing of the tissue and selection of pieces of tissue which are not too large to prevent rapid freezing.

Other problems specific to frozen sections mainly occur during cutting the sections with the microtome: for example chattering of the blade produces parallel lines in the section and the thickness of the section may be somewhat variable.

FIVE

Intra-operative Differential Diagnosis

The differential diagnosis of central nervous system tumours depends on their clinical, radiological, surgical and pathological features. Although this book is concerned primarily with the intra-operative pathological diagnosis, it is important to have as much information as possible from these other sources available when a biopsy is submitted for intra-operative diagnosis. Biopsy specimens from each patient should be accompanied by a request form which summarizes the following:

1. Clinical features –
   age
   sex
   nature and duration of symptoms
   relevant family history
   relevant medical history, particularly details of previous neurosurgery, neuropathological diagnosis and treatment

2. Neuroradiology –
   site and approximate size of lesion
   contrast enhancement on CT and MRI scans
   characteristics of tumour margins
   relative tissue density
   effect on adjacent structures including oedema

3. Surgical findings –
   precise location and size of lesion
   appearance of the lesion and its margins
   presence of necrosis, haemorrhage, calcification or cysts
   associated lesions
   stereotactic target number

Neuropathologists will readily appreciate that not all the above information will always be available on the request form and personal contact with the neuroradiologists and clinicians concerned with the case is invaluable in obtaining essential information. In some instances it may be helpful to inspect the CT and MRI scans personally, although this is not practical in every case. Advance warning of particularly complex cases is also helpful, although most neuropathologists will have had the experience of suddenly being confronted with highly unusual lesions from patients with atypical clinical histories and neuroradiological findings which are difficult to interpret.

It is a useful practice to evaluate the clinical and neuroradiological features on each case using the information available from the request form and the relevant clinicians before the specimen is sampled and microscopy carried out. In this way, a provisional differential diagnosis can be established which is then modified in light of the macroscopic and microscopic features, allowing a diagnosis in most cases. The information required to begin the process of differential diagnosis, as indicated above, is not complex and should be available without undue difficulty in all cases.

5.1. Clinical features

Age and sex differences are of major importance in forming differential diagnosis. Whilst most neuroepithelial tumours occur at a higher incidence in males, the reverse is true for meningeal and nerve sheath tumours. The sex of the patient obviously influences the likely primary sites for metastatic lesions, particularly for breast carcinoma which is so commonly a cause of cerebral metastases. The age of the patient has an even greater impact on differential diagnosis, and detailed neuropathological investigations of brain tumours over a wide period of time and from many different countries have helped establish age-related incidence trends for intracranial tumours. These are summarized in Table 5.1, although the usefulness of this information must always be tempered by the knowledge that age is seldom a contra-indication to any diagnosis, particularly in children. Certain CNS tumours occur in the context of well-defined genetic disorders (*see* Table 5.2) and an accurate clinical and family history is of great importance in such conditions, particularly with patients with atypical clinical features. It is also recognized that neuroepithelial tumours in particular may occur in families who have none of these specific genetic disorders, the underlying basis for which is not yet established. Occasionally the diagnosis of a genetic disorder may be made only on investigation of the case in hand, for example a diagnosis of neurofibromatosis type II in a patient with bilateral acoustic Schwannomas. New mutations causing genetic disease may occasionally present as apparently sporadic disorders and a full family history is not always available in every patient.

It is critical to establish whether a patient has suffered from a previous tumour in the CNS, preferably in advance of the surgery so that any earlier histological material may be reviewed in advance of the intra-operative diagnosis. There is an increasing clinical

Table 5.1

Relative frequency of intracranial tumours in relation to age (commonest tumours at heads of columns)

Age (years)			
<3	3–15	15–65	>65
Medulloblastoma	Pilocytic astrocytoma	Glioblastoma	Metastatic carcinoma
Pilocytic astrocytoma	Medulloblastoma	Anaplastic astrocytoma	Glioblastoma
Ependymoma	Ependymoma	Astrocytoma	Anaplastic astrocytoma
Choroid plexus tumours	Astrocytoma	Meningioma	Meningioma
Teratoma	Choroid plexus tumours	Pituitary tumours	Acoustic Schwannoma

Table 5.2

Genetic disorders associated with CNS neoplasms

Disorder	Neoplasm
Neurofibromatosis type I	Pilocytic astrocytoma of optic nerve and chiasm
	Spinal neurofibroma
	Astrocytoma of cerebellum, brainstem or spinal cord
	Meningioma
Neurofibromatosis type II	Bilateral acoustic Schwannomas
	Multiple meningiomas
	Spinal Schwannoma
	Astrocytoma of spinal cord, brainstem and cerebellum
Tuberous sclerosis	Giant cell subependymal astrocytoma
Li-Fraumeni syndrome	Medulloblastoma
	PNET
Turcot's syndrome	Medulloblastoma
	Glioblastoma
	Astrocytoma
Gorlin's syndrome	Medulloblastoma
von Hippel-Lindau syndrome	Haemangioblastoma of cerebellum, spinal cord and retina
Familial retinoblastoma	Retinoblastoma
	Pineoblastoma

Table 5.3

Intraventricular tumours listed by site

Lateral ventricle	Third ventricle	Fourth ventricle
Ependymoma	Ependymoma	Ependymoma
Choroid plexus tumours (children)	Choroid plexus tumours (children)	Choroid plexus tumours (adults)
Central neurocytoma	Pilocytic astrocyoma	Subependymoma
Subependymal giant cell astrocytoma	Colloid cyst	Medulloblastoma
Subependymoma	Germ cell tumours	Pilocytic astrocytoma
Meningioma	Pineal cell tumours	Meningioma

Table 5.4

Regional intracranial tumours

Pituitary region	Skull base
Pituitary adenoma	Chordoma
Meningioma	Chondrosarcoma
Craniopharyngioma	Meningioma
Metastatic carcinoma	Acoustic Schwannoma
Astrocytoma	Carcinoma of paranasal sinuses
Germinoma	Glomus jugulare tumour
Rathke's cleft cyst	Olfactory neuroblastoma
Orbit (with intracranial extension)	**Cerebellopontine angle**
Meningioma	Acoustic Schwannoma
Optic nerve pilocytic astrocytoma	Meningioma
Lymphoma	Epidermoid cyst
Adenoid cystic carcinoma	Choroid plexus papilloma
Plexiform neurofibroma	Ependymoma
Malignant melanoma	Metastatic carcinoma

Table 5.5

Spinal cord tumours

Extradural	Intradural	
	Extramedullary	Intramedullary
Prolapsed intervertebral disc	Schwannoma	Astrocytoma
Metastatic carcinoma	Neurofibroma	Myxopapillary ependymoma
Lymphoma	Meningioma	Ependymoma
Plasmacytoma/multiple myeloma	Metastatic carcinoma	Oligodendroglioma
Bone and soft tissue tumours	Cysts (enterogenous, arachnoidal)	Haemangioblastoma
Bacterial abscess	Bacterial abscess	Paraganglioma
Tuberculosis	Metastatic PNET, glioblastoma, ependymoma	Multiple sclerosis

trend to re-biopsy recurrent brain tumours in order to establish an accurate diagnosis and give the most appropriate treatment and prognosis in both children and adults. It should also be borne in mind that CNS neoplasms occur at a higher incidence as second neoplasms in individuals with malignancies at other sites in the body, for example cerebral PNET occurring as a second malignancy in children who have been treated for leukaemia. This emphasizes the need to have full clinical information on previous neoplasms, even if they do not relate to the CNS and are apparently unassociated with the current clinical problem. It is also important to establish the nature of any treatment given for previous disorders, particularly radiotherapy and chemotherapy. The changes induced by radiotherapy in the brain are complex and may occasionally be mistaken for recurrent tumour or tumour progression e.g. astrocytoma to anaplastic astrocytoma. In particular, the vascular changes occurring as a consequence of irradiation can be mistaken for the endothelial hypoplasia which occurs in malignant gliomas; this difficulty can be anticipated when full background clinical details are available. It is important to know the sites of any other neoplasms in the body when biopsy of a suspected intracranial metastasis is carried out, although it is recognized that metastatic deposits within the brain may bear only a limited histological resemblance to the primary lesion.

5.2. NEURORADIOLOGY

Neuroradiological information is invaluable in the differential diagnosis of intracranial tumours, not only for the accurate delineation of the site, size and apparent margins of the neoplasm (Figs 5.1–5.2; Tables 5.3–5.5), but for the accurate recognition of tissue changes occurring in and around the lesion including calcification, necrosis and haemorrhage (Table 5.6) and cystic change within the lesion (Table 5.7). It is becoming increasingly possible to identify specific tissue constituents, e.g. adipose tissue, within CNS lesions and this is obviously

helpful for the neuropathologist. One of the most useful pieces of information from the neuroradiologist in addition to the above is the pattern of contrast enhancement on both CT and MRI scans following the administration of an intravenous contrast agent. In general, tumours arising outside the brain and spinal cord exhibit a uniform pattern of contrast enhancement, e.g. in meningiomas, since there is no blood-brain barrier to impair the spread of the contrast agent. However, a similar pattern can be seen in intrinsic tumours which are

Table 5.6

Macroscopic tumour abnormalities identifiable at surgery

Necrosis	Haemorrhage
Glioblastoma	Glioblastoma
Metastatic tumours	Metastatic tumours (particularly malignant melanoma)
Lymphoma	Haemangioblastoma
Anaplastic oligodendroglioma	Anaplastic oligodendroglioma
Anaplastic ependymoma	Anaplastic ependymoma
Medulloblastoma	Malignant teratoma and choriocarcinoma
PNET	Intracerebral haematoma
Choroid plexus carcinoma	Cerebral infarct
Malignant teratoma	

Calcification	
Extracerebral	Intracerebral
Meningioma	Oligodendroglioma
Craniopharyngioma	Pilocytic astrocytoma
Epidermoid and dermoid cysts	Astrocytoma
Pineal cysts and tumours	Choroid plexus papilloma
Pituitary adenoma	Subependymoma
	Ganglion cell tumours
	Subependymal giant cell astrocytoma
	Central neurocytoma

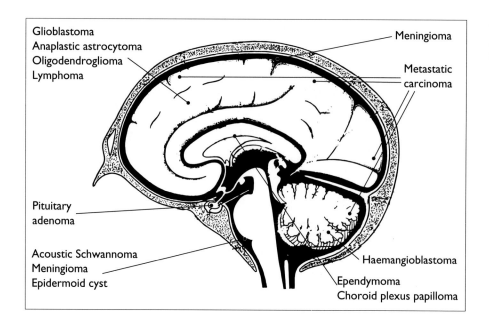

Figure 5.1
Anatomical distribution of the commonest CNS tumours in adults

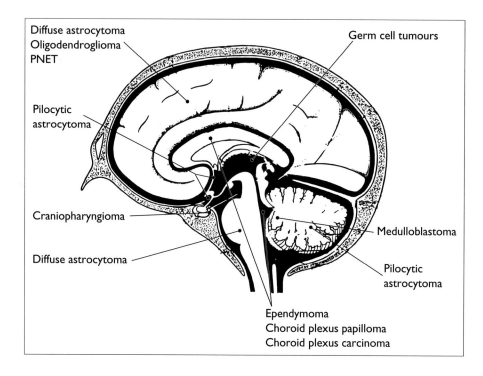

Figure 5.2
Anatomical distribution of the commonest CNS tumours in children

Table 5.7
Cystic CNS lesions

Extracerebral	Intracerebral	Spinal
Craniopharyngioma	Pilocytic astrocytoma	Myxopapillary ependymoma
Epidermoid and dermoid cysts	Haemangioblastoma	Pilocytic astrocytoma
Meningeal cysts (arachnoidal, glioependymal, enterogenous)	Ependymoma	Ependymoma
Pineal glial cyst	Colloid cyst	Haemangioblastoma
Rathke cleft cyst	Choroid plexus tumours	Syringomyelia
Pleomorphic xanthoastrocytoma		
Schwannoma		
Meningioma		

Table 5.8

Tumour enhancement patterns on CT/MRI scans

Lesion	Pattern of enhancement
Pilocytic astrocytoma	Diffuse enhancement with cystic change
Astrocytoma	Non-enhancing
Anaplastic astrocytoma	Variable, non-homogenous
Glioblastoma	Ring enhancement around necrotic foci
Oligodendroglioma	Non-enhancing with foci of calcification
Ependymoma	Solid portions show enhancement; cystic change and haemorrhage are common
Medulloblastoma	Variable, non-homogenous
Lymphoma	Densely enhancing with indistinct margins. Ring enhancement and multiple lesions may occur
Haemangioblastoma	Low density cyst with enhancing vascular nodule; solid enhancing vascular masses may occur
Metastatic tumours	Non-homogenous, with ring enhancement around necrotic lesions. Multiple lesions may occur
Pituitary adenoma	Homogenous
Craniopharyngioma	Non-homogenous enhancement with cystic change and calcification
Meningioma	Homogenous enhancement; extra-axial mass with associated skull hyperostosis
Schwannoma	Intense enhancement: extra-axial mass which expands the internal auditory canal

highly vascular e.g. haemangioblastomas. For neuroepithelial tumours, the presence of ring enhancement with contrast is a very helpful piece of information in differential diagnosis (Table 5.8), although this is by no means specific for such lesions and may be encountered in benign or reactive conditions. The knowledge of a neuroradiologist's opinion on the investigations performed in each case is most helpful and this frequently generates a differential diagnosis list which can be used as the starting point for pathological differential diagnosis. The neuroradiological features in each case are also important in relation to tumour undergoing stereotactic biopsy, where several targets may be sampled from different regions of the tumour. It is important to establish which targets come from neuroradiologically distinct areas of the tumour, e.g. tumour margin, tumour centre, necrotic region, etc. In this way, an accurate assessment of the cytological and histological features can be made in relation to the tumour architecture and this is of particular importance when neurosurgical resection is to be considered. Neuroradiology will also give information of immense value in lesions arising from adjacent structures to the brain and spinal cord, including the spinal extradural space, skull, vertebral column, paranasal sinuses and blood vessels. Digital subtraction angiography is available in many neuroradiological centres, and this provides additional information which is of value to the neuropathologist, particularly when the vascular characteristics or blood supply of a particular lesion are in question, or its relationship to major blood vessels.

5.3. OPERATIVE FINDINGS

A succinct account of the operative findings will in many cases aid neuropathological differential diagnosis, although it is recognized that this information is not applicable to stereotactic biopsy specimens. In other circumstances, the knowledge of the precise location of the lesion, its colour, shape, margin and relationship with other structures will provide useful information. The presence of cystic change within the lesion, necrosis or haemorrhage can all be readily identified at surgery; calcification may also be recognized during biopsy, even when it is not evident on MRI scans (Tables 5.6–5.7). In larger lesions where multiple biopsies have been performed it is important to establish the site of each biopsy in relation to the characteristics of the tumour, particularly in relation to the tumour margin. The biopsy of a cystic lesion frequently results in collapse of the cyst and this occasionally makes for difficulty in clinicopathological correlation. Most neurosurgeons will biopsy a mural nodule within a cyst, as this will often contain viable tumour which will give diagnostic information if sampled. Finally, it is important for the surgeon to confirm the anatomical location of the biopsy samples as this knowledge will influence the neuropathological interpretation not only of any reactive or neoplastic elements within the biopsy specimen, but will also make allowances for the wide variation in the normal cytological and architectural constituents of the brain (see Chapter 3).

Table 5.9
Differential diagnosis of cytological features in CNS tumours

Multinucleate cells	Neuronal or ganglion cells
Glioblastoma	Ganglion cell tumours
Gemistocytic astrocytoma	Pineocytoma
Ganglion cell tumours	Infiltrated cerebral grey matter and cerebellar cortex.
Pilocytic astrocytoma	Cortical dysplasia
Pleomorphic xanthoastrocytoma	Differentiated PNET/ medulloblastoma
Subependymal giant cell astrocytoma	Teratoma
Choriocarcinoma and malignant teratoma	Hypothalamic hamartoma
Tuberculosis	
Progressive multifocal leukoencephalopathy	
Fungal infections	
Prominent capillary blood vessels	**Perivascular lymphocytic cuffing**
Glioblastoma	Viral encephalitis
Anaplastic astrocytoma	Multiple sclerosis
Pilocytic astrocytoma	Lymphoma
Haemangioblastoma	Ganglion cell tumours
Lymphoma	Recent infarction
Pituitary adenoma	Glioblastoma
Myxopapillary ependymoma	Anaplastic astrocytoma
Edge of cerebral infarct	Pleomorphic xanthoastrocytoma
Arteriovenous malformation	
Radiation damage	
Small rounded tumour cells	**Small poorly differentiated tumour cells**
Oligodendroglioma	Medulloblastoma/PNET
Pituitary adenoma	Ependymoblastoma
Central neurocytoma	Pineoblastoma
Lymphoma	Neuroblastoma
DNET	Metastatic small cell anaplastic carcinoma
Germinoma	Glioblastoma
Pineocytoma	Malignant teratoma
Epithelial cells	
Metastatic carcinoma	
Choroid plexus tumours	
Epidermoid and dermoid cysts	
Craniopharyngioma	
Pituitary adenoma	
Rathke cleft cyst	
Teratoma (malignant and mature)	
Enterogenous cyst	

Table 5.10
Benign lesions which may be mistaken for CNS neoplasms at intra-operative diagnosis (see also Chapter 3)

Benign lesion	Misdiagnosis
Reactive astrocytosis	Astrocytoma
Cerebral infarct	Necrotic glioblastoma
Vascular malformation	Glioblastoma
Pineal glial cyst	Pineocytoma, astrocytoma
Pyogenic abscess	Glioblastoma
Viral encephalitis	Lymphoma
Multiple sclerosis	Lymphoma, Glioblastoma
Progressive multifocal leukoencephalopathy	Glioblastoma

Table 5.11
Low grade CNS neoplasms which may be mistaken for high grade tumours at intra-operative diagnosis

CNS neoplasm	Misdiagnosis
Pilocytic astrocytoma	Fibrillary astrocytoma, anaplastic astrocytoma
Giant cell subependymal astrocytoma	Glioblastoma
Pleomorphic xanthoastrocytoma	Glioblastoma
Central neurocytoma	Oligodendroglioma
DNET	Oligodendroglioma Ganglioglioma
Desmoplastic infantile ganglioglioma	Meningeal sarcoma Glioblastoma
Haemangioblastoma	Pilocytic astrocytoma Metastatic renal carcinoma
Choroid plexus papilloma	Metastatic papillary adenocarcinoma

5.4. NEUROPATHOLOGICAL DIFFERENTIAL DIAGNOSIS

Neuropathological differential diagnosis begins once the information on the clinical request form has been read and assimilated, and the biopsy specimen is inspected macroscopically. In larger biopsy specimens there will be a number of sites available for sampling for smear preparations and it will also be helpful in many cases to perform examination of the tissue by cryostat section. The tissue sampled for both smear and cryostat section examination should include suspected neoplasm, whilst taking care to avoid areas which appear totally necrotic or haemorrhagic, or tissue which is completely calcified or contains fragments of bone and cartilage which are not amenable to examination by either smear preparations or cryostat sections. Many biopsies are composed of tissue which is too firm for smear examination (see Chapter 18) but in most cases, particularly in intrinsic neuroepithelial tumours, the tissue is soft enough to make adequate smear preparations and these alone may be satisfactory for diagnosis (see Chapter 3). The interpretation of the cellular constituents in smear preparations and cryostat sections has already been covered in Chapters 3 and 4, but identification of specific cellular or architectural features can in turn establish a differential diagnosis which is finally resolved by the recognition of other (sometimes more subtle) histological features.

Without being comprehensive, it is helpful to establish differential diagnosis lists for certain cytological features which are commonly encountered in intra-operative diagnosis (Table 5.9). This complex question of differential diagnosis may be reduced in essence to three main considerations:

1. Is the tissue normal?
2. If the tissue is abnormal, does it contain:
   (a) reactive changes only? (Table 5.10).
   (b) neoplastic tissue and if so, what type? (Table 5.11).

Not infrequently, there may be normal, reactive and neoplastic elements contained within a single biopsy specimen and it is clearly important for the neuropathologist to distinguish between them, when present both in combination and singly (see subsequent chapters for specific tumour entities).

5.5. CONCLUSION

It is clear that a wide range of clinical, neuroradiological, operative and histological information is necessary for differential diagnosis in order to arrive at a definitive intra-operative diagnosis. It is hoped that the information summarized in the text and tables above will facilitate this process, although considerable experience in intra-operative diagnosis has not diminished our amazement over the years at the wide spectrum and variety of histological changes encountered in smear and cryostat preparations of intracranial tumours. Having said that, it is also important to remember that 'common things occur commonly' and that one should never feel forced into making an intra-operative diagnosis on material which is not sufficient or satisfactory for this purpose or which has not been sampled adequately. Neuropathologists have an important role to play in patient management by providing an accurate diagnosis to the neurosurgeon at the time of surgery. This important role requires the neuropathologist to act as a member of the team involved in the care and the investigation of the patient, and the importance of adequate communication between the team members cannot be over-emphasized, particularly at the time of intra-operative diagnosis.

SIX

ASTROCYTIC TUMOURS

Taken together as a group the astrocytic tumours are the commonest primary brain tumours. The unifying feature of these tumours is their resemblance to astrocytes, most notably due to their possession of cytoplasmic processes and immunoreactivity for GFAP. In the WHO classification (1992) there are three entities – astrocytoma, anaplastic astrocytoma and glioblastoma – which can essentially be regarded as different grades of malignancy of 'ordinary' astrocytic tumours. In addition, the WHO classification includes three other astrocytic tumours which are uncommon but which are important to recognize because they are distinct clinicopathological entities associated with a relatively good prognosis – pilocytic astrocytoma, pleomorphic xanthoastrocytoma and subependymal giant cell astrocytoma. It can be a challenge to identify these latter three tumours intra-operatively as some of their features, such as nuclear atypia and vascular proliferation may, inappropriately, suggest that the tumour is of high grade. The importance of an awareness of the clinical context, particularly the age of the patient and the anatomical location of the tumour, in correctly identifying these tumours cannot be over-emphasized.

THE ASTROCYTOMA, ANAPLASTIC ASTROCYTOMA, GLIOBLASTOMA SPECTRUM

Tumours of the astrocytoma, anaplastic astrocytoma, glioblastoma spectrum may occur at any location within the central nervous system. Clinical presentation is usually as a consequence of the mass effect of the tumour, with seizures or with focal neurological deficits. They are typically diffusely infiltrating tumours, with ill-defined margins, and consequently complete excision is usually impracticable. Grading of astrocytic tumours is associated with a number of problems and imposes artificial and somewhat arbitrary divisions of what may be a continuous spectrum of malignancy. Historically there have been numerous different grading systems and this has led to some confusion with respect to nomenclature and application of numbers to the different grades. A practical problem with grading arises as a consequence of two factors: firstly, there is an increasing trend towards provision of very small samples of tumour acquired by stereotactic surgery; secondly, astrocytic tumours are frequently non-uniform in their histological features. As a result there may be uncertainty about how representative the sample of tissue obtained is of

the lesion as a whole. An additional problem is that the natural history of astrocytic tumours is to evolve over a period of time in their degree of malignancy. As a consequence of these factors it is appropriate to regard the histological grade assigned to a particular tumour biopsy as the minimum grade of the tumour as a whole. It is often appropriate to combine the information from a biopsy with that obtained from imaging studies, particularly with respect to the identification of necrosis and contrast enhancement. The presence of contrast enhancement correlates reasonably well with the vascular changes which indicate that a tumour is of high grade. Despite the drawbacks, both real and potential which are outlined above, in practice the grading of astrocytic tumours provides a useful guide to prognosis and to appropriate therapy. Of particular relevance to a discussion of intra-operative diagnosis, information at the time of operation about the grade of an astrocytic tumour may help to guide the neurosurgeon in the extent of surgery.

Assignation of an 'ordinary' astrocytic tumour to one of the three categories of the WHO classification (astrocytoma, anaplastic astrocytoma and glioblastoma) essentially is based on the presence or absence of four variables: nuclear atypia, mitotic figures, endothelial cell hyperplasia and tumour necrosis. In practice there should be little difficulty in identifying these features, whether in smear preparations or in frozen sections at the time of the neurosurgical operation.

6.1. ASTROCYTOMA

Astrocytoma represents the low-grade end of the spectrum of 'ordinary' astrocytic tumours (WHO grade 2) and is defined by the absence of mitotic figures, absence of endothelial cell hyperplasia and absence of tumour necrosis. Nuclear atypia is usually present.

6.1.1. CLINICAL AND RADIOLOGICAL FEATURES

The archetypal astrocytoma arises in the cerebral hemispheres of a young adult. However astrocytomas may occur at any location in the central nervous system, including grey and white matter in the cerebrum, brainstem, cerebellum or spinal cord and over a broad range of age. By far the commonest variant is the fibrillary astrocytoma which is typically centred on cerebral white matter. The much less common protoplasmic astrocytoma has a tendency to be superficially located, involving cerebral cortical grey matter. CT scans show an ill-defined low density lesion without contrast enhancement. MR shows an ill-defined area of low signal in T1 weighted images, although the lesion often appears to be better circumscribed on T2 weighted images. Astrocytomas, including those in the spinal cord, may be associated with a fluid-filled cyst. The mean survival of patients presenting with astrocytoma is 5–8 years with conversion to glioblastoma a common terminal event.

6.1.2. SURGICAL FINDINGS

Astrocytomas may be difficult to distinguish at operation from the surrounding central nervous tissue. This is due in part to their homogeneous appearance and the similarity in the colour of the tumour to the surrounding brain. Diffuse infiltration of pre-existing structures, for example expansion of cortical gyri, ensures that a tumour margin is usually not identifiable macroscopically. The neurosurgeon may report that the tumour is recognizable by a difference in texture, being relatively firm in comparison with the surrounding brain.

6.1.3. INTRA-OPERATIVE PATHOLOGY

Smear cytology

As a consequence of the difficulty described above in defining the margins of astrocytic tumours selection of the appropriate areas to smear from a large specimen may be problematic. However, the solid areas of tumour are usually abnormally firm and may contain cysts. Astrocytomas usually smear easily. The low-power appearance of smear preparations shows a tumour of low to moderate cellularity in which the cells are often arranged in irregular clusters around blood vessels giving

a somewhat papillary pattern. The margins of the cell clusters usually appear rather ill-defined as they are formed from cytoplasmic processes which are typically abundant. In some tumours the cells are less cohesive and smear out individually. The tumour cell nuclei may be round, oval or somewhat elongated with an irregular profile and coarsely stippled chromatin. The cytoplasm is usually scanty. The cytoplasmic processes are metachromatic in smears stained with toluidine blue and eosinophilic with haematoxylin and eosin staining. Mitotic figures are absent, blood vessels are thin-walled, and tumour necrosis is not identified. When smears are made from the diffusely infiltrating margin of an astrocytoma the neoplastic astrocytes may be scattered among neurons and oligodendrocytes with the background being formed from finely textured neuropil rather than entirely from coarser astrocytic tumour cell processes as seen in smears of solid astrocytoma. On occasion tumours may consist only of a focus of diffusely infiltrated brain with no solid tumour being present (diffuse cerebral astrocytoma).

Frozen sections

There is usually little difficulty in recognizing astrocytomas on frozen sections and they show cytological features similar to those described above. The neoplasm is recognized as being astrocytic in nature by the morphology of the nuclei and the abundant cytoplasmic processes. The cellularity is usually low to moderate. Mitotic figures and necrosis are absent. Blood vessels are thin-walled. Microcysts are a common feature of astrocytoma. Diffuse infiltration of tumour cells at the margin of an astrocytoma is usually distinguishable from normal or reactive central nervous tissue by the increased cellularity and the nuclear pleomorphism.

Protoplasmic astrocytoma is an uncommon variant in which the tumour cell nuclei are typically uniform and rather spherical and cytoplasmic processes are scanty

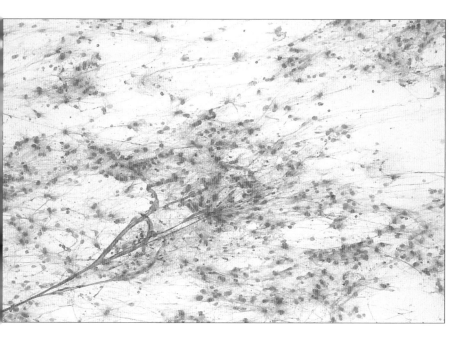

Fig. 6.1
Astrocytoma. Male aged 33 years, frontal tumour. Astrocytomas are usually of low to moderate cellularity in smear preparations. As shown in this example the cells are often loosely aggregated around blood vessels which do not exhibit endothelial hyperplasia. The cells are uniform and a background of cytoplasmic processes is visible even at low power. There is no tumour necrosis. Smear preparation, haematoxylin eosin, ×350.

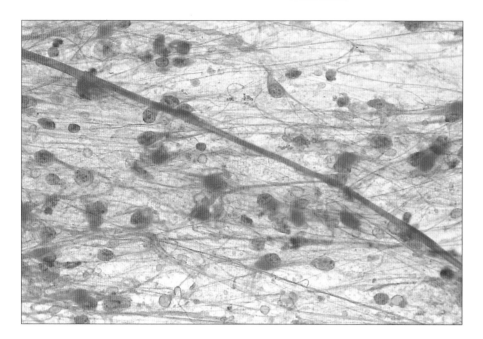

Figure 6.2
Astrocytoma. Male aged 33 years, frontal tumour. The same tumour as illustrated in Fig. 6.1. The cells have uniform round or ovoid nuclei, scanty cytoplasm and abundant coarse cytoplasmic processes. Mitoses are not identified. A thin-walled blood vessel crosses the field. Smear preparation, haematoxylin eosin, ×1400.

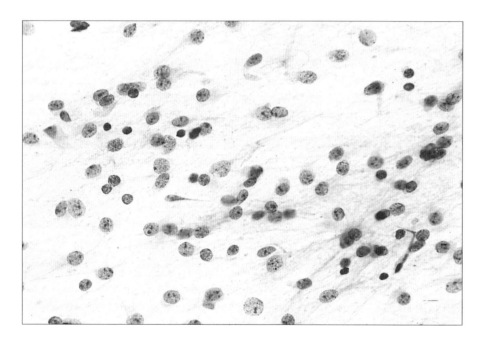

Figure 6.3
Astrocytoma. Female aged 40 years, parietal tumour. In smears stained with toluidine blue the cytoplasmic processes are often less distinct than with H&E, but the nuclear detail is more clearly seen. The nuclei are round or ovoid in shape, in some cases with a slightly irregular profile, with coarsely stippled chromatin and relatively indistinct nucleoli. The overall appearance resembles that of a potato. Smear preparation, toluidine blue, ×1400.

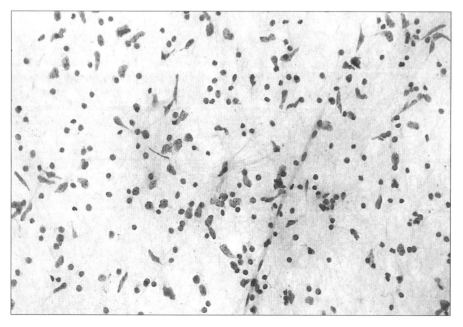

Figure 6.4
Astrocytoma. Female aged 31 years, cerebral tumour. This smear is from the diffusely infiltrating margin of an astrocytoma and has the appearance of hypercellular central nervous tissue. The population of cells is heterogeneous and includes cells with small round nuclei, probably oligodendrocytes, together with larger irregularly shaped astrocytic nuclei. The textureless blue-stained background represents pre-existing neuropil rather than the more coarse cytoplasmic processes of astrocytes. It may be difficult or impossible to be certain whether this appearance represents diffusely infiltrating astrocytoma or reactive gliosis. Smear preparation, toluidine blue, ×700.

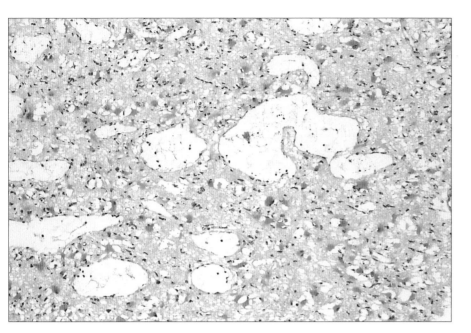

Figure 6.5
Astrocytoma. Male aged 47 years, cerebral tumour. Frozen sections show an astrocytic tumour of low cellularity. Although there is a degree of cellular pleomorphism mitoses are not identified, blood vessels are thin-walled and there is no tumour necrosis. The eosinophilic background is composed of cytoplasmic processes of the tumour cells. Microcysts, as seen in this example, are generally a feature of low grade astrocytic tumours. Frozen section, haematoxylin eosin, ×700.

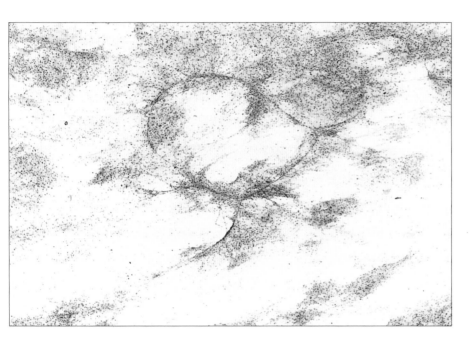

Figure 6.6
Protoplasmic astrocytoma. Male aged 31 years, frontal tumour. This variant shows the low power appearance typical of an astrocytic tumour with tumour cells aggregating around thin-walled blood vessels. However, even at this power the blue-stained background formed from tumour cell processes has an unusually fine texture for an astrocytoma. Smear preparation, toluidine blue, ×90.

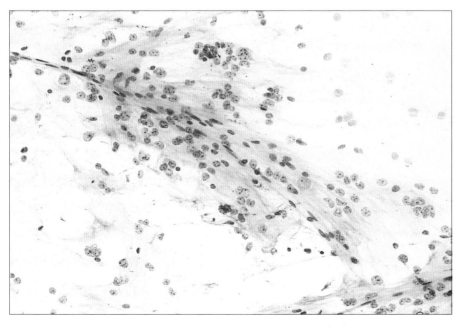

Figure 6.7
Protoplasmic astrocytoma. Male aged 31 years, frontal tumour. The same tumour as illustrated in Fig. 6.6. In contrast to the more common (fibrillary) astrocytomas illustrated above the cells have spherical nuclei and very fine cytoplasmic processes giving a rather mucinous appearance to the background. Smear preparation, toluidine blue, ×700.

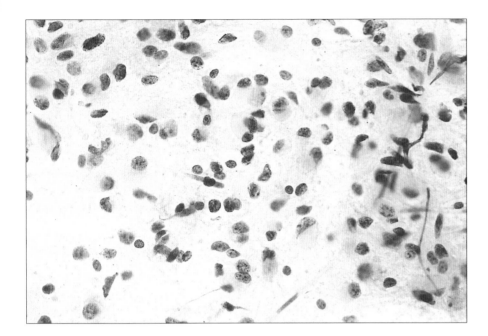

Figure 6.8
Gemistocytic astrocytoma. Male aged 37 years, cerebral tumour. In gemistocytic astrocytomas the majority of cells have abundant cytoplasm. This feature can be difficult to appreciate in smears stained with toluidine blue as the cytoplasm is pale. The cells generally exhibit less cohesion than other astrocytomas presumably because they tend to have fewer processes. Smear preparation, toluidine blue, ×1400.

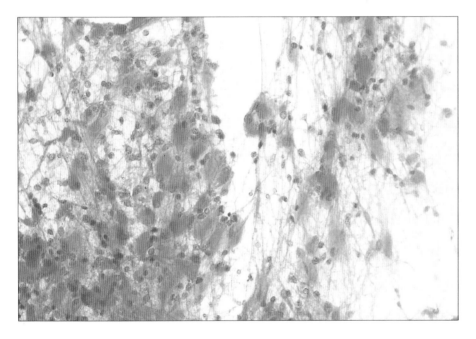

Figure 6.9
Gemistocytic astrocytoma. Female aged 27 years, cerebral tumour. The abundant cytoplasm of gemistocytic astrocytomas is intensely eosinophilic in smears stained with H&E. Cytoplasmic processes are also apparent. The nuclei are often more spherical than in other astrocytic tumours and lie eccentrically in the cells. Smear preparation, haematoxylin eosin, ×700.

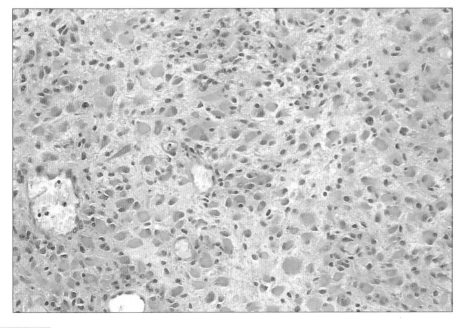

Figure 6.10
Gemistocytic astrocytoma. Female aged 27 years, cerebral tumour. The same tumour as illustrated in Fig. 6.9. Frozen sections show a tumour of moderate cellularity in which the majority of cells have gemistocytic morphology. Although there are no mitoses, blood vessels are thin-walled and there is no tumour necrosis, gemistocytic astrocytomas have a poorer prognosis than other forms of low grade astrocytoma. Frozen section, haematoxylin eosin, ×700.

and very fine, sometimes giving a mucinous appearance to the background. In **gemistocytic astrocytoma** a large proportion of the tumour cells have abundant cytoplasm and typically rather scanty processes. The nuclei are usually situated eccentrically within the cells. Perhaps because of the relative paucity of their processes the cells of gemistocytic astrocytoma have less of a tendency to form clusters with a greater tendency for the cells to smear individually. The importance of identifying gemistocytic astrocytoma is because of its propensity to undergo relatively rapid anaplastic transformation and association with a relatively short survival. However, recognition of the protoplasmic and gemistocytic variants of astrocytoma is likely to be of relatively limited importance at the time of operation and such refinements are probably best left to examination of the paraffin histology.

6.1.4. DIFFERENTIAL DIAGNOSIS

The clinical and radiological differential diagnosis of astrocytoma includes reactive gliosis, pilocytic astrocytoma, anaplastic astrocytoma, mixed tumours in which astrocytoma is a component, particularly oligoastrocytoma, and ependymoma.

Distinction between a low-grade astrocytic neoplasm and **reactive hypertrophy and proliferation of astrocytes** may represent a challenge at the time of operation and the distinction clearly is likely to be of use to the neurosurgeon. One helpful feature is that hypertrophic reactive astrocytes tend to have abundant cytoplasm, and although this is also the case with the cells of a gemistocytic astrocytoma, reactive astrocytes usually have more abundant processes. With certain exceptions, such as the bizarre cells seen in progressive multifocal leucoencephalopathy, reactive astrocytes are more uniform in nuclear and cytoplasmic morphology than neoplastic astrocytes. Microcysts, which may be identified in frozen sections but not clearly in smears, are rarely a feature of reactive gliosis. **Infarction** and **demyelination**, particularly if subacute, may produce appearances which are difficult to distinguish from astrocytoma although these reactive processes generally include other types of cells such as lymphocytes and macrophages. Reactive changes adjacent to a slowly growing non-astrocytic tumour or a non-neoplastic lesion can cause a problematic differential diagnosis and this may be a particular problem in the spinal cord from which the tissue sample provided is usually very small.

It may be impossible to distinguish with certainty an astrocytoma from a **pilocytic astrocytoma** at the time of operation and the distinction is unlikely to modify greatly the neurosurgical procedure. An awareness of the characteristic anatomical locations of pilocytic astrocytoma and the age range of the patients affected is important in raising the possibility of this diagnosis.

At times the neurosurgeon may experience difficulty in defining macroscopically the tumour margin and may request serial smears or frozen sections to aid in this process. Microscopic identification of the tumour margin may be equally problematic, due to the diffusely infiltrating nature of these tumours, and rests essentially on assessment of the increased cellularity of otherwise preserved grey or white matter. During this process the difference which can be made by the thickness of the smear preparation or frozen section to the apparent cellularity of the tissue must be appreciated.

Once the astrocytes have been recognized as neoplastic there are relatively few situations in which they may occur outside the context of pure astrocytic tumours. Of particular note with regard to the mixed tumours that may contain an astrocytic component is **oligoastrocytoma** which may not be recognized as such if a predominantly astrocytic area is examined intra-operatively. **Dysembryoplastic neuroepithelial tumour**, which typically presents with intractable seizures and is located in the temporal lobe, may contain foci of astrocytic differentiation. In addition, **astrocytic differentiation in a primitive neuroectodermal tumour** may occur rarely and may be so pronounced as to mimic astrocytoma.

Oligodendroglioma can usually be readily distinguished from astrocytoma by the tendency of the cells to spread apart in smears and by the spherical shape of the nuclei. However because of the nuclear morphology protoplasmic astrocytoma, in particular, may be confused with oligodendroglioma.

Ependymoma is an important differential diagnosis with a paraventricular or spinal cord lesion. The cells of ependymoma in smear preparations are less cohesive than those of astrocytoma, the nuclei are more spherical and cytoplasmic processes are usually less abundant. Perivascular pseudorosettes can often be recognized in smear preparations, but if there is doubt about their presence then frozen sections should be examined. In the spinal cord, ependymoma is the principal differential diagnosis and the importance in its recognition at the time of surgery is related to the relatively well-demarcated margin of ependymoma, in comparison with astrocytoma, allowing for an attempt at complete macroscopic excision.

6.2. ANAPLASTIC ASTROCYTOMA

Anaplastic astrocytoma (WHO grade 3) is intermediate in histological grade and biological behaviour between astrocytoma and glioblastoma. Mean post-operative survival is in the region of two years. Likewise the ages of the patients in which these tumours occur typically lie between those of the young adult with astrocytoma and the middle aged to elderly individuals with glioblastoma. CT and MR scans show a lesion resembling an astrocytoma, without contrast enhancement or evidence of necrosis. The presence of these latter features on imaging may suggest that the lesion is in reality a glioblastoma although, as a result of sampling bias, a biopsy shows only sufficient microscopic features to permit a diagnosis of anaplastic astrocytoma. At operation the appearance is that of an astrocytic tumour without the haemorrhage and necrosis seen in glioblastoma.

6.2.1. INTRA-OPERATIVE PATHOLOGY

In the WHO classification anaplastic astrocytoma is by definition a tumour with nuclear atypia and mitotic figures but without endothelial cell hyperplasia or necrosis. The appearances of anaplastic astrocytoma show considerable variability. Some tumours warranting this diagnosis resemble astrocytoma in their cell density and degree of differentiation, but contain a few mitotic figures, whereas others are densely cellular and poorly differentiated tumours with considerable cellular pleomorphism and numerous mitotic figures. The volume of tumour examined in smears or frozen sections is very small and it must always be recognized that features not present may be included in the remainder of the surgically removed tissue which will subsequently be processed for paraffin histology. It may therefore be appropriate to report to the neurosurgeon that smears or frozen sections showing nuclear atypia and mitotic figures alone represent a 'high grade astrocytic tumour' with the understanding that subsequent paraffin histology will clarify whether the tumour is an anaplastic astrocytoma or a glioblastoma.

6.2.2. DIFFERENTIAL DIAGNOSIS

There is usually little difficulty in distinguishing an anaplastic astrocytoma from a reactive astrocytic

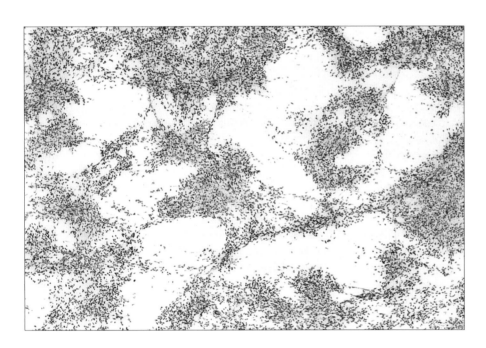

Figure 6.11
Anaplastic astrocytoma. Male aged 41 years, cerebral tumour. This tumour has smeared into irregular clusters to give a low power appearance typical of an astrocytic tumour. However, even at this power the cellularity is more dense than is usually the case with low grade astrocytomas. Smear preparation, toluidine blue, ×175.

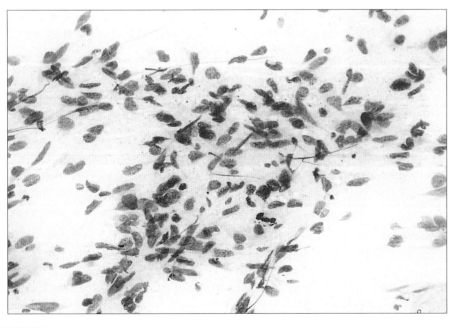

Figure 6.12
Anaplastic astrocytoma. Male aged 41 years, cerebral tumour. The same tumour as illustrated in Fig. 6.11 is seen at higher power. The tumour appears not very well differentiated: the nuclei are large and rather irregular and cytoplasmic processes are not prominent. A mitotic figure is identifiable (below right of centre). In this case endothelial hyperplasia and necrosis were not present in the smears or in the material subsequently processed for paraffin histology. Smear preparation, toluidine blue, ×700.

process. An exception to this is **progressive multifocal leucoencephalopathy** (PML) in which the astrocytes are typically pleomorphic and bizarre. PML is distinguishable by the presence of macrophages and enlarged oligodendrocyte nuclei and it is particularly important to be aware of the clinical context: PML occurs almost exclusively in immunosuppressed individuals, including those with AIDS.

The most common differential diagnosis is that of **glioblastoma** in which, by chance, the vascular changes and necrosis that are the defining features of glioblastoma were not included in the sample of tumour examined intra-operatively.

6.3. GLIOBLASTOMA

6.3.1. CLINICAL AND RADIOLOGICAL FEATURES

By far the most common primary CNS tumour is glioblastoma (WHO grade 4) which represents the high grade end of the spectrum of 'ordinary' astrocytic tumours. Glioblastoma may occur at all ages and at all locations in the central nervous system. However, most commonly it presents as a tumour in the cerebral hemispheres of middle-aged or elderly individuals with a short history of symptoms. There is evidence to suggest that it may arise in one of two different ways. Firstly, it may arise by evolution from an astrocytoma or anaplastic astrocytoma in which case there may be a prolonged clinical and radiological history. Previous neurosurgical operations may have been performed and material may be available from these for comparison. Secondly, glioblastoma may arise *de novo* as a rapidly growing and highly malignant tumour. Imaging studies typically show a central low density area with 'ring'

enhancement and oedema of surrounding tissue. In these respects it resembles an abscess which is an important clinical and radiological differential diagnosis. Glioblastomas may appear well circumscribed on imaging and the possibility that the lesion represents a metastasis may have been considered.

The macroscopic appearance of glioblastoma at operation is typically of firm greyish-brown tissue with areas of haemorrhage and whitish-yellow areas of necrosis. At operation these tumours may appear well-circumscribed but this is misleading as there is always diffuse infiltration of surrounding structures and even when a macroscopically complete removal is performed glioblastomas recur rapidly. Glioblastoma may also disseminate via the CSF pathways and form discrete deposits of tumour elsewhere in the central nervous system – usually superficially, sometimes in relation to the leptomeninges or nerve roots. Metastasis outside the central nervous system is exceptionally unusual. Glioblastoma is a highly malignant and rapidly growing tumour which is associated with a very poor prognosis – mean survival following diagnosis is typically less than one year.

6.3.2. INTRA-OPERATIVE PATHOLOGY

Glioblastomas are usually readily diagnosed on smear preparations or on frozen sections. This tumour is defined by the presence of nuclear atypia and mitoses together with endothelial cell hyperplasia and/or tumour necrosis. The appearances of glioblastoma vary widely with some lesions being composed of well-differentiated, albeit malignant astrocytes with abundant cytoplasmic processes which on smear preparations show the arrangement of tumour cells around blood vessels which is also seen in lower grade astrocytic tumours. At the other end of the spectrum are poorly differentiated tumours in which there is little cohesion

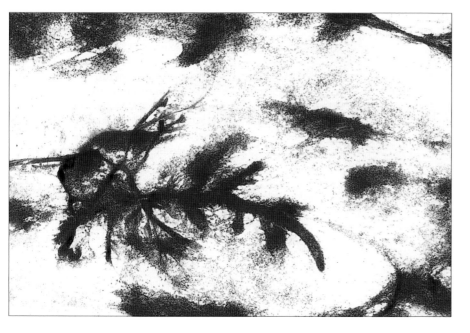

Figure 6.13
Glioblastoma. Female aged 54 years, frontal tumour. At low power the tumour has smeared into a pattern typical of a glial tumour with clustering of cells around blood vessels. The indistinct appearance to the margins of the cell clusters is due to the presence of cytoplasmic processes. Even at this power the blood vessels appear hyperplastic. Smear preparation, toluidine blue, ×90.

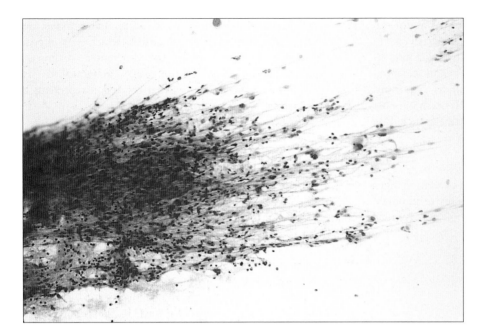

Figure 6.14
Glioblastoma. Male aged 48 years, cerebral tumour. At higher power the ill-defined appearance of the margin of the cell clusters is seen to be largely a consequence of the cytoplasmic processes. The tumour is densely cellular in comparison with the low grade astrocytomas illustrated above. Smear preparation, toluidine blue, ×350.

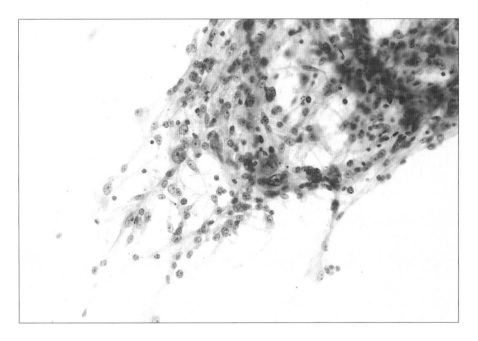

Figure 6.15
Glioblastoma. Male aged 48 years, cerebral tumour. The same tumour as illustrated in Fig. 6.14. The cells are pleomorphic with large nuclei, scanty cytoplasm and coarse cytoplasmic processes. Many of the cells have prominent nucleoli. Smear preparation, toluidine blue, ×700.

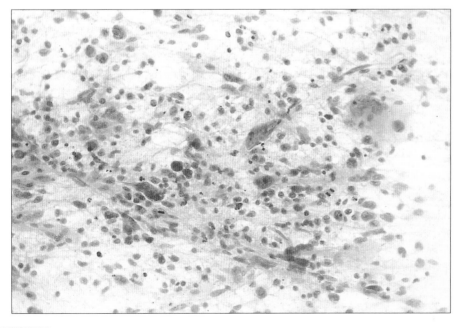

Figure 6.16
Glioblastoma. Female aged 68 years, corpus callosum tumour. In some examples of glioblastoma the cells are small and relatively uniform whereas in other tumours, as in this case, there is marked variation in size and shape. Although this tumour was rather degenerate the eosinophilic cytoplasmic processes can still be seen. Smear preparation, haematoxylin eosin, ×700.

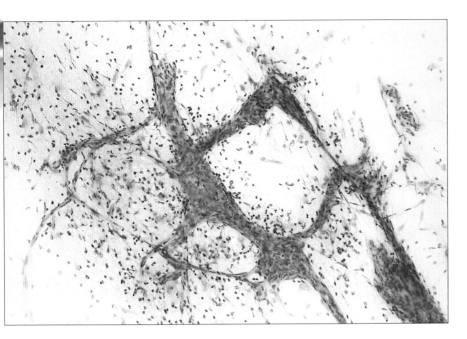

Figure 6.17
Glioblastoma. Male aged 75 years, parietal tumour. This smear is from the diffusely infiltrating edge of a glioblastoma. The vessels show prominent endothelial cell hyperplasia standing out against the background which is relatively sparsely cellular compared with the solid tumour. Endothelial cell hyperplasia is one of the defining features of glioblastoma. Smear preparation, toluidine blue, ×700.

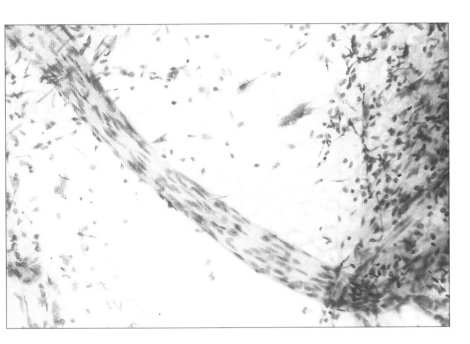

Figure 6.18
Glioblastoma. Male aged 42 years, cerebral tumour. A high power view of a vessel exhibiting endothelial cell hyperplasia. Pleomorphic astrocytic tumour cells are present in the background. Smear preparation, toluidine blue, ×1400.

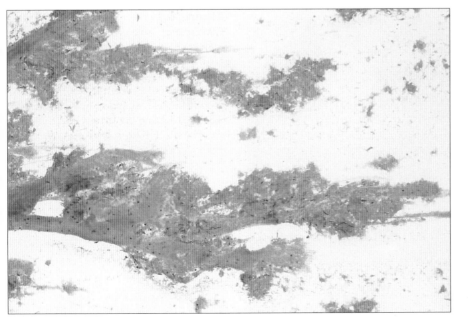

Figure 6.19
Glioblastoma. Male aged 58 years, cerebral tumour. Even though most of the material in this smear preparation was necrotic the low power architecture of an astrocytic tumour is retained. Viable tumour cells were present elsewhere in the smear to permit an intra-operative diagnosis of glioblastoma. Smear preparation, haematoxylin eosin, ×350.

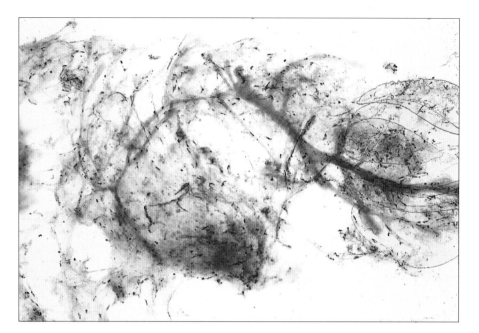

Figure 6.20
Glioblastoma. Male aged 58 years, cerebral tumour. The same tumour as illustrated in Fig. 6.19. This is the appearance of necrotic glioblastoma in smears stained with toluidine blue. As in the previous figure the characteristic low power architecture of the tumour is retained. The degenerate blood vessels appear to have been hyperplastic. Smear preparation, toluidine blue, ×350.

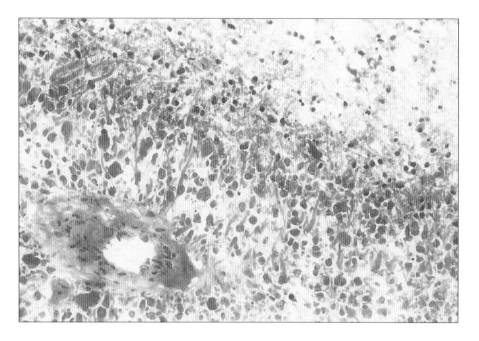

Figure 6.21
Glioblastoma. Female aged 73 years, cerebral tumour. This frozen section of glioblastoma shows pleomorphic tumour cells with pseudo-palisading of cells adjacent to an area of tumour necrosis (top). The tumour is rather degenerate and relatively few cytoplasmic processes are visible. Frozen section, haematoxylin eosin, ×700.

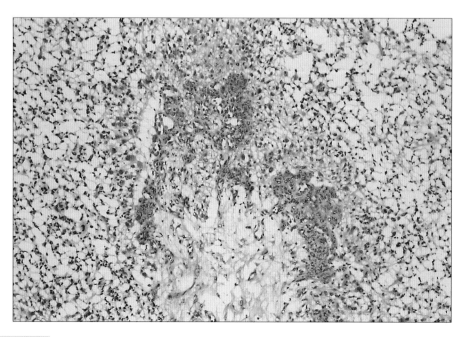

Figure 6.22
Glioblastoma. Male aged 63 years, cerebral tumour. This tumour is composed of relatively small and uniform cells. However mitotic figures were identified and there were numerous clusters of hyperplastic endothelial cells, as shown in the centre of this field, defining the tumour as a glioblastoma. Frozen section, haematoxylin eosin, ×350.

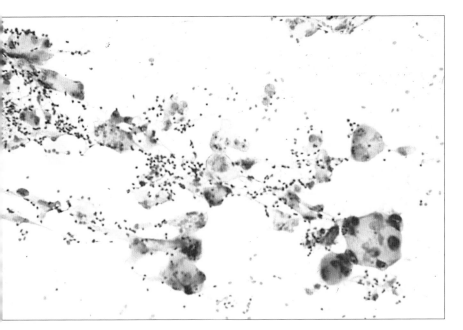

Figure 6.23
Giant cell glioblastoma. Male aged 46 years, cerebral tumour. Giant cell glioblastoma contains very large, bizarre and pleomorphic tumour cells. Numerous multinucleated giant tumour cells are present in this low power view. There is usually little doubt as to the glial nature of this tumour although cytoplasmic processes may be relatively sparse. Few other tumours have such large and bizarre cells. Smear preparation, toluidine blue, ×350.

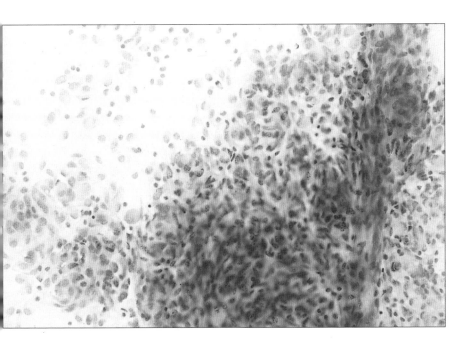

Figure 6.24
Gliosarcoma. Male aged 45 years, superficial frontal tumour. Gliosarcoma is a tough tumour which generally smears poorly to reveal a densely cellular malignant tumour. Although the softer glial component of this biphasic tumour is more likely to be selected for smearing in this example the tumour cells are poorly differentiated and it is unclear which component is represented here. The diagnosis of gliosarcoma was not made intra-operatively but on the basis of subsequent paraffin histology. Smear preparation, toluidine blue, ×700.

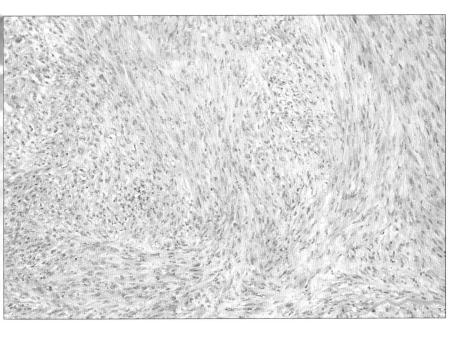

Figure 6.25
Gliosarcoma. Female aged 64 years, superficial cerebral tumour. This frozen section shows a sarcomatous appearance with malignant spindle-shaped cells arranged in ill-defined fascicles. Subsequent paraffin histology showed biphasic tumour with cytologically malignant mesenchymal and glial components. Frozen section, haematoxylin eosin, ×350.

of the cells – instead they smear out individually, and there are few cytoplasmic processes. Such tumours may be very difficult or impossible at the time of operation to distinguish from other poorly differentiated tumours – such as metastases. It is worth noting that true vascular endothelial cell hyperplasia, which is readily recognizable in smears, rarely occurs outside the context of glioblastoma – it is occasionally seen in metastases, particularly of bronchial carcinoma, and is common in pilocytic astrocytoma. In some cases there may be no uncertainty concerning the astrocytic nature of the tumour, but there is doubt about the interpretation of vascular changes or identification of necrosis. In this situation it may be appropriate, as suggested above, to inform the neurosurgeons that the lesion is a 'high grade astrocytic tumour' with more precise classification to follow when the paraffin histology has been examined.

Giant cell glioblastoma is a variant in which there are very large, bizarre and pleomorphic tumour cells. Often there are cells with very numerous nuclei and abundant cytoplasm. Cytoplasmic processes are usually easily identifiable but may be relatively scanty. Some studies have suggested that the outlook for this variant of glioblastoma is slightly less gloomy.

It is unlikely that a firm diagnosis of **gliosarcoma** will be made intra-operatively on the basis of the small amounts of tumour sampled by smear or frozen section. This tumour contains both malignant glial and malignant mesenchymal components. Identification of this variant does not significantly alter the patient's prognosis. Gliosarcomas are often superficially situated and firm in texture and may be mistaken clinically and radiologically for meningioma. The glial component usually resembles a typical glioblastoma whereas the sarcomatous component resembles a malignant mesenchymal tumour formed from spindle-shaped cells. As the sarcomatous component is relatively tough it is likely that in making smear preparations the glial component will be preferentially selected. Confident diagnosis of a gliosarcoma is likely to require waiting for paraffin histology with its benefits of wider sampling of the tumour, stains for reticulin and immunohistochemistry. Even when this additional information is available there are no clear guidelines for distinguishing gliosarcoma from a glioblastoma with florid proliferation of reactive mesenchymal elements.

6.3.3. DIFFERENTIAL DIAGNOSIS

An important differential diagnosis of glioblastoma from the clinical and radiological point of view is that of an **abscess**. There is usually little difficulty making the distinction intra-operatively by smear or frozen section. However, on occasions this may be problematic due to reasons of sampling. Not infrequently the specimen initially obtained from the centre of a glioblastoma is entirely necrotic. The necrotic areas of a glioblastoma usually contain very few inflammatory cells, whereas the

pus from an abscess comprises abundant and often degenerate or necrotic acute inflammatory cells. It is, however, unwise to make the diagnosis of glioblastoma on this basis without definite recognition of neoplastic astrocytes. In this situation the neurosurgeon should be asked to supply more tissue before the operation is completed and warned that without it there can be no guarantee that a diagnosis will be forthcoming. If doubt remains then material should be obtained for microbiological analysis. On the other hand, the often florid reactive astrocytosis at the margin of an abscess should not be confused with glioblastoma. In addition to abscess some other florid reactive processes may be mistaken for glioblastoma, most notably progressive multifocal leucoencephalopathy.

Poorly differentiated glioblastoma in which there are few cytoplasmic processes and in which the cells smear out individually may well be impossible to confidently distinguish from any **other poorly differentiated neoplasm**, such as a metastatic carcinoma or melanoma. In this situation the neurosurgeon should be informed that the lesion is a malignant neoplasm and that further classification must await paraffin histology with its benefits of more extensive sampling and immunohistochemistry. In some examples of **lymphoma** there may be a florid reactive gliosis which may be mistaken for glioblastoma. Clearly it is important to determine whether the astrocytes or the lymphocytes in the lesion exhibit malignant cytological factors. Examination of the blood vessels is often helpful in difficult cases: in a glioblastoma the blood vessels are cellular as a result of proliferation of endothelial cells which appear elongated, whereas in a lymphoma there is infiltration of blood vessel walls by neoplastic lymphocytes with spherical nuclei.

Distinction between glioblastoma and **anaplastic astrocytoma** may be difficult with the small samples of tumour used for intra-operative diagnosis. Indeed, as discussed above it may be inappropriate to make the distinction as more material will subsequently become available which may show additional histological features.

There is usually little difficulty in making the diagnosis of giant cell glioblastoma intra-operatively. Even if there is relatively little in the way of astrocytic differentiation there are few tumours which exhibit such bizarre cytology, although it may be appropriate to consider the possibility of **choriocarcinoma** in a woman of reproductive age.

Gliomatosis cerebri may be regarded as representing the extreme end of the spectrum of an infiltrating astrocytic neoplasm. There is widespread diffuse infiltration of the central nervous system by neoplastic glial cells without a solid focal tumour mass. Gliomatosis cerebri is rare and the diagnosis is usually made at autopsy in a patient who has been intensively investigated by neurologists for a progressive disorder of the central nervous system, often without clear localizing signs. Neurosurgeons are relatively infrequently involved as no focal lesion for biopsy is identifiable on imaging. However diffuse abnormalities may be detected on imaging consisting of areas of high signal intensity on T2 weighted images. Smear preparations and frozen sections show diffusely infiltrating astrocytic tumour cells. The distinction between gliomatosis cerebri and the diffusely infiltrating edge of an astrocytic neoplasm cannot be made without full awareness of clinical and radiological features. The cytological features of the neoplastic cells vary considerably from case to case and from one anatomical location to another within one case. The abnormality may consist of mildly hypercellular central nervous tissue with mild cellular pleomorphism and be difficult or impossible to distinguish from reactive gliosis. Alternatively, the cells may exhibit marked cellular pleomorphism with readily identifiable mitotic figures.

OTHER ASTROCYTIC TUMOURS

6.4. PILOCYTIC ASTROCYTOMA

6.4.1. CLINICAL AND RADIOLOGICAL FEATURES

Pilocytic astrocytomas occur most frequently in children and young adults. Their anatomical location is largely restricted to specific regions within the central nervous system namely the cerebellum, the optic nerves and chiasm, the region of the third ventricle, the brain stem and spinal cord. The importance in the recognition of these tumours is that despite the presence of some microscopic features which may suggest a high grade tumour, they are tumours with a very low potential for growth (WHO grade 1). Post-operatively they tend not to recur and they do not have the tendency for anaplastic transformation seen in fibrillary astrocytomas.

The clinical presentation clearly relates to the anatomical location of the tumour with, for example, optic nerve lesions causing loss of vision. The history of symptoms may be relatively long, indicating the slow growth rate of this tumour.

Imaging typically shows a relatively well-circumscribed lesion which may contain cysts and form exophytic protrusions from the surface of the neuraxis. Pilocytic astrocytomas show enhancement with contrast unlike fibrillary astrocytomas. The signal intensity on T1 weighted MRI is often high. Pilocytic astrocytomas of the visual system are usually associated with expansion of the optic nerve and/or chiasm. Tumours at other locations typically comprise a well-circumscribed spherical or lobulated mass which may contain a single cyst or multiple cysts. Some tumours appear as mural nodules within a large cyst. Hypothalamic tumours may appear to lie within the third ventricle. Cerebellar tumours may lie across the midline or within one hemisphere and commonly show evidence of leptomeningial involvement. Pilocytic astrocytomas of the spinal cord may produce diffuse enlargement of the cord extending over several segments.

6.4.2. SURGICAL FINDINGS

The surgeon typically encounters a well-circumscribed tumour which may be forming lobulated exophytic nodules protruding from the surface of the neuraxis. Cerebellar tumours frequently involve the leptomeninges overlying the surface of the cerebellum. A single cyst or multiple cysts containing clear fluid may be encountered. The texture of the tumour is typically tough and rubbery. The well-demarcated margin of the tumour presents the surgeon with a plane of cleavage not seen with fibrillary astrocytoma.

Pilocytic astrocytomas, even if incompletely removed, are associated with very long post-operative survival often with little or no evidence of recurrence. As these tumours grow very slowly radiotherapy is of little or no benefit.

6.4.3. INTRA-OPERATIVE PATHOLOGY

Smear cytology

Pilocytic astrocytomas may be relatively tough and rubbery, however smear preparations are usually readily made. Of key importance in the recognition of this tumour is the suspicion raised by the clinical setting – of particular significance are the young age of the patient and the characteristic locations of the tumour as described above. Without this suspicion the presence of certain microscopic features, principally the often marked cytological atypia and the presence of vascular proliferation, may lead to the temptation to designate this as a high grade astrocytoma. The appearance on smear preparations is of a tumour which is typically astrocytic in character. The tumour cells often vary considerably in shape and size and in intensity of staining. The cytoplasm is typically scanty whereas cytoplasmic processes are often very abundant. The tumour cells have the characteristic tendency of astrocytomas to cluster around the blood vessels and may form ill-defined fascicles with the cytoplasmic processes forming parallel arrays. The 'hair-like' morphology of the cell which gives this tumour its name is often seen clearly in smear preparations. This cell has an elongated rod-shaped nucleus, scanty cytoplasm and bipolar cytoplasmic processes. However, such cells are not always identifiable in smear preparations and may not even be seen in paraffin sections – conversely, cells with similar morphology may at times be seen in 'ordinary' astrocytic tumours, particularly glioblastomas. Some pilocytic astrocytomas are composed predominantly of cells with round nuclei and relatively sparse processes. Blood vessels are frequently thickened and hypercellular, leading to the temptation to interpret the appearances as representing the endothelial cell hyperplasia which is a characteristic feature of glioblastoma. Mitotic figures and necrosis are not a feature of pilocytic astrocytoma. It is particularly reassuring as evidence of the very low grade nature of the tumour to identify Rosenthal fibres and/or spherical granular bodies. When present, Rosenthal fibres are readily identifiable as well-circumscribed elongated, often carrot-shaped or multilobulated, structures which are stained purplish-brown with toluidine blue and bright orange-red with haematoxylin and eosin. The density of Rosenthal fibres usually varies considerably from place to place in pilocytic astrocytomas and they may well not be present in the samples of tumour selected for the smear preparation. If there is doubt at the time of operation as to whether an astrocytic tumour is pilocytic or fibrillary in nature the neurosurgeon may well be sufficiently reassured to know that a mass in the cerebellum of a child is an astrocytic tumour rather than a medulloblastoma, and that more precise classification will follow.

Frozen sections

Frozen sections are likely to show the characteristic architecture of pilocytic astrocytoma with at low power a biphasic appearance having compact fibrillary areas intermingled with more sparsely cellular or microcystic areas. Sections which include the pial surface may show it to be breached by tumour cells with tumour in the subarachnoid space. This is a characteristic feature of pilocytic astrocytoma and should not be interpreted as evidence of malignancy or that the tumour has the potential to disseminate via the cerebrospinal fluid. The typical cellular pleomorphism and vascular proliferation are usually identifiable as discussed above. As in smear preparations it is reassuring to identify Rosenthal fibres or granular eosinophilic bodies.

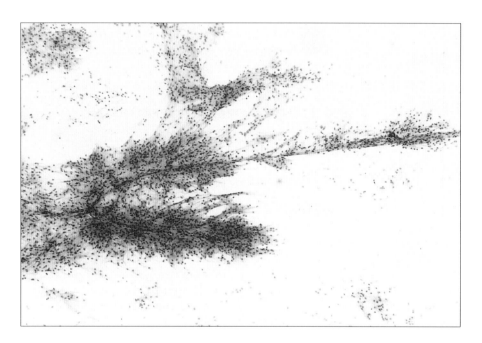

Figure 6.26
Pilocytic astrocytoma. Female aged 11 years, cerebellar tumour. Although they are often tough, satisfactory smears can usually be made from pilocytic astrocytomas. The smears show the typical low power architecture of an astrocytic tumour with clustering of the tumour cells around blood vessels. The clusters have ill-defined margins as a consequence of the presence of cytoplasmic processes. Smear preparation, toluidine blue, ×90.

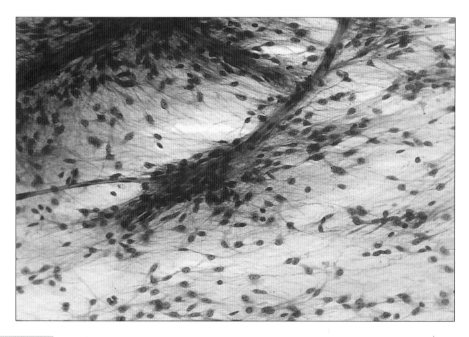

Figure 6.27
Pilocytic astrocytoma. Male aged 2 years, cerebellar tumour. The tumour cells are loosely arranged around blood vessels. There are abundant cytoplasmic processes which are metachromatic with toluidine blue. Smear preparation, toluidine blue, ×700.

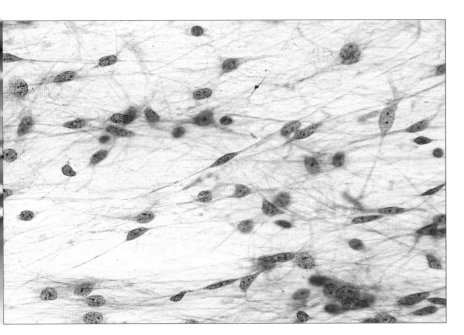

Figure 6.28
Pilocytic astrocytoma. Male aged 2 years, cerebellar tumour. The same tumour as illustrated in Fig. 6.27. In most examples of this tumour high power examination reveals the characteristic 'pilocytic' morphology of the cells. Several of the cells in this field, including one in the centre, have the typical elongated nuclei and coarse bipolar process. Smear preparation, toluidine blue, ×1400.

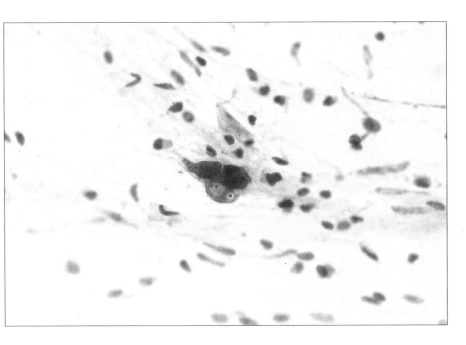

Figure 6.29
Pilocytic astrocytoma. Female aged 4 years, cerebellar tumour. Rosenthal fibres, as seen in the centre of this field, are a characteristic feature of pilocytic astrocytoma and provide reassurance that the tumour is of very low grade. They may also be seen in a long standing reactive gliosis. Rosenthal fibres are elongated structures often carrot-shaped and multinodular. They are purplish-brown in smears stained with toluidine blue and brightly eosinophilic with H&E. Smear preparation, toluidine blue, ×1400.

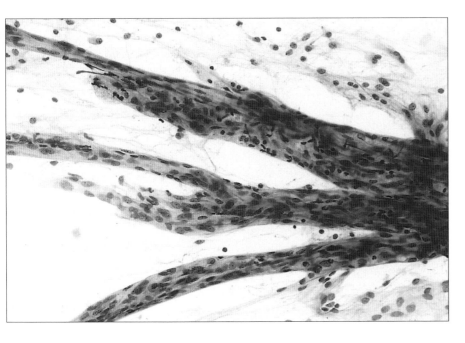

Figure 6.30
Pilocytic astrocytoma. Female aged 4 years, cerebellar tumour. The same tumour as illustrated in Fig. 6.29. Vascular proliferation is often a prominent feature of pilocytic astrocytomas and may resemble the endothelial hyperplasia seen in glioblastomas. As the cells of pilocytic astrocytoma are often pleomorphic, these two features may make distinction between pilocytic astrocytoma and glioblastoma difficult. Attention to the age of the patient and the site of the tumour is usually helpful. Smear preparation, toluidine blue, ×1400.

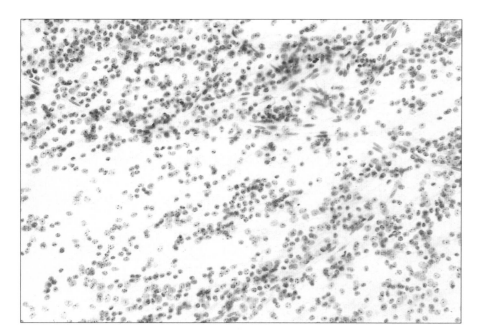

Figure 6.31
Pilocytic astrocytoma. Male aged 31 years, cerebellar tumour. Pilocytic astrocytomas may have areas composed of cells with round nuclei and scanty processes as illustrated here. Indeed, some tumours contain this pattern exclusively. In this example the characteristic features of pilocytic astrocytoma were subsequently identified in the tissue processed for paraffin histology. Smear preparation, toluidine blue, ×350.

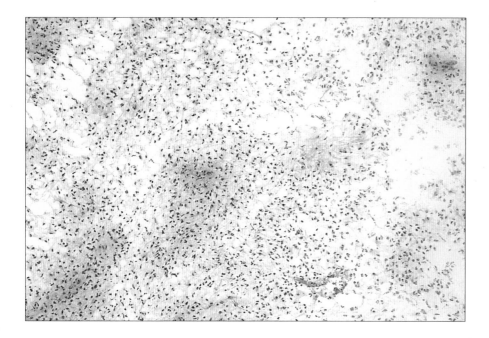

Figure 6.32
Pilocytic astrocytoma. Female aged 4 years, cerebellar tumour. Frozen sections may show the characteristic low power architecture of pilocytic astrocytoma with intermingled cystic and compact areas as illustrated in this field. Frozen section, haematoxylin eosin, ×350.

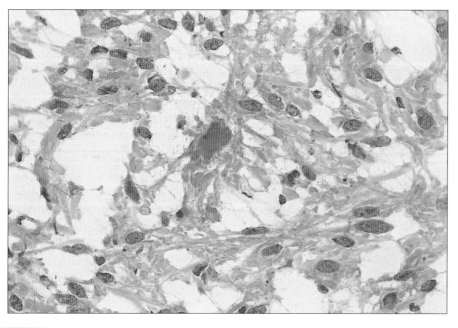

Figure 6.33
Pilocytic astrocytoma. Male aged 14 years, cerebellar tumour. A frozen section seen at high power shows the elongated nuclei of the tumour cells although the cytoplasmic processes are not seen as clearly as in smear preparations (see Fig. 6.28). Microcysts are present. There is a Rosenthal fibre in the centre of the field. Frozen section, haematoxylin eosin, ×1400.

6.4.4. DIFFERENTIAL DIAGNOSIS

As described above a pilocytic astrocytoma may be erroneously interpreted as a **high grade astrocytic tumour** on the basis of cellular atypia and vascular proliferation. The importance of an awareness of the clinical and radiographic features of this tumour are again stressed. If the smear preparations or frozen sections show an astrocytic tumour without 'hair-like' cells, Rosenthal fibres or granular bodies it may not be possible at the time of operation to discriminate between a pilocytic and a fibrillary astrocytoma. Biopsies from the optic nerve, brain stem and spinal cord may present a particular challenge owing to the small size of the samples of tissue which are likely to be obtained from these regions. Indeed in this situation it may be appropriate, in consultation with the surgeon, to fix all of the tissue obtained and process it for paraffin histology without even attempting an intra-operative diagnosis. The distinction may still not be possible on subsequent paraffin histology and in this situation the radiographic and clinical features assume over-riding importance. In view of the presence of cytological atypia and vascular proliferation in these tumours it may even be difficult to distinguish them from anaplastic astrocytoma or glioblastoma when presented with a small biopsy. In this situation a search for Rosenthal fibres, granular bodies and mitotic figures is of particular importance.

An important differential diagnosis is that of a **long-standing reactive process**. A chronic reactive process can lead to proliferation of astrocytes with abundant processes and Rosenthal fibres. It is important to recognize that the presence of Rosenthal fibres and granular bodies indicates a long-standing lesion, but does not help to discriminate between a pilocytic astrocytoma and a non-neoplastic process. For example, the chronic gliosis forming the wall of fluid-filled cyst in the cerebellum induced by a small mural haemangioblastoma, the reaction around a craniopharyngioma or the wall of a syrinx in the spinal cord, may all be a challenge to distinguish from pilocytic astrocytoma.

Pleomorphic xanthoastrocytoma may resemble pilocytic astrocytoma in that it presents in a young patient and may be associated with a cyst. In this situation the characteristic anatomical location of pilocytic astrocytomas is emphasized. Pleomorphic xanthoastrocytomas tend to be more cellular and exhibit a greater degree of pleomorphism than pilocytic astrocytoma. If this uncertainty arises it is appropriate to await paraffin histology for the definite diagnosis.

6.5. PLEOMORPHIC XANTHOASTROCYTOMA

Pleomorphic xanthoastrocytoma, which typically has a superficial location in the cerebral hemispheres, microscopically is noted to have marked cellular pleomorphism and xanthomatous change, and is characterized by a relatively favourable course.

6.5.1. CLINICAL AND RADIOLOGICAL FEATURES

Pleomorphic xanthoastrocytoma occurs usually in children and young adults and presents most commonly with a history of seizures or less often with the features of an expanding space-occupying lesion. Most of these neoplasms are supratentorial and the typical location is the temporal lobe. A characteristic feature of this tumour is its superficial situation, forming a mass within or adjacent to the leptomeninges. There is often an underlying cyst and there may be involvement of the underlying brain by tumour.

As a result of the relative rarity of this neoplasm, its biological behaviour has to be regarded with some uncertainty. However, in general this is a low grade neoplasm (WHO grade 2) – prolonged survival is likely and a cure following surgical excision seems a possibility. In particular it is important to recognize that the relatively benign nature of the tumour seems out of keeping with the marked cellular pleomorphism. Despite the typically benign behaviour of this lesion malignant transformation has been described.

6.5.2. SURGICAL FINDINGS

The neurosurgeon encounters a firm and often well-circumscribed mass lying on the surface of the cerebrum. As indicated above, there is often an underlying fluid-filled cyst. There may be involvement of the underlying brain by tumour.

6.5.3. INTRA-OPERATIVE PATHOLOGY

Smear cytology

Smear cytology reveals a strikingly pleomorphic astrocytic tumour. The cells vary considerably in shape and size and have round, irregular or elongated nuclei. There is considerable variation in the amount of cytoplasm – some cells have abundant cytoplasm which may form elongated masses. Astrocytic cytoplasmic processes are noted. A characteristic feature of this tumour is the presence of lipid droplets in the tumour cell cytoplasm. This is a variable feature and may be a prominent feature in some tumours and barely noticeable in others. In the setting of such a strikingly pleomorphic astrocytic tumour mitotic figures, endothelial cell proliferation and necrosis are notable by their absence. A sometimes prominent feature of the tumour is infiltration by lymphocytes. Spherical granular bodies may be noted and are an indication that this is a slowly-growing tumour.

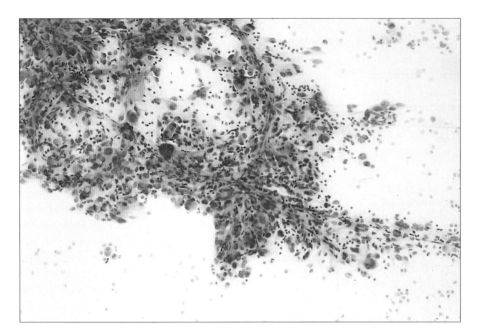

Figure 6.34
Pleomorphic xanthoastrocytoma. Female aged 28 years, superficial temporal lobe tumour. At low power in smear preparations pleomorphic xanthoastrocytoma has the architecture of a glial tumour with aggregation of tumour cells around blood vessels. However even at this power the pleomorphism of the tumour cells is apparent. Smear preparation, toluidine blue, ×90.

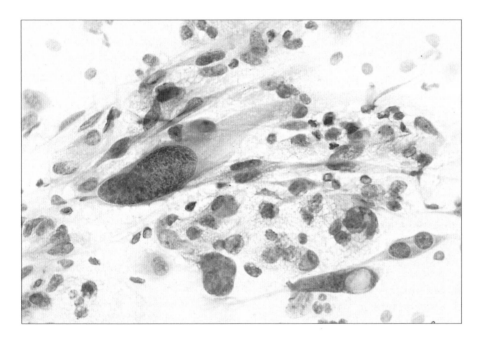

Figure 6.35
Pleomorphic xanthoastrocytoma. The same case as illustrated in Fig. 6.34. The cells are markedly pleomorphic, have varying amounts of cytoplasm and processes which are rather sparse in this field. Several of the cells illustrated have vacuolated (xanthomatous) cytoplasm. The very large and bizarre cells might easily tempt a diagnosis of a high grade tumour, however mitoses are not seen, there is no endothelial cell hyperplasia and no tumour necrosis. There is likely to be a long history of seizures which would be unusual for a high grade neoplasm. Smear preparation, toluidine blue, ×1400.

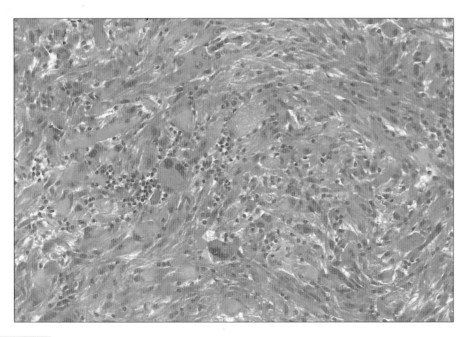

Figure 6.36
Pleomorphic xanthoastrocytoma. Male aged 17 years, temporal lobe tumour. Frozen sections show a pleomorphic astrocytic tumour. Many of the cells have abundant cytoplasm and a few of these are elongated. Xanthomatous change is not a prominent feature of this example although one large cell (top centre) has multiple small intracytoplasmic vacuoles. Lymphocytes are commonly encountered in these tumours. They were scattered throughout this example, most noticeably to the left of centre in this field. Frozen section, haematoxylin eosin, ×700.

Frozen sections

Frozen sections may reveal the characteristic superficial location of the tumour, lying within the subarachnoid space overlying the surface of the brain. There may be involvement of the underlying brain in an infiltrative manner more reminiscent of a fibrillary astrocytoma. The strikingly pleomorphic astrocytic tumour cells may have an elongated appearance and may be arranged in ill-defined fascicles. As described above the important features of this neoplasm are xanthomatous change, a lymphocytic infiltrate and granular eosinophilic bodies with absence of mitoses, vascular endothelial cell hyperplasia and necrosis.

6.5.4. DIFFERENTIAL DIAGNOSIS

Recognition of this neoplasm depends upon an awareness of the clinical setting and radiological features. The marked cellular pleomorphism of the tumour may lead to the temptation to suggest a diagnosis of **glioblastoma** – however, glioblastoma is rare within the age range encompassed by pleomorphic xanthoastrocytoma and closer examination reveals the absence of the other microscopic features found in a rapidly growing astrocytic neoplasm. It should be noted that lipidization of tumour cell cytoplasm may occasionally be identified in glioblastoma. The presence of granular bodies generally indicates a slowly growing tumour and these are unlikely to be seen in a glioblastoma. A potentially confounding feature of pleomorphic xanthoastrocytoma is the lack of the specific defining features if the tumour involves the underlying brain.

It should be noted that tumours designated pleomorphic xanthoastrocytoma have been described which do contain mitotic figures and small foci of necrosis and the implication of these findings for the biological behaviour of the tumour is as yet uncertain. If the clinical and radiological setting are not entirely typical it is probably wise to inform the neurosurgeon that the tumour is astrocytic in type and that further characterization must await paraffin histology. The well-circumscribed appearance of the tumour and the presentation with fits in a young patient may prompt the suggestion of a **ganglion cell tumour** or **dysembryoplastic neuroepithelial tumour**. Indeed some of the tumour cells may resemble abnormal neurons, particularly in their nuclear features, and the distinction between astrocytic and neuronal differentiation may require immunohistochemistry.

Pilocytic astrocytoma is usually readily differentiated by the characteristic anatomical locations in which this tumour arises and the relatively mild degree of nuclear pleomorphism.

Malignant fibrous histiocytoma is a further potential differential diagnosis and again the distinction between this and pleomorphic xanthoastrocytoma may not be possible intra-operatively but may need to await immunohistochemistry.

6.6. SUBEPENDYMAL GIANT CELL ASTROCYTOMA

Subependymal giant cell astrocytoma is a low grade intraventricular tumour which occurs most commonly, although not exclusively, in children and young adults with tuberous sclerosis.

6.6.1. CLINICAL AND RADIOLOGICAL FEATURES

This neoplasm most commonly presents with the features of raised intracranial pressure due to hydrocephalus in a patient with tuberous sclerosis. The tumour may also occur in individuals in whom the other features of tuberous sclerosis are not present. Radiological investigations identify a well-circumscribed mass arising from the wall of the lateral ventricle close to the foramen of Munro which becomes obstructed. The mass is often calcified and hamartomatous ependymal nodules, from which the tumour is presumed to arise, may be identifiable nearby. At operation the tumour presents a lobulated surface protruding into the lateral ventricle. The mass is generally firm, may be calcified, and is attached to the wall of the lateral ventricle. The lesion is usually well demarcated without significant infiltration of the adjacent brain. This tumour has little potential for growth. The long-term outcome is favourable and surgical resection may result in a cure.

6.6.2. INTRA-OPERATIVE PATHOLOGY

Smear cytology

Subependymal giant cell astrocytoma may not smear easily as the tumours tend to be tough and sometimes contain calcification. Smear preparations show a tumour composed of large cells with astrocytic morphology. The cells often have abundant cytoplasm, sometimes giving elongated strap-like morphology, and cytoplasmic processes. The nuclei may be rather large and vesiculated with prominent nucleoli resembling those of neurons. The degree of cytological pleomorphism may prompt consideration of a high grade tumour. However, mitotic figures are absent or scanty, vascular endothelial cell hyperplasia is not seen and necrosis is absent. Calcospherites are often present.

Frozen sections

Frozen sections show large and pleomorphic cells with astrocytic morphology. The tumour cells often have abundant eosinophilic cytoplasm in which the nucleus is located eccentrically giving an appearance similar to gemistocytic astrocytes. A proportion of the cells may be spindle shaped. The background is composed of cytoplasmic processes. In some cases the cells may be orientated

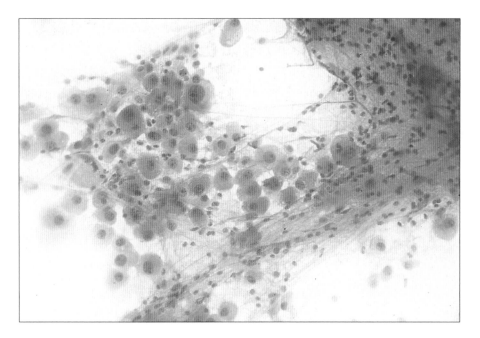

Figure 6.37
Subependymal giant cell astrocytoma. Male aged 16 years with tuberous sclerosis, tumour in wall of lateral ventricle. This smear preparation shows small astrocytic tumours cells with a fibrillar matrix. Also included are numerous very large bizarre cells with large round pale nuclei, prominent nucleoli and abundant well-demarcated cytoplasm without readily apparent cytoplasmic processes. These large cells bear some resemblance to ganglion cells and immunocytochemically may express both neuronal and glial antigens. Smear preparation, haematoxylin eosin, ×700.

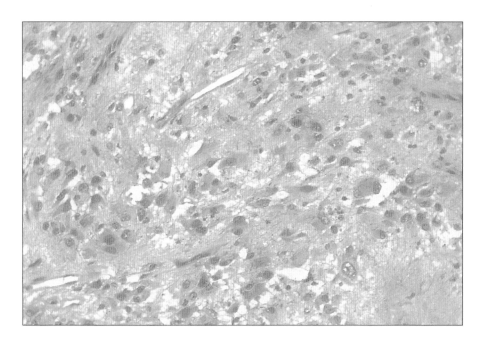

Figure 6.38
Subependymal giant cell astrocytoma. The same tumour as illustrated in Fig. 6.37. Frozen sections show a tumour with a matrix of cytoplasmic processes and pleomorphic cells. The striking pleomorphism might mislead into a diagnosis of a high grade tumour, however mitoses are not seen, there is no endothelial cell hyperplasia and no tumour necrosis. The characteristic site of the tumour and the usual, although not invariable, setting in the context of tuberous sclerosis are helpful pointers to the correct diagnosis. Frozen section, haematoxylin eosin, ×350.

around blood vessels in a manner somewhat reminiscent of the perivascular pseudorosettes of ependymoma.

6.6.3. DIFFERENTIAL DIAGNOSIS

In the absence of knowledge of the clinical setting and the radiological features of the tumour the possibility of a subependymal giant cell astrocytoma may not even be considered when an intra-operative diagnosis is requested. In particular, **gemistocytic astrocytoma** may

well be confused with this neoplasm. However, gemistocytic astrocytoma is a neoplasm that arises within the parenchyma of the cerebrum and possesses an infiltrating margin, in contrast to the relatively well-circumscribed appearance and intraventricular location of subependymal giant cell astrocytoma. The possibility that the lesion constitutes a **ganglion cell tumour** may well be considered at the time of operation and definite classification may need to await subsequent paraffin histology with its more extensive sampling and the potential for immunohistochemistry.

SEVEN

OLIGODENDROGLIAL TUMOURS

7.1. CLINICAL AND RADIOLOGICAL FEATURES

Oligodendrogliomas are uncommon neoplasms which represent around 5–7% of all intracranial gliomas, occurring most frequently in adults in the fourth and fifth decades of life, with a slight predominance in males. However, these tumours can occur across a wide age range and are well recognized in childhood. They arise most frequently in the white matter of the cerebral hemispheres in the frontal and parietal regions, but may extend to involve the corpus callosum and occasionally the contralateral hemisphere. These tumours are infrequently sited in the posterior fossa and occur only very rarely in the spinal cord.

Neuroradiological studies of oligodendrogliomas usually reveal supratentorial tumours with focal calcification in around 60% of cases, which is most evident on CT scans. Calcification within these tumours may also occur in a gyriform pattern, in addition to the commoner non-random distribution. MRI studies of low grade oligodendrogliomas often show little peritumoural oedema with hypodensity on T1-weighted sequences and hyperdensity on T2-weighted sequences. Gadolinium enhanced MRI studies usually reveal a poorly-enhancing peripheral margin in low-grade tumours. Extensive infiltration of the cerebral white matter may mimic gliomatosis cerebri on radiology. Cystic degeneration and haemorrhage can be identified particularly in T1-images, particularly in anaplastic oligodendrogliomas. Anaplastic oligodendrogliomas and mixed gliomas in which the astrocytic component is anaplastic will often be accompanied by haemorrhage and will therefore demonstrate more marked peripheral or ring enhancement on MRI and CT scans. Superficially located low grade tumours with a relatively long duration of illness may be accompanied by radiological evidence of pressure erosion of the inner table to the skull, but meningeal infiltration is uncommon at the time of primary investigation and diagnosis.

Patients with oligodendrogliomas usually present with the signs and symptoms of an infiltrative expanding intracranial neoplasm, although many patients experience a long history of seizures (durations of 5 years and over are not uncommon) prior to the onset of headache and other signs and symptoms of raised intracranial pressure. Tumours occurring around the thalamus may cause obstructive hydrocephalus, and therefore present at an early stage with the signs and symptoms of raised intracranial pressure. Anaplastic oligodendrogliomas pursue a more aggressive clinical course.

7.2. SURGICAL FINDINGS

Oligodendrogliomas are characteristically diffuse neoplasms of gelatinous consistency with an ill-defined tumour margin. Cystic change with mucin formation is occasionally encountered, and although most of the calcification within these tumours is microscopic, occasional neoplasms have large aggregates of calcification which can be detected at surgery. Occasional oligodendrogliomas will project into the ventricular system, particularly the lateral or third ventricles, producing obstructive hydrocephalus. Oligodendrogliomas arising in the posterior fossa may also involve the fourth ventricle, producing hydrocephalus; this occurs most frequently in children. Infiltration of the cerebral cortex may be apparent on inspection of the internal cortical surface which can appear discoloured and abnormally smooth. Invasion into the subarachnoid space may also be detected in occasional cases, with thickening and discolouration of the pia-arachnoid.

Anaplastic oligodendrogliomas are more frequently associated with haemorrhage, resulting in a heterogenous appearance at surgery. Cystic change appears to occur more frequently in these neoplasms, which are more liable to haemorrhage upon surgical resection. Foci of necrosis may be encountered in anaplastic oligodendrogliomas, appearing as yellow-white softened areas within the tumour. The infiltrating margin of these anaplastic tumours is ill-defined, despite an apparently circumscribed margin on neuroradiological examination.

7.3. INTRA-OPERATIVE PATHOLOGY

Smear cytology

Most oligodendrogliomas are soft enough to make good smear preparations, on which a diagnosis can be made if the characteristic cytological appearances are present. In typical oligodendrogliomas, a low-power examination of the smear preparations shows a fine branching capillary network, usually with little evidence of the endothelial hypoplasia commonly encountered in astrocytic gliomas. The neoplastic cells are aggregated around these blood vessels, but usually spread from the vessels in a uniform manner, forming a monolayer sheet with no evidence of cellular aggregation.

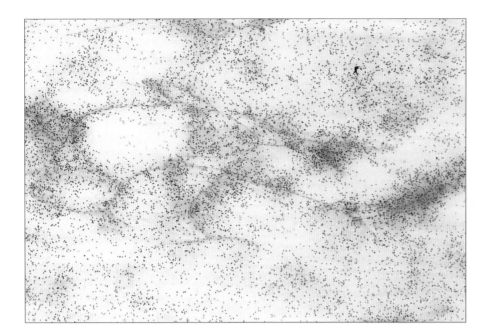

Figure 7.1
Oligodendroglioma. Female aged 26 years, left frontal lobe. The finely branching vascular pattern of oligodendrogliomas is evident at low power magnification in smear preparations, with tumour cells spreading from the capillary structures. Smear preparation, haematoxylin eosin, ×70.

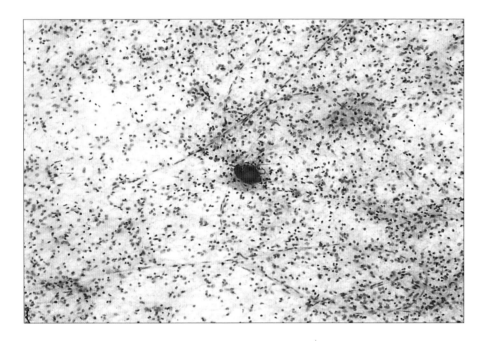

Figure 7.2
Oligodendroglioma. Male aged 36 years, central white matter. Calcification (centre) is a common feature of oligodendrogliomas, but it is by no means specific and may occur in a variety of other CNS tumours (see Chapter 5), Smear preparation, toluidine blue, ×140.

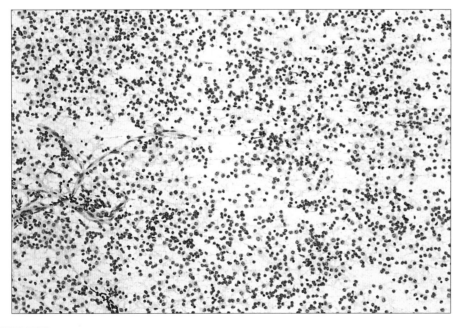

Figure 7.3
Oligodendroglioma. Male aged 18 years, right temporal lobe. The tumour cell nuclei in oligodendrogliomas are small, rounded and relatively uniform. The absence of a gliofibrillary matrix may cause confusion with a cerebral lymphoma or even a pituitary adenoma on low power examination. Smear preparation, toluidine blue, ×140.

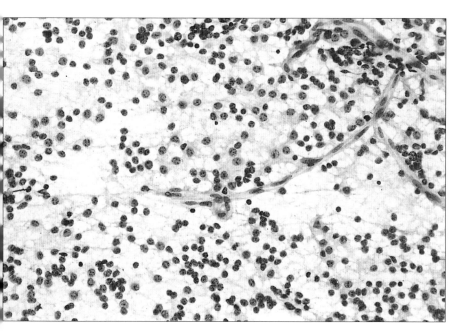

Figure 7.4
Oligodendroglioma. Male aged 29 years, left frontal lobe. The finely branching capillary network in oligodendrogliomas is thin-walled and lacks the hyperplasia characteristic of astrocytic tumours. Smear preparation, toluidine blue, ×350.

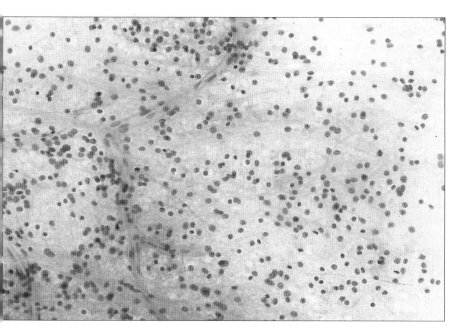

Figure 7.5
Oligodendroglioma. Female aged 15 years, right temporal lobe. The tumour cells in oligodendrogliomas spread readily in a monolayer, with little cellular cohesion and no gliofibrillary matrix around the capillaries within the tissue. Smear preparation, haematoxylin eosin, ×350.

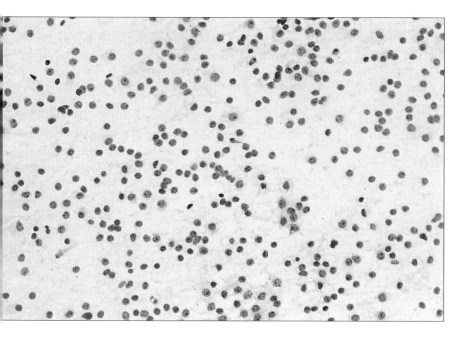

Figure 7.6
Oligodendroglioma. Male aged 16 years, central white matter. The tumour cells characteristically contain uniform nuclei with little cytoplasm and no cell processes. Mitotic figures are usually absent in oligodendrogliomas. Smear preparation, toluidine blue, ×350.

Nuclear pleomorphism is not a prominent feature in typical oligodendrogliomas, and in toluidine blue preparations the nucleus is characterized by a clear margin with irregular speckled chromatin. Nucleoli are inconspicuous and mitotic activity is not readily identified. There is usually little evidence of haemorrhage, but calcification is readily identified in smear preparations and occasionally may be detected whilst the smear preparation is being made by a gritty sensation between the glass slides. Staining with haematoxylin and eosin shows similar cytological features, and emphasizes the scanty pale-staining cytoplasm present in the typical tumour cell. The nucleus is usually eccentric in location, and the cells body appears rounded, with no fibrillary processes on either the cells or around the blood vessels. Reactive astrocytosis occurs at the infiltrating margin of oligodendrogliomas; this may result in interpretative difficulty if the tumour margins are sampled for smear preparations, when the presence of enlarged astrocytic cells and a gliofibrillary matrix may be misinterpreted as an astrocytoma or part of a mixed glioma. Oligoastrocytomas vary in their appearances in smear preparations according to the relative proportions of the two populations of neoplastic cells. In our experience, the oligodendroglial component usually predominates and is variably mixed with neoplastic astrocytic cells. The latter are accompanied by a patchy gliofibrillary matrix and vascular endothelial hyperplasia, in contrast to typical oligodendrogliomas.

Frozen sections

Cryostat sections of oligodendrogliomas are often helpful in establishing a diagnosis. The typical finely-branching capillary network is often evident and foci of calcification are readily identifiable. The neoplastic cells in cryostat sections do not exhibit the perinuclear haloes which are characteristically present in paraffin sections (representing a tissue fixation and processing artefact). Instead, the cells appear rounded with ill-defined cytoplasmic boundaries and a variable quantity of pale staining eosinophilic cytoplasm. Prominent cell processes and a gliofibrillary matrix are absent in oligodendrogliomas and this helps distinction from well-differentiated astrocytomas, although difficulties may arise if the tumour margin is sampled and exhibits reactive astrocytosis. Aggregation of neoplastic cells to form palisaded clusters is sometimes identifiable in cryostat sections of oligodendrogliomas, as is the cystic change in tumours which produce abundant mucin. Mitotic figures are not usually present in cryostat sections of oligodendrogliomas.

Anaplastic oligodendrogliomas exhibit a wider range of nuclear pleomorphism than typical tumours in cryostat sections and this is usually accompanied by an increase in the number of blood vessels, with endothelial hyperplasia and frequent haemorrhage. The neoplastic cells contain more abundant cytoplasm than in typical oligodendrogliomas, and this may be intensely eosinophilic. Although cell processes are not identified in anaplastic tumours, the more abundant cytoplasm often displaces the nucleus towards the periphery of the cell. Small areas of necrosis can occasionally be identified in anaplastic oligodendrogliomas and this may cause confusion with glioblastoma multiforme. Reactive astrocytes may also be identified within anaplastic oligodendrogliomas and may be misinterpreted as part of an astrocytic component to the neoplasm, raising the possibility of a mixed glioma. Oligoastrocytomas contain a variable proportion of neoplastic astrocytic cells and hyperplastic vascular endothelium, which are irregularly distributed within the tumour tissue. It is frequently difficult to establish the relative proportion of the astrocytic component of mixed gliomas in cryostat sections; paraffin sections are required for the adequate assessment of this question.

7.4. GRADING AND MALIGNANCY

Oligodendrogliomas exhibit a clinical and pathological spectrum of malignancy, although in contrast to astrocytic tumours absolute criteria for grading are somewhat poorly defined. Most oligodendrogliomas are slow-growing low grade tumours, but there is increasing awareness of the existence of anaplastic oligodendrogliomas which exhibit increased nuclear pleomorphism and a higher cell density than typical tumours, often with mitotic activity and occasional areas of necrosis. The spectrum of cellular morphology in anaplastic oligodendrogliomas extends from the classical 'fried egg' oligodendroglioma cell to a smaller cell which contains more abundant eosinophilic cytoplasm, the so-called gliofibrillary oligodendrocyte or 'baby gemistocyte'. Such cells usually exhibit strong positivity for glial fibrillary acidic protein on immunocytochemistry and can readily be recognized in both smear and cryostat preparations of oligodendroglioma. Oligodendrogliomas may evolve into glioblastomas over a period of years; conversely, oligodendroglioma-like areas are occasionally found in glioblastomas. The presence of an anaplastic component in an oligodendroglioma should therefore be suspected if cells corresponding to gliofibrillary oligodendrocytes are identified which exhibit conspicuous nuclear pleomorphism, with identifiable mitotic activity accompanied by vascular endothelial proliferation and frequently haemorrhage. Oligodendrogliomas may infiltrate extensively into surrounding grey and white matter and also into the subarachnoid and subpial space, the latter is *per se* not an indication of anaplasia, which is better diagnosed on the cytological and architectural features mentioned above. It is evident that both smear and cryostat preparations are helpful in establishing a diagnosis of anaplastic oligodendroglioma, the former for cytological features and the latter for architectural details, particularly vascular endothelial abnormalities and necrosis.

7.5. DIFFERENTIAL DIAGNOSIS

The clinical and radiological differential diagnosis of intracranial oligodendrogliomas includes other gliomas,

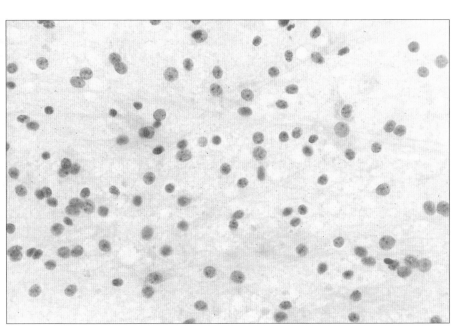

Figure 7.7
Oligodendroglioma. Female aged 29 years, right frontal lobe. The nuclear chromatin in oligodendrogliomas is faintly speckled, without prominent nucleoli. This pattern is clearly distinguishable from cerebral lymphoma and pituitary adenoma. Smear preparation, haematoxylin eosin, ×700.

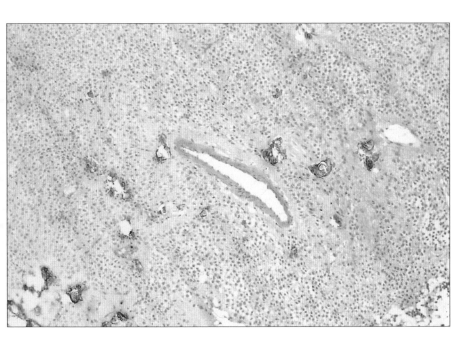

Figure 7.8
Oligodendroglioma. Female aged 24 years, left temporal lobe. Occasional thick-walled blood vessels are present in oligodendrogliomas, but the fine branching capillary network is not always apparent in cryostat sections. Several foci of calcification are present in this tumour. Cryostat section, haematoxylin eosin, ×70.

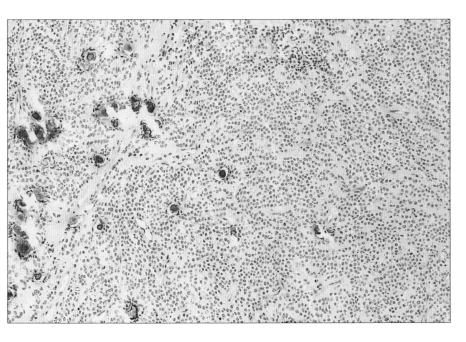

Figure 7.9
Oligodendroglioma. Male aged 38 years, right frontal lobe tumour. The tumour cells are arranged in solid sheets containing several foci of calcification. The cytoplasm does not exhibit the characteristic perinuclear haloes present in paraffin sections, but is scanty and pale-staining. Cryostat section, haematoxylin eosin, ×140.

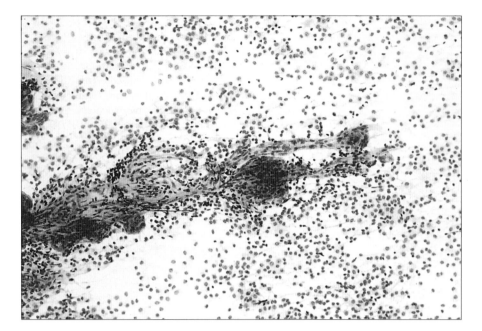

Figure 7.10
Anaplastic oligodendroglioma. Female aged 44 years, left parietal lobe. The vascular network comprises hyperplastic endothelial structures which branch irregularly, resembling those in malignant astrocytic gliomas. Smear preparation, toluidine blue, ×70.

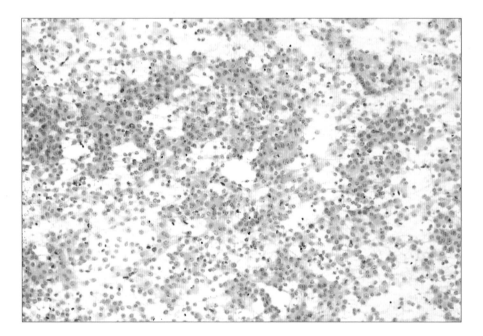

Figure 7.11
Anaplastic oligodendroglioma. Male aged 38 years, central white matter. The tumour cells tend to disperse from the blood vessels in irregular clusters. A variable quantity of cytoplasm is present within the cells, in contrast to low grade oligodendrogliomas. Smear preparation, haematoxylin eosin, ×350.

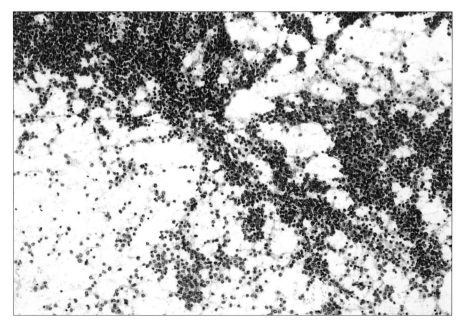

Figure 7.12
Anaplastic oligodendroglioma. Male aged 46 years, left temporal lobe. Although a true gliofibrillary matrix is absent, the neoplastic cells may aggregate around the hyperplastic endothelium, with little spread away from the blood vessels. Smear preparation, toluidine blue, ×140.

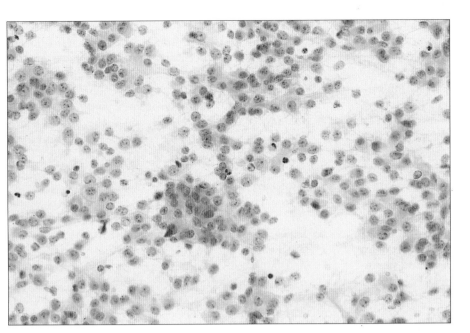

Figure 7.13
Anaplastic oligodendroglioma. Female aged 28 years, right frontal lobe. The tumour cells contain pleomorphic nuclei and a variable quantity of pale staining cytoplasm. Apoptotic cells are often present, and occasional mitotic figures can be identified. Smear preparation, haematoxylin eosin, ×700.

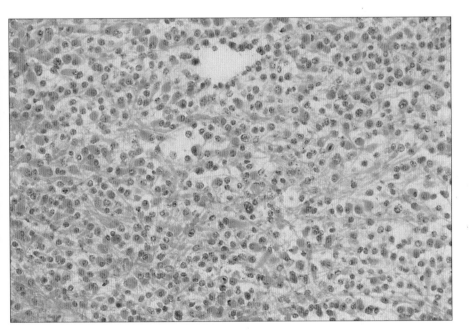

Figure 7.14
Anaplastic oligodendroglioma. Male aged 42 years, central white matter. The pleomorphic tumour cell population often contains cells with intensely eosinophilic cytoplasm and a rounded cell body, corresponding to 'gliofibrillary oligodendrocytes'. Occasional cyst-like structures are present within the tumour. Cryostat section, haematoxylin eosin, ×350.

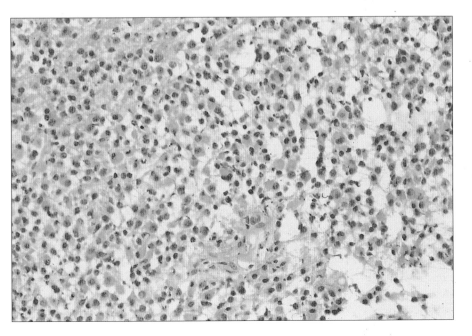

Figure 7.15
Anaplastic oligodendroglioma. Male aged 28 years, left temporal lobe. Tumour cells are present in irregular clusters in a mucinous matrix. Occasional apoptotic cells are present, but no necrosis was identified in this case. Cryostat section, haematoxylin eosin, ×350.

particularly **astrocytomas**, **ependymomas** if the tumour is located near a ventricle, and **central neurocytomas** for intraventricular lesions. The diffuse infiltration of the cerebral white matter can resemble a primary **lymphoma** of the brain, and more extensively infiltrating tumours may be confused with **gliomatosis cerebri**. Oligodendrogliomas in the posterior fossa can be confused radiologically with **medulloblastomas** and **ependymomas**; **pilocytic astrocytomas** usually have a less homogenous appearance on neuroradiological investigations than oligodendrogliomas and calcification is unusual in these astrocytic tumours. Calcification is by no means specific for oligodendrogliomas, and can of course be encountered in many other types of intrinsic and extrinsic brain tumours including **astrocytomas**, **choroid plexus tumours**, **ependymomas**, **central neurocytomas** and **meningiomas** (*see* Chapter 5).

A distinction from **astrocytomas** is usually straightforward on both smear and crytostat sections, aided by the presence of cell processes and a gliofibrillary matrix in astrocytic tumours, the relationship of the tumours to the blood vessels and the characteristic nuclear morphology of oligodendroglial tumours. Calcification is not uncommonly present in well-differentiated astrocytomas within the cerebral hemispheres and hence cannot be considered specific for oligodendroglioma. A more difficult question is the presence of an astrocytic component in a tumour with oligodendroglioma-like features. The difficulties in interpreting **reactive astrocytosis** in tumour margin biopsies and occasionally at more deep seated locations within the tumour are discussed above, but the identification of a neoplastic astrocytic component raises the possibility of a **mixed glioma**. The guidelines for diagnosis of mixed glioma are somewhat ill-defined, but a general guidance indicates that if the astrocytic component is neoplastic and accounts for at least 20% of the tumour cell population, then the neoplasm should be considered as a mixed glioma. The neoplastic astrocytic component of mixed gliomas can be identified in both smear preparations and cryostat sections in most cases; however, the presence and nature of the astrocytic component within oligodendrogliomas is best investigated in paraffin sections.

Oligodendrogliomas may occasionally be confused in cytological terms with other tumours in which small rounded cells with relatively uniform nuclei and scanty cytoplasm predominate, including **pituitary adenomas** and **pineal neoplasms** if a deep-seated central tumour is biopsied, **central neurocytoma** if an intraventricular tumour is sampled, **lymphoma** if there is extensive infiltration of the white matter, and **dysembryoplastic neuroepithelial tumours** (DNET) in cortical lesions in children and young adults.

For centrally-located tumours, distinction between oligodendroglioma and **pituitary adenoma** is usually possible on the basis of the nuclear features, with multiple nucleoli usually being present in pituitary tumours and the tendency of pituitary tumours and smear prepa-

rations to form sheets of cohesive cells rather than the single cells usually encountered in oligodendrogliomas. Calcification can occur in pituitary tumours, but the vascular pattern in these adenomas is different from oligodendrogliomas, with extensively branching thick-walled vessels. Distinction from a **pineal parenchymal tumour** is usually possible, since the pineal region tumours usually show evidence of astrocytic or neuronal differentiation, or occasionally both. Focal calcification may occur in pineocytomas, but the finely branching vascular pattern of oligodendrogliomas is not encountered in these lesions. **Pineal germinomas** are the only variety of primary intracranial germ cell tumours which are likely to be confused with oligodendrogliomas in smears and cryostat sections. The neoplastic cells in germinomas are larger than those in oligodendrogliomas and contain more abundant pale-staining cytoplasm around the large vesicular nucleus, with its prominent nucleolus. Germinomas may contain a finely branching capillary network, similar to that in oligodendrogliomas, but their vessels are frequently surrounded by a prominent population of reactive lymphocytes, which are uncommon on oligodendrogliomas. Calcification may also occur in germinomas, which may cause further diagnostic difficulties, although it is not usually present in a widespread distribution within the tumour.

Distinction between an intraventricular oligodendroglioma and a **central neurocytoma** is, however, more problematic. There are occasional subtle differences in smear preparations, with the nuclei of central neurocytomas usually having diffuse or finely granular chromatin, and the vascular pattern tends to be less extensively branching than in oligodendrogliomas. However, this distinction is not so readily maintained on cryostat sections, and paraffin section histology with immunocytochemistry may be required to establish a final diagnosis. Oligodendrogliomas may be distinguished from **supratentorial PNET and cerebral neuroblastomas** by their relatively uniform cellularity, lack of mitotic activity and necrosis, and typical capillary network.

Oligodendrogliomas can be differentiated from primary brain **lymphomas** in view of the wider spectrum of nuclear morphology usually present in lymphomas, which are most often high grade tumours showing appreciable mitotic activity. Lymphomas often contain thick-walled blood vessels which are infiltrated by tumour cells, rather than the finely branching capillary network of oligodendrogliomas. In the posterior fossa, **medulloblastomas and ependymoblastomas** may be distinguished from oligodendrogliomas because of their more elongated nuclei which may appear carrot-shaped in smear preparations, the wider spectrum of cellular morphology (which in medulloblastomas may include cells with neuronal and astrocytic differentiation) and the absence of the typical oligodendroglioma vascular pattern. Calcification is less common in medulloblastomas than in oligodendrogliomas. Oligodendrogliomas can readily be distinguished from **ependymomas** because of the gliofibrillary matrix and process-bearing

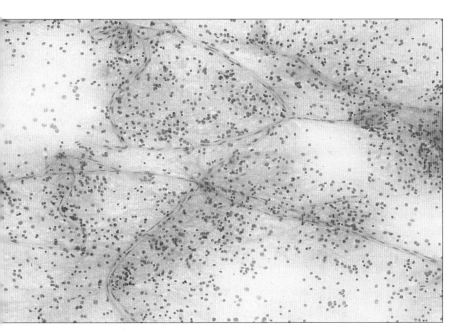

Figure 7.16
Oligoastrocytoma. Female aged 27 years, right frontal lobe. A gliofibrillary matrix is present around the finely branching capillary network in mixed gliomas, from which the small rounded oligodendroglial cells spread in a monolayer. Smear preparation, haematoxylin eosin, ×70.

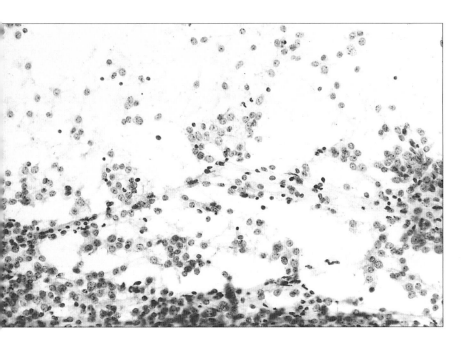

Figure 7.17
Oligoastrocytoma. Male aged 15 years, right frontal lobe. The dual population of neoplastic cells comprises the small rounded oligodendroglial cells with scanty cytoplasm and the larger astrocytic cells with more abundant cytoplasm and cell processes which form a perivascular gliofibrillary matrix. Smear preparation, toluidine blue, ×350.

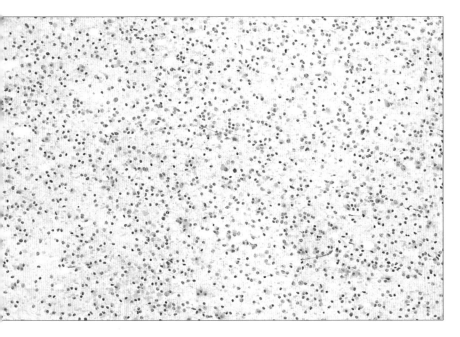

Figure 7.18
Oligoastrocytoma. Female aged 25 years, right frontal lobe. The oligodendroglial population predominates in this tumour, but there is a significant subpopulation of neoplastic astrocytic cells which are larger and contain more densely eosinophilic cytoplasm. Vascular endothelial proliferation is absent in this low grade tumour.
Cryostat section, haematoxylin eosin, ×140.

cells characteristically present in ependymal tumours around blood vessels, which are usually thick-walled rather than the characteristic thin-walled vessels present in oligodendroglioma.

The cytological appearances of **DNET** may be confused with oligodendroglioma, but the former usually contain an admixture of glial and neuronal cells, and cryostat sections are helpful in the identification of the characteristic architecture and 'floating neurones' in DNET. In many cases, the diagnosis of DNET will require paraffin section histology and immunocytochemistry. It must be emphasized that DNET is a complex clinicopathological entity, and this diagnosis should not be entertained in the absence of a characteristic clinical history and neuroradiological findings.

Oligodendrogliomas can usually be distinguished easily from **metastatic carcinomas** by their uniform cellularity, a tendency to smear in a monolayer with little cellular cohesion, the typical vascular network and a relative absence of mitotic activity and necrosis, which are common in metastatic deposits. Finally, it should be remembered that oligodendroglioma-like areas can be encountered in other CNS tumours, including ependymomas, medulloblastomas and glioblastomas. In these cases, the resemblance is often superficial and detailed inspection will reveal the features of the main neoplastic component, allowing accurate diagnosis. With limited sampling of neoplasms for intra-operative diagnosis by the increasing use of stereotaxy, this can sometimes produce difficulties which may only be resolved finally on paraffin histology and immunocytochemistry.

EPENDYMAL TUMOURS

8.1. TYPICAL EPENDYMOMA AND ITS MALIGNANT FORMS

8.1.1. CLINICAL AND RADIOLOGICAL FEATURES

Ependymomas often arise in topographical relation to the ventricular cavities but they may be sited anywhere in the neuraxis. They occur most frequently in the fourth ventricle, arising from the floor or roof, and at this site they are most likely to be tumours of infancy or childhood, presenting with obstructive hydrocephalus. Supratentorial examples usually fill one or other lateral ventricular cavity and may present in children or adults, usually with clinical evidence of mass effect or with seizures. Less commonly, they can arise in the posterior third ventricle, presenting clinically and radiologically as a pineal region mass. Deep intracerebral ependymomas, apparently quite separate from the ventricular cavity and its lining, are rare tumours of younger age groups which are nearly always large and rapidly growing. In the spinal canal, ependymomas are most often cauda equina lesions of myxopapillary type (see below), but typical ependymomas may also occur, usually as intramedullary tumours in the cervical or lumbosacral region. Spinal ependymomas usually present in adulthood, often with a long history of back pain.

Radiologically, ependymomas are iso- or hyperdense with brain in CT scans and show rather patchy contrast enhancement. Calcification is quite common, especially in the posterior fossa tumours. MR scans emphasize the circumscribed margins of most ependymomas, an especially important feature in their distinction from diffusely infiltrating astrocytomas within the spinal cord. Ependymomas are usually isodense with brain in T1 weighted images, but hyperdense in T2 weighted sequences, with variably intense gadolinium enhancement. Cysts may be visible within the supratentorial tumours, and intramedullary spinal cord examples are often associated with a syrinx cavity.

8.1.2. SURGICAL FINDINGS

At operation, ependymomas typically appear as firm, lobulated masses of reddish-grey colour. Ventricle-related tumours project into the ventricular cavity, which may be entirely obliterated. In surgical terms, one of the most important features of ependymomas is their demarcation from adjacent brain tissue. Even at their point of origin there is usually a good surgical plane, which becomes more marked where the tumour is pressing against an expanded ventricular lining. Such circumscription is also a property of entirely intra-parenchymal ependymomas in the cerebral hemisphere or spinal cord. This may not be immediately apparent to the surgeon, however, especially in the initial stages of surgery, and intra-operative distinction from diffusely infiltrating lesions such as astrocytomas is frequently of great importance in guiding the extent of excision. Ependymomas of the fourth ventricle are frequently gritty when cut because of calcification, and larger examples may grow out of the CSF foramina to fill the cisterna magna and envelope the medulla. In the spine, intramedullary ependymomas produce a fusiform expansion of the cord. They are usually well circumscribed, sausage-shaped masses which are sited centrally, deep to the pial surface, and may extend over several anatomical segments.

8.1.3. INTRA-OPERATIVE PATHOLOGY

Smear cytology

Most ependymomas are soft enough to make good smear preparations, and in typical cases a diagnosis can normally be reached using cytology alone. As always, however, it is important to examine as many fields of smeared tissue as possible. With the less epithelial variants of ependymoma, especially those in adults, many areas of the smear can appear superficially similar to astrocytic tumours, and ependymomatous features may be missed if they are not specifically looked for. The most important clue is the formation of organized papillary masses around blood vessels. These are the equivalent of the perivascular pseudorosettes seen in histological sections, but in smears they are not often visible in cross section because the blood vessels are orientated longitudinally. Instead, there are dense palisades of tumour cell nuclei, sometimes several layers deep, which are arranged either side of the vessels. The nuclei are loosely orientated away from the axis of the vessel, and a characteristic fibrillar zone can often be seen separating them from the underlying vessel wall. If the tissue is thickly smeared, however, this zone may be masked because a layer of cells lies all around the papillary structure within the depth of the preparation. In larger clumps of smeared tissue, the relationship of tumour cells to blood vessels may not be apparent at all, leaving simply an impression of loose palisading or radial orientation of nuclei around the margins of the tissue.

There is usually a very obvious glial fibrillary stroma in ependymoma smears, most clearly visible around blood vessels and at the edges of the larger papillary masses. In some cases, the stroma may be the predominating feature, but in contrast to astrocytic tumours, metachromasia of toluidine blue staining and Rosenthal fibres are not often seen in smears of typical ependymomas. Despite the fibrillary matrix, the tumour cells in ependymomas also show less cohesion than those of astrocytomas, and individual cells tend to smear out quite easily from the margins of perivascular structures and larger clumps of tissue. When isolated in this way, the cells are often seen to have circumscribed perinuclear cytoplasm and tapering processes, either with a stellate or unipolar configuration. The tumour cell nuclei are larger and rounder than those typically seen in astrocytic tumours, with pale, stippled chromatin and one or more prominent nucleoli. Ependymal cell rosettes are only rarely visible in smear preparations, and the presence of distinct tubular structures should arouse suspicion of an epithelial neoplasm such as metastatic carcinoma.

Frozen sections

Most typical ependymomas are easily recognized in cryostat sections, and these should be prepared if there is any doubt as to the smear diagnosis. This is particularly important where a diffusely infiltrating astrocytic tumour cannot be entirely excluded using cytology and the surgeon needs to know whether to expect a clean surgical plane at the margins of the lesion. Frozen sections can also be very useful where malignant transformation is suspected, demonstrating features such as focal necrosis and vascular endothelial proliferation (see below). The sections should be examined at quite low magnification in the first instance, or the typical architecture of the tumour may not be apparent. Perivascular

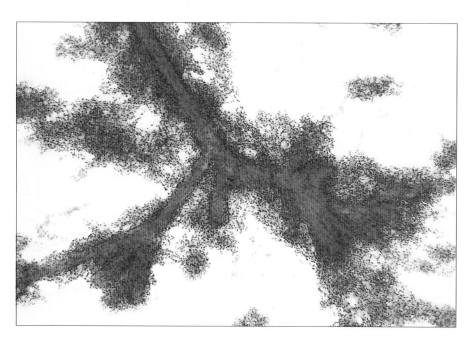

Figure 8.1

Ependymoma. Male aged 30 years, lumbar spinal cord. Smears of typical ependymomas usually show some areas where the tissue forms a distinct papillary pattern around blood vessels. Even at low magnification, these papillary masses tend to appear more organized than those associated with astrocytic tumours. A narrow perivascular cuff of densely packed tumour cell nuclei is visible here, running either side of the branching central vessels. More loosely adherent cells lie outside this, smeared out away from the vessels. Smear preparation, haematoxylin eosin, ×45.

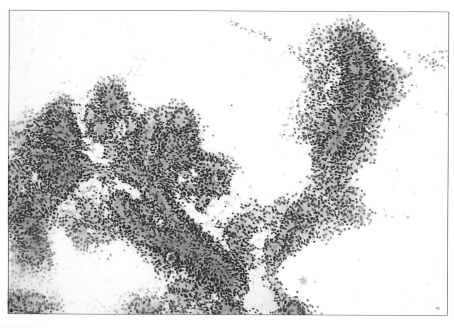

Figure 8.2

Ependymoma. Female aged 8 years, lumbar spinal cord. The branching blood vessels are arranged longitudinally and flanked either side by dense palisades of tumour cell nuclei, giving the impression of organized papillary fronds of tissue. More peripheral cells smear individually out from the margins of the frond-like masses. Gliofibrillar matrix is not apparent at this magnification, but a narrow anucleate central zone is identifiable immediately adjacent to the vessel wall. Smear preparation, toluidine blue, ×90.

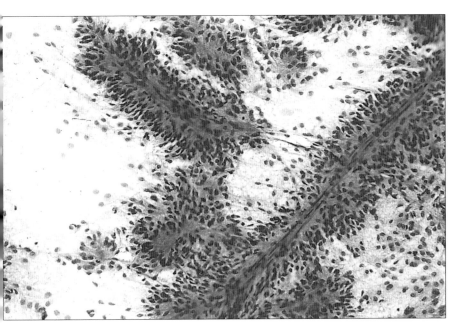

Figure 8.3
Ependymoma. Female aged 31 years, fourth ventricle. Blood vessels flanked by palisades of tumour cell nuclei, sometimes several layers thick, are the smeared equivalent of perivascular pseudorosettes, seen transversely cut in tissue sections. In this smear, the tumour cell nuclei are orientated away from the axis of the vessel and an inner zone of fibrillar stroma is clearly visible. Individually smeared cells are again a prominent feature in between the papillary masses. Smear preparation, toluidine blue, ×175.

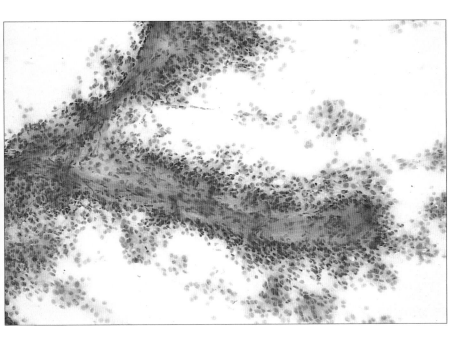

Figure 8.4
Ependymoma. Male aged 26 years, lumbar cord. This case shows very similar features to those illustrated in the toluidine blue-stained example in Fig. 8.3. Isolated clumps of tumour cells with rather indistinct perinuclear cytoplasm lie in between the fronds of more cellular, perivascular tissue with palisade nuclei. The central blood vessels can be clearly identified in both this case and the previous one. Smear preparation, haematoxylin eosin, ×175.

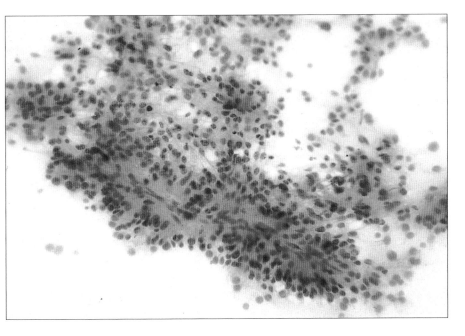

Figure 8.5
Ependymoma. Another view from the same case illustrated in Fig. 8.4. In very thinly smeared areas, the tumour cells may lie individually or in small groups, sometimes producing elongate, rosette-like clusters around fragments of capillary vessel, like that seen here. The background cytoplasm is rather ill-defined and not very obviously fibrillar in this example. Smear preparation, haematoxylin eosin, ×220.

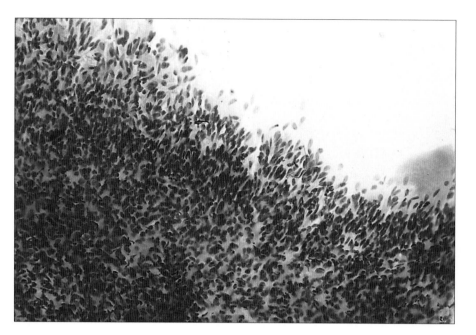

Figure 8.6
Ependymoma. Male aged 45 years, cervical spinal cord. Where the tumour is thickly smeared into dense papillary masses, the central blood vessels can be entirely obscured by cellular tissue. At the margins of these thick clumps where the tissue is more attenuate, however, the tumour cell nuclei often give at least a hint of a palisade arrangement, as seen here. The impression of hypercellularity in this example is largely caused by the thickness of the preparation. Smear preparation, toluidine blue, ×175.

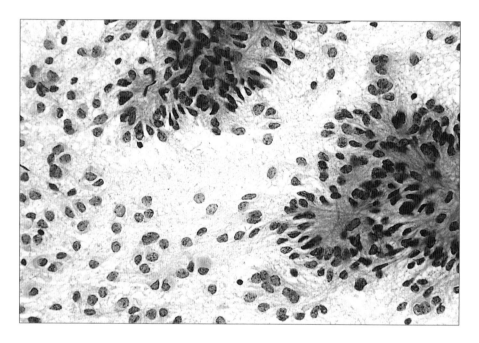

Figure 8.7
Ependymoma. Female aged 31 years, fourth ventricle. At higher magnification, the fibrillar nature of the background stroma can be appreciated. The tumour cells are again showing a characteristic tendency to smear out individually from the edges of clumps of tissue, where their cytological features are best appreciated. The nuclei of ependymoma cells are typically quite large, with a rounded profile, pale chromatin and one or more distinct nucleoli. Smear preparation, toluidine blue, ×350.

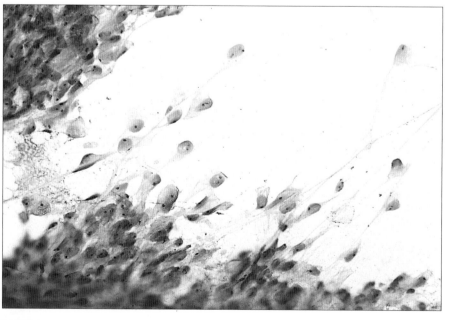

Figure 8.8
Ependymoma. Female aged 72 years, cervical spinal cord. Another case showing the tendency of ependymoma cells to smear out individually around the margins of larger masses of tumour. The nuclei are characteristically rounded with pale chromatin and prominent nucleoli. In this smear, the isolated tumour cells have clearly defined, elongate cytoplasmic processes. The unipolar appearance of some of these cells is a typical cytological feature of ependymomas in smear preparations. Smear preparation, toluidine blue, ×350.

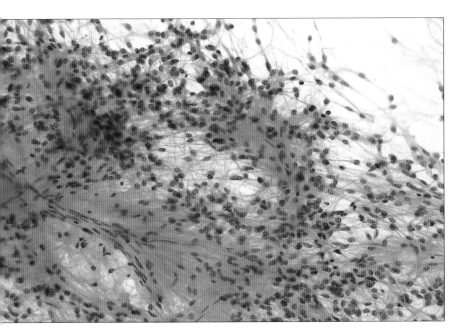

Figure 8.9
Ependymoma. Male aged 42 years, lumbar spinal cord. Smear preparations of some ependymomas show a very abundant and prominent fibrillar stroma, with the potential for confusion with astrocytic tumours. This is particularly the case with adult ependymomas and those sited in the spinal cord, where the intra-operative distinction between astrocytoma and ependymoma is of considerable clinical importance. Even in the field illustrated here, however, radiating fibrillar architecture, loose nuclear palisades and separately smeared cells with individual cytoplasmic processes all help to identify the tumour as ependymoma. Smear preparation, haematoxylin eosin, ×175.

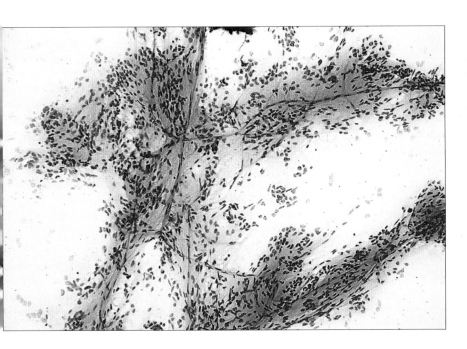

Figure 8.10
Ependymoma. Male aged 9 years, lateral ventricle. This is another case where the fibrillar background stroma was very prominent in smear preparations, especially around the branching blood vessels. The layer of tumour cell nuclei surrounding the vascular fronds is incomplete, but some stretches of nuclear palisading adjacent to the fibrillar cores are still apparent. Smear preparation, toluidine blue, ×110.

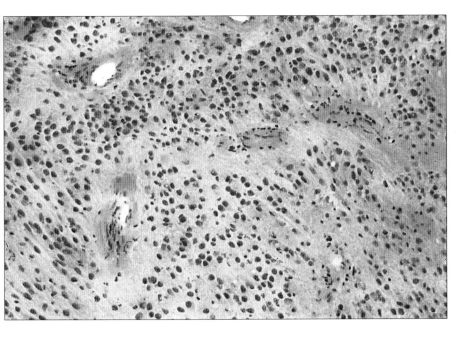

Figure 8.11
Ependymoma. Male aged 57 years, cervical spinal cord. The characteristic architecture of ependymomas is best appreciated at relatively low magnification in frozen sections, allowing the perivascular pseudorosettes to be more easily identified. Where the radiating fibrillar architecture of these rosettes is not obvious, as in this example, it is important to be sure that tumour stroma as well as vessel wall elements separate the vascular lumen from the surrounding nuclei. The intervening tumour tissue here has a characteristic monotonous appearance, with homogeneous sheets of rounded nuclei. Frozen section, haematoxylin eosin, ×175.

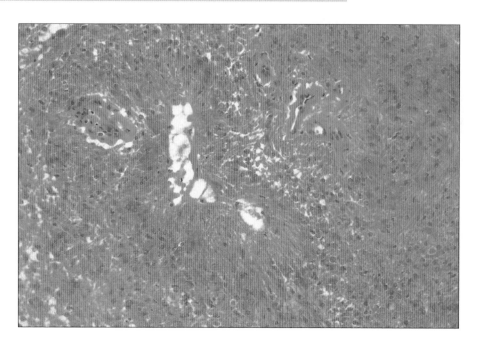

Figure 8.12
Ependymoma. Female aged 45 years, fourth ventricle. The background stroma in this case is coarsely fibrillar in nature, and the radiating architecture of the large perivascular pseudorosette in the centre is clearly apparent. Confident diagnosis of ependymoma in frozen sections usually relies on the identification of such structures, since true tubular rosettes and epithelial-lined canals are only present in a relatively small proportion of ependymomas (see Fig. 8.16). It should be noted that pseudorosette formation is much less obvious around the two smaller blood vessels in this field, where it could easily be missed on superficial examination. Frozen section, haematoxylin eosin, ×175.

pseudorosettes in particular may be quite subtle in cryostat sections, and can sometimes be difficult to appreciate at higher magnifications. Cell density varies greatly, for example between a rapidly growing posterior fossa ependymoma of childhood and a sparsely cellular adult spinal cord tumour. Nevertheless, all ependymomas tend to show a distinctive homogeneity of cellularity, which sets them apart from most astrocytic tumours. If true ependymal rosettes are present, this obviously helps matters considerably, but it should be remembered that they are a relatively uncommon histological feature in routine practice, most likely to be encountered in posterior fossa tumours in childhood.

8.1.4. GRADING AND MALIGNANCY

Ependymomas exhibit a clinical and pathological spectrum of malignancy in a similar fashion to astrocytic tumours, although the grading system is perhaps rather more controversial. Approximately 20% of all cases are overtly malignant in pathological terms, and for the purposes of intra-operative diagnosis, it is worth remembering that the vast majority of these are posterior fossa or deep intracerebral ependymomas of infancy or childhood. In smear preparations, the features suggesting that an ependymoma is a malignant (anaplastic) lesion are similar to those seen in smears of other types of glial neoplasm. A significant mitotic rate is the most reliable cytological indicator, and the presence of more than very occasional mitoses in the smear should arouse the pathologist's suspicion, especially in a child. Other findings suggesting malignancy are increased cellularity, which obviously needs careful interpretation in terms of the thickness of the tissue smeared, and vascular budding or thickened, hypertrophied vessels. Cytological pleomorphism is also a worrying feature, although in contrast to astrocytic tumours, childhood posterior fossa ependymomas may often prove to be histologically malignant without

significant nuclear pleomorphism, cytological atypia or giant cell formation. Focal necrosis is again by no means a pre-requisite for malignancy in ependymomas, but is obviously significant when seen. Frozen sections may be helpful in confirming features such as significant hypercellularity, focal necrosis and vascular endothelial proliferation if there is doubt as to the grade of the lesion in smear preparations.

Ependymoblastomas are a primitive, malignant variant of ependymomas which are essentially primitive neuroectodermal tumours (PNETs) with evidence of ependymal differentiation. They are nearly all large, rapidly growing cerebral hemispheric tumours of infancy and have similar cytological appearances to other PNETs. Using smear preparations, there may be papillary masses with perivascular palisades in some cases, but much of the tissue usually smears out into a diffuse monolayer of cells with quite pleomorphic nuclei. The cells have indistinct perinuclear cytoplasm and tend to show nuclear moulding where they press against each other. Mitotic figures are always present and are often numerous. Where there are no ependymomatous features in the smear, it may not be possible to make an intra-operative diagnosis more specific than that of PNET. Frozen sections may be helpful if multilayered, ependymoblastic rosettes can be identified. In practice, however, this refinement of the diagnosis is rarely going to be of any real importance to the intra-operative management of the patient.

8.1.5. DIFFERENTIAL DIAGNOSIS

The clinical and radiological differential diagnosis of intracranial ependymomas includes many other types of tumour occurring at intraventricular or paraventricular sites. In the lateral ventricles, obvious examples are **choroid plexus tumours**, **intraventricular meningiomas** and **metastases**. The latter two are only likely in older

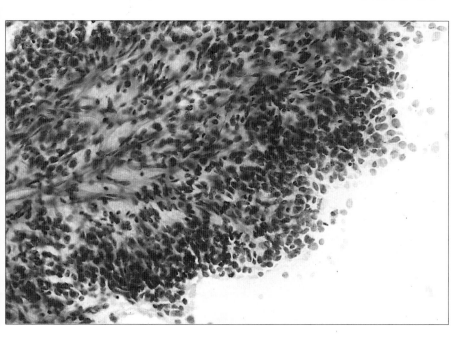

Figure 8.13

Anaplastic ependymoma. Female aged 12 years, intracerebral lesion. The papillary masses of smeared tissue in this case appear genuinely hypercellular, with very thick cuffs of tumour cell nuclei around their margins. There is an impression of nuclear palisading, but this is much less organized than might be expected in a well differentiated ependymoma. There is also quite marked vascular proliferation, and a plexus of branching blood vessels occupies the core of the papillary structure in this field. Smear preparation, toluidine blue, ×220.

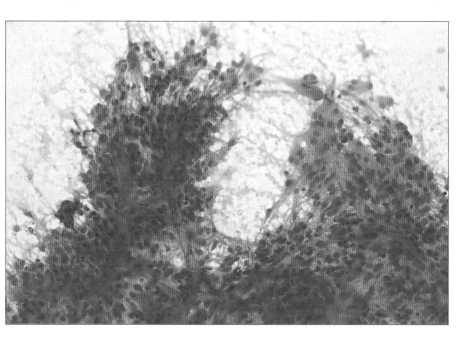

Figure 8.14

Anaplastic ependymoma. Female aged 3 years, fourth ventricle. Hypercellularity and proliferated blood vessels are again a feature in this case, and even at this magnification a degree of nuclear pleomorphism is apparent. The diagnosis of ependymal rather than astrocytic tumour is suggested both by the relationship of tumour cell nuclei to blood vessels and the tendency of cells to smear out individually at the tissue margins. Smear preparation, haematoxylin eosin, ×175.

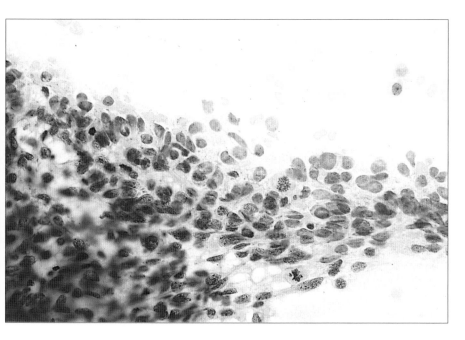

Figure 8.15

Anaplastic ependymoma. A higher magnification view of a smear from the same case as illustrated in Fig. 8.13. Tumour cell nuclei show a significant degree of moulding and pleomorphism. Mitotic figures can be easily seen. Smear preparation, toluidine blue, ×350.

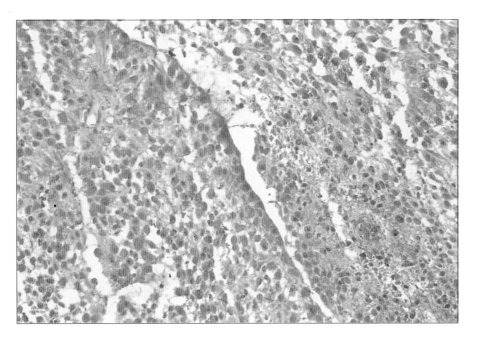

Figure 8.16
Anaplastic ependymoma. Male aged 7 years, fourth ventricle. Perivascular pseudorosettes are rather ill-defined in this cryostat section, but one can be recognized at the top left of the field. The tumour is quite epithelial in nature and an ependymal lined canal is also present. Malignancy is suggested by the degree of nuclear hyperchromatism and pleomorphism, and also by the focal area of necrosis seen at the bottom right. Frozen section, haematoxylin eosin, ×220.

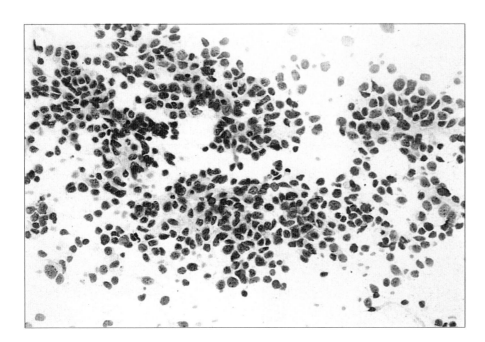

Figure 8.17
Ependymoblastoma. Male aged 17 years, intracerebral lesion. The tumour cells have smeared out into a thin monolayer with little evidence of cohesion and no obvious papillary structures. There is a faintly stained and rather ill-defined background stroma, but individual cell cytoplasm is not discernible. The tumour cell nuclei are pleomorphic and show moulding against each other. Mitoses were easily found at higher magnification. The cytological appearance is indistinguishable from smears of other types of primitive neuroectodermal tumour. Smear preparation, toluidine blue, ×220.

age groups and are usually easy to recognize in smear preparations, even if the diagnosis is not suggested radiologically or at operation. Choroid plexus tumours are distinguishable by their uniform, bright contrast enhancement in CT or MR scans, and often have an obvious surgical origin from the choroid plexus root. They are also much more vascular than most ependymomas, and this will again be apparent to the surgeon while operating. For the pathologist, benign examples have very distinctive, epithelial features and usually show obvious similarities to normal choroid plexus tissue in both smears and frozen sections (*see* Chapter 9). Malignant choroid plexus tumours may cause more difficulty if the regular epithelial arrangement of tumour cells around blood vessels is lost. As with metastatic adenocarcinomas, the main cytological differences from anaplastic ependymomas are the tendency of the cells to clump together in an epithelial

fashion with discreet perinuclear cytoplasm, and the complete absence of a glial fibrillary background. The epithelial nature of these two lesions is usually even more apparent on frozen sections.

Deep hemispheric ependymomas need to be distinguished from **infantile glioblastomas**. Both are likely to show obvious evidence of glial lineage and malignancy using smear preparations, but circumscribed unipolar cytoplasm and the formation of distinct perivascular pseudopalisades will help to identify an intraparenchymal ependymoma, assuming the diagnosis is kept in mind at this rather unusual site. A much rarer possibility is an **astroblastoma**, which typically occurs in infancy, is radiologically and surgically circumscribed and has a predominantly intra- or paraventricular location. Using smears, the monotonous cytology of astroblastomas and their tendency to form perivascular palisades may easily cause confusion with ependymomas. Frozen sections can present a similar difficulty, but there is a subtle difference between the two types of perivascular rosette. Those of astroblastomas have a ring of broad cytoplasmic plates around the blood vessel wall, rather than the anuclate zone of radiating, finely fibrillar processes seen in ependymomas.

In the third ventricle, a **central neurocytoma** needs to be considered if the lesion is anteriorly located, and a **pineocytoma** if it is sited in the posterior recesses. In smear preparations, either lesion may have a perivascular papillary pattern with filamentous stroma, and confident distinction from a third ventricle ependymoma may sometimes be impossible. Frozen sections will reveal an absence of ependymal-type perivascular pseudorosettes in both cases, but pineocytomas may still be confused with ependymomas because of the large pineocytomatous rosettes. On close inspection, however, these structures lack either radial fibrillar orientation or a central blood vessel. If true tubular rosettes are seen in frozen sections, these will again help to distinguish an ependymoma.

In the fourth ventricle, the most important differential diagnoses of ependymomas are **choroid plexus tumours** (see above) and **medulloblastomas**. Using smear preparations, ependymomas differ from most medulloblastomas in showing an obvious gliofibrillary stroma. They also form cohesive clumps of tissue and perivascular palisades, rather than smearing out into a diffuse monolayer like the cells of medulloblastomas. Posterior fossa ependymomas are frequently malignant, but the pronounced pleomorphism and nuclear moulding typical of medulloblastomas are not usually seen. If there is doubt, frozen sections will be needed to confirm the presence of ependymal perivascular pseudorosettes. Tubular rosettes are most likely to be present in posterior fossa ependymomas of childhood and may also be of value in the distinction from medulloblastoma, but it should be remembered that they are not usually visible in smear preparations.

With intramedullary spinal cord lesions, the most important differential diagnosis lies between ependymoma and **astrocytoma**. Both may be associated with an elongate, syrinx-like cavity, although in an astrocytoma the cyst is likely to contain golden yellow proteinacious fluid rather than the clear CSF typically found in an ependymoma-related syrinx. Ependymomas are likely to show more radiological contrast enhancement than low grade astrocytomas, but this will not be of benefit if the astrocytoma has undergone malignant transformation. For the surgeon, the importance of distinguishing between the two tumour types at the time of operating lies in the very different potential for complete resection. Astrocytomas are usually diffusely infiltrating lesions which blend into functioning cord tissue at their margins, whereas ependymomas tend to be well circumscribed with a good surgical plane. This may not be apparent when entering abnormal tumour tissue early in the procedure, however, and hence the value of intra-operative pathology. Using

smear preparations, it is important to look for the organized perivascular palisades of ependymoma, and to remember that these are sometimes most apparent at quite low magnifications. In astrocytic tumours, the vascular papillary patterns are not associated with nuclear palisading, and are simply the result of a non-specific tendency of astrocytic cells to cling to blood vessels. Other useful distinguishing features are the larger, rounder nuclei of ependymoma cells and the way in which they smear individually away from tissue masses, often revealing circumscribed, unipolar cytoplasm. If there is any doubt, frozen sections should be prepared to look for ependymal-type perivascular pseudorosettes. True tubular rosettes are rather uncommon in intramedullary spinal cord ependymomas.

8.2. MYXOPAPILLARY EPENDYMOMA

8.2.1. CLINICAL AND RADIOLOGICAL FEATURES

This is a distinctive variant of ependymoma which is almost exclusively confined to the cauda equina region of the spinal canal, where it accounts for 50% of all ependymal tumours. Uncommonly, myxopapillary ependymomas may also arise ectopically in the soft tissues of the parasacral region, and very rare examples present as intra-abdominal masses. The typical cauda equina lesions occur most frequently in young adults and usually present with a long history of low back pain, sometimes with additional evidence of lumbosacral radiculopathy.

Radiologically, these lesions are best seen using MR scans, where they characteristically appear as well defined, elongate masses, isodense to cord in T1-weighted images and hyperdense with T2 weighting. They usually show moderate contrast enhancement and larger tumours may be associated with erosion of the bony canal.

8.2.2. SURGICAL FINDINGS

At surgery, cauda equina myxopapillary ependymomas are distinctive, sausage-shaped tumours with a smooth, lobulated surface, lying separate from the spinal cord in the lumbosacral canal. Cauda equina nerve roots are usually displaced to either side, but in some cases they may be enveloped within the tumour mass. The cut section often shows evidence of old or recent haemorrhage, but gritty calcification is not so prominent a feature as in typical ependymomas.

8.2.3. INTRA-OPERATIVE PATHOLOGY

Like typical ependymomas, the myxopapillary variant is usually soft enough to make good smear preparations, and the highly distinctive cytological features permit a fairly straightforward intra-operative diagnosis in most cases. The smears show numerous organized papillary structures, with multilayered cuffs of tumour cell nuclei around blood vessels. In contrast to typical ependymomas, however, the gliofibrillar stroma is partially replaced by an amorphous, myxoid matrix. This is most easily identified using toluidine stained preparations, because it is strongly metachromatic and has a striking purple colour. Using HE staining, the matrix is faintly eosinophilic and may incorporate more intensely stained, blob-like structures. Myxoid matrix is visible both around blood vessels and at the edges of smeared masses of tissue. Sometimes there is no central blood vessel, and the tissue smears out as circular rosettes with solid myxoid cores cuffed by tumour cells. The cells of myxopapil-

lary ependymomas have large, round nuclei with pale chromatin and prominent nucleoli, similar to those in typical ependymomas. Discreet perinuclear cytoplasm is much less apparent in myxopapillary lesions, however, even at the edges of the papillary fronds where the cells smear out individually. Using frozen sections, myxoid rosettes are again distinctive features to look for. Most strikingly, the radial fibrillar architecture of typical ependymal pseudorosettes is replaced by a loose, myxoid expansion of the perivascular spaces. In some examples there may also be sheets of well-organized, myxoid rosettes lacking a central vessel, but this appearance is perhaps less commonly encountered. The characteristic myxopapillary architecture may be focally obscured by prominent secondary degenerative changes, including fibrous scarring, old haemorrhage and fibrin deposition.

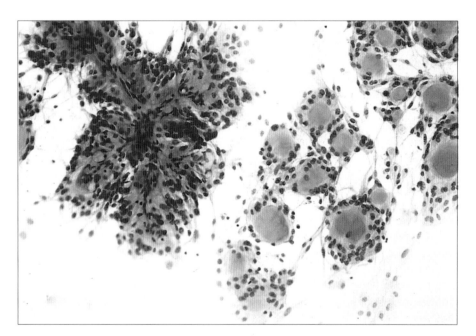

Figure 8.18
Myxopapillary ependymoma. Male aged 15 years, cauda equina. Smear preparations typically show numerous, highly organized papillary structures like those illustrated here. Some are arranged longitudinally around central blood vessels, as in smears of classic ependymomas. Others lack central vessels and smear out as circular rosettes, like those to the right of this field. The myxoid stroma is very striking in toluidine blue stained preparations because of intense violacious metachromasia, and is present both around the vessels and in the centre of the solid rosettes. Smear preparation, toluidine blue, ×175.

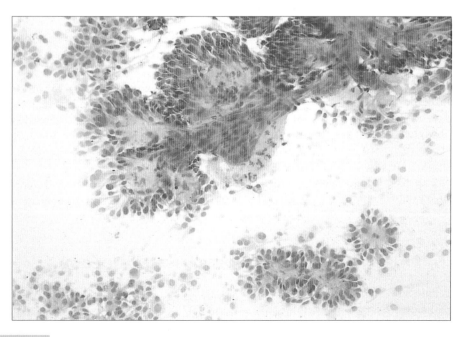

Figure 8.19
Myxopapillary ependymoma. Female aged 17 years, lumbosacral spinal cord. Another case showing well-organized examples of both perivascular papillary structures and solid, circular rosettes. The myxoid stroma in both these is less visually striking than in toluidine blue stained preparations, but again lacks the fibrillary texture of typical ependymomas. Smear preparation, haematoxylin eosin, ×175.

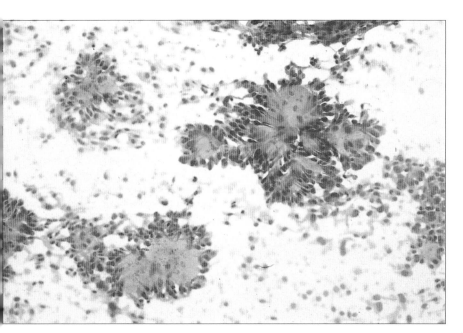

Figure 8.20

Myxopapillary ependymoma. Same case as in Fig. 8.19, showing several of the solid rosette-like structures. They are filled with abundant myxoid matrix, which is mostly rather pale stained but includes occasional brightly eosinophilic blobs. The nuclear morphology is similar to that of typical ependymomas and the tumour cells show the same tendency to smear out individually from the edges of the papillary formations. Smear preparation, haematoxylin eosin, ×175.

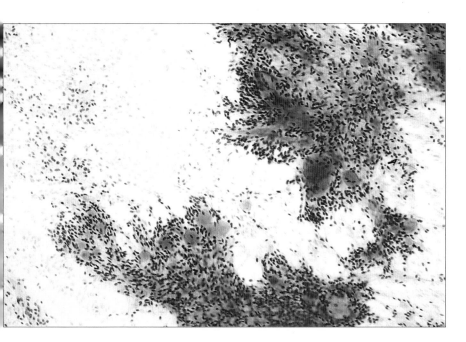

Figure 8.21

Myxopapillary ependymoma. Male aged 63 years, cauda equina. Well preserved myxopapillary rosettes are not an obvious feature of this smear, but their myxoid, brightly metachromatic cores are easy to identify amongst the more cellular areas of tissue. Metachromatic matrix can also be seen in the centre of perivascular papillary structures. Smear preparation, toluidine blue, ×110.

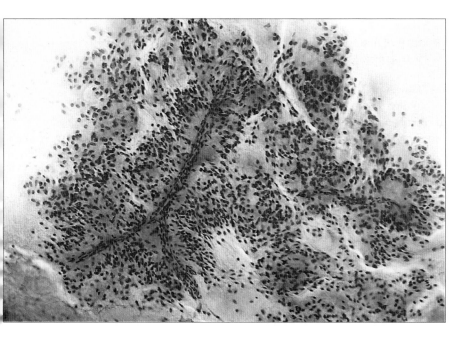

Figure 8.22

Myxopapillary ependymoma. Female aged 16 years, lumbosacral spinal cord. In this example, even the myxoid cores of solid rosettes are absent, but there is abundant metachromasia of the background matrix and an obvious ependymomatous perivascular architecture. The myxopapillary nature of this particular tumour would perhaps be more difficult to appreciate in an H&E-stained preparation. Smear preparation, toluidine blue, ×110.

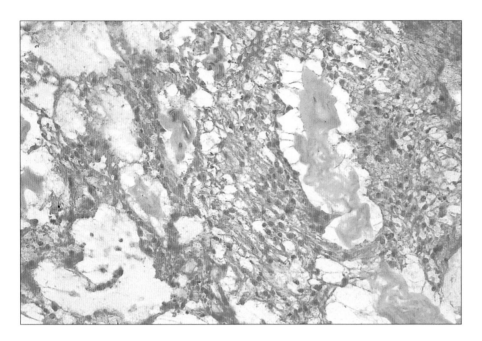

Figure 8.23
Myxopapillary ependymoma. Male aged 35 years, lumbosacral spinal cord. Whilst frozen sections may sometimes show sheets of highly organized, epithelial rosettes containing myxoid material, it is perhaps more usual to be confronted by an image similar to that shown here. Numerous, irregular spaces are present, separated by ependymal nuclei embedded in a loose, fibrillar background. Some of the cystic cavities represent perivascular spaces expanded by eosinophilic myxoid material, although the central vessel is often hard to discern. Others are solid rosettes, but mostly lack an organized surrounding layer of nuclei. Frozen section, haematoxylin eosin, ×175.

8.2.4. MALIGNANCY

Myxopapillary ependymomas are tumours of very low biological grade and do not undergo anaplastic transformation. Some examples, especially those in ectopic sites, may behave in a locally invasive or recurrent fashion, but mitotic figures and other pathological features of malignancy are not seen in smear preparations or frozen sections.

8.2.5. DIFFERENTIAL DIAGNOSIS

The differential diagnosis of cauda equina myxopapillary ependymoma is that of circumscribed tumours lying within the lumbosacral spinal canal. **Paragangliomas** and **Schwannomas** may be difficult to exclude surgically, but are not likely to present an intra-operative problem for the pathologist. The 'twisted rope' appearance of interlacing fascicles seen in Schwannomas will normally identify them using smears (*see* Chapter 13). Paragangliomas are mostly too tough to smear well and require frozen sections, which will show their typical alveolar architecture. In neither case is there any myxoid matrix like that of myxopapillary tumours. However, a similar matrix, also metachromatic with toluidine blue staining, is present in **chordomas** and **cartilaginous tumours**. Clinically, these are both likely to show significant involvement of the adjacent bony structures, but this may also be the case with some very large myxopapillary tumours, including those arising ectopically in parasacral tissues. Cartilaginous tumours will not smear at all and show an obvious lacunar architecture in frozen sections. Chordomas, by contrast, may smear out quite well, with a prominent mucinous background. There are no ependymoma-like papillary structures, however, and the cells of chordomas usually show obvious pleomorphism and physaliperous change, both in smear preparations and frozen sections.

Metastatic adenocarcinomas of the cauda equina region may be easily confused with myxopapillary ependymomas both radiologically and surgically, and can produce a similar mucinous papillary appearance in smear preparations. The main cytological difference is the epithelial cohesion exhibited by most carcinomas, which tend to smear as clumps of closely grouped cells with discreet perinuclear cytoplasm. Cytological features of malignancy should also warn against the diagnosis of myxopapillary ependymoma. Finally, CSF seedlings from **choroid plexus tumours** may present as circumscribed, papillary, masses in the cauda equina region, although the primary tumour is usually apparent clinically before this occurs. Depending on the state of differentiation of the tumour, smears and frozen sections will either show similarities to normal choroid plexus or frankly carcinomatous features, but without the prominent mucinous stroma of myxopapillary ependymomas.

8.3 SUBEPENDYMOMA

8.3.1. CLINICAL AND RADIOLOGICAL FEATURES

Only about half of all subependymomas are symptomatic tumours, the remainder being small lesions found coincidentally at autopsy or on radiological examination. Larger subependymomas present clinically in older age groups, mostly over the age of 40 years. A majority arise from the floor of the fourth ventricle and produce features of obstructive hydrocephalus, brainstem compression (including respiratory disturbances) or lower cranial nerve palsies. Less commonly they may be attached to the lateral ventricular walls or the intraventricular septum, causing obstruction of the foramina of Monroe, or occur in an intramedullary location in the cervical cord. They are slow growing tumours and there is usually quite a long clinical history.

Radiologically, subependymomas appear as solid, isodense masses in CT scans. Contrast enhancement is inconstant and often entirely absent, but calcification is often visible, especially in the posterior fossa tumours. With MR scanning, they are usually hypodense in T1-weighted images, hyperdense with T2 weighting, and again do not generally show contrast enhancement.

8.3.2. Surgical findings

The intraventricular tumours are sessile or polypoid masses which project into the ventricular cavity. They have a smooth, domed or lobulated surface and are very firm tumours with a markedly tough texture. The cut section is often gritty due to calcification and may show cysts or evidence of old haemorrhage. In the spinal cord, the tumours arise deep to the pial surface, causing a fusiform expansion over several segments like that seen with typical ependymomas. Subependymomas are mostly extremely well circumscribed lesions, but are inevitably firmly adherent to their sites of origin, especially in the fourth ventricle. In this location, correct intra-operative identification is vital, since overzealous attempts to secure a radical excision can easily cause lethal damage to the respiratory centres in the ventricular floor. It is our experience that excision of fourth ventricular subependymomas is best limited to partial debulking and decompression of the CSF obstruction, especially bearing in mind the extremely slow growth and otherwise benign outcome of these tumours.

8.3.3. Intra-operative pathology

Subependymomas are generally too tough to make good smear preparations, and frozen sections are nearly always necessary to make a definitive intra-operative diagnosis. If smears are attempted, they show dense, thick masses of fibrillar material, which are often twisted around each other to enclose large spaces. The tissue shows little tendency to smear more thinly at the edges, and the tumour cell nuclei are frequently distorted by squeeze artefact. Using frozen sections, examination at low magnification is needed in order to appreciate the typical architecture of subependymomas. The cell nuclei are grouped together in separate clusters, widely separated by large areas of dense gliofibrillary stoma. There are frequently prominent degenerative changes, including calcification, vascular hyalinization, fibrin deposition and evidence of old haemorrhage. The cell nuclei are rounded, uniform and ependymal in appearance. There are no distinct perivascular pseudorosettes in true subependymomas, and these lesions are always of very low grade, without mitoses or any other evidence of malignancy. It should be noted, however, that some of the larger tumours, especially those in the fourth ventricle, merge with areas of typical ependymoma. The biological behaviour and prognosis of these mixed lesions is that of a typical ependymoma, and the presence of pseudorosettes or other typical ependymomatous features in some parts of the frozen section will thus carry considerable intra-operative implications for the surgeon.

8.3.4. Differential diagnosis

The lack of radiological contrast enhancement in subependymomas will help set them apart pre-operatively from a number of other intraventricular tumours, including **meningiomas, choroid plexus tumours** and **medulloblastomas**. At surgery, subependymomas differ from these lesions in their tough, avascular texture and unsuitability for smearing, and they should be easily distinguishable when frozen sections are prepared. **Subependymal giant cell astrocytomas** may occur in the

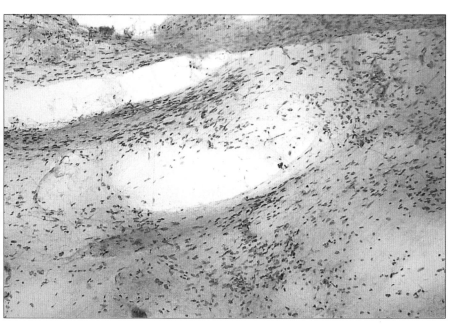

Figure 8.24
Subependymoma. Male aged 53 years, anterior third ventricle. The tissue is usually too tough to make good smear preparations, which generally show thick masses of fibrillar tissue, often twisted around each other to enclose empty areas. In contrast to typical ependymomas, tumour cells do not smear out from the edges of the tissue masses, and cytological features are hard to discern. The tumour may give the impression of being sparsely cellular, but this will depend on the thickness of the smeared clumps. Squeeze artefact of the nuclei is not uncommon because of the toughness of the tissue. Smear preparation, toluidine blue, ×90.

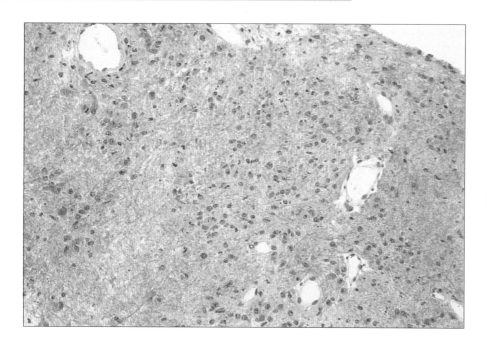

Figure 8.25
Subependymoma. Male aged 72 years, fourth ventricle. Frozen sections typically show an abundant fibrillar stroma, in which loose clusters of tumour cell nuclei are embedded. In 'pure' subependymomas like this one, the nuclei are randomly arranged without the perivascular pseudorosettes typical of other types of ependymal tumour. Some larger tumours, however, may show areas with features of typical ependymoma, and such mixed lesions are often associated with local invasion and a poorer prognosis. Frozen section, haematoxylin eosin, ×175.

absence of other stigmata of tuberose sclerosis and typically present as tough, partly calcified circumscribed masses projecting into the lateral ventricles. They are again usually strongly enhancing lesions, however, and their pilocytic nature will hopefully be apparent in smears or frozen sections, even if the characteristic giant cells are not seen. Particularly in the fourth ventricle, it is important to exclude a **typical ependymoma**, remembering that some tumours may present a mixed pattern with subependymoma. Pure ependymomas are likely to smear easily and show characteristic perivascular palisades, whilst mixed tumours where subependymoma predominates will be tougher and more often require frozen sections. An ependymomatous component should be suspected if areas with distinct perivascular pseudorosettes are seen, even if the remainder of the section appears clearly subependymomatous.

Metastases may mimic subependymomas clinically at any site, and must always be kept in mind as a diagnostic possibility, particularly because of the older age of presentation of subependymomas. Even if a metastatic tumour is too tough to smear, it should be easy to distinguish from a benign, sparsely cellular subependymoma in frozen sections. Third ventricular and cerebellar **pilocytic astrocytomas** differ from subependymomas in their location and age at presentation, and usually show contrast enhancement in radiological scans. They also smear quite easily, exhibiting typical pilocytic cytology. Using frozen sections, a microcystic architecture will also help identify a pilocytic astrocytoma, but many areas can have a solid fibrillar background similar to that of subependymomas, and Rosenthal fibres can be a feature of either tumour. In the cervical spinal cord, both astrocytomas, including those of pilocytic type, and typical ependymomas need to be considered in the differential diagnosis of subependymoma. Spinal **Schwannomas** may also occur in an intramedullary location, and if tough, can make similarly unsatisfactory smear preparations to subependymomas. As always, however, there should be no real difficulty here so long as the pathologist requests frozen sections and refrains from trying to over-interpret a thick, non-diagnostic smear.

CHOROID PLEXUS TUMOURS

9.1. CHOROID PLEXUS PAPILLOMA

9.1.1. CLINICAL AND RADIOLOGICAL FEATURES

The majority of choroid plexus papillomas arise in infancy and childhood, with about 50% presenting in the first year of life. Some are congenital tumours, diagnosed at birth or picked up on antenatal screening. The infantile and congenital tumours most often arise in the trigone region of one or other lateral ventricle, but may also involve the third ventricle and spread to the lateral ventricle on the opposite side. Affected infants typically present with clinical features of progressive hydrocephalus, often accompanied by head enlargement. Choroid plexus papillomas which present in adult life are usually sited in the fourth ventricle, although they may extend out through the lateral CSF exit foramina and present as CP angle lesions. The signs and symptoms are again usually those of hydrocephalus, although the clinical history tends to be more protracted than in childhood cases.

Radiologically, choroid plexus papillomas appear as lobulated intraventricular masses in CT scans, and may be either isodense or hyperdense to brain tissue. They tend to have a homogenous background signal intensity but frequently show brightly speckled calcification. There is consistent and very intense signal enhancement after administration of intravenous contrast media. With MR scanning, papillomas again show an obvious intraventricular location with a well defined, lobulated outline. Unlike CT scans, the presence of calcification produces a characteristic non-homogeneity of signal. The tumour tissue is iso- or hypo-intense in T1-weighted images but hyper-intense using T2 weighting, and strong contrast enhancement with gadolinium is an invariable feature. Either type of scan will also show accompanying hydrocephalus in the vast majority of cases. This usually has obstructive features if the lesion is in the fourth ventricle, but may be of communicating type in some lateral ventricular examples.

9.1.2. SURGICAL FINDINGS

The vascularity of choroid plexus papillomas is an impressive intra-operative feature, and profuse haemorrhage is to be expected regardless of the extent of the surgical procedure. In some cases, meticulous and complete resection is necessary before the bleeding can be properly controlled. The tumours are pinkish in colour and have a characteristic tufted or fronded surface, which has been likened to that of a cauliflower. The tissue has a friable, granular texture and may be gritty due to calcification. The cut surfaces often show areas of old blood staining or more recent haemorrhage. The extraparenchymal nature of the lesion is nearly always apparent, with a clear demarcation from adjacent brain tissue. A vascular pedicle may be found in some instances, which usually relates to the tela choroida of the trigone region if the tumour is in a lateral ventricle. Fourth ventricular and CP angle papillomas are most likely to have an attachment in one of the lateral recesses of the ventricular cavity.

9.1.3. INTRA-OPERATIVE PATHOLOGY

Smear cytology

Choroid plexus papillomas make distinctive smear preparations, and in most cases the intra-operative diagnosis should be fairly straightforward. Similarities with normal choroid plexus tissue are usually apparent, although the tissue tends to smear out more easily because it is not as tough or cohesive in nature. In typical cases, smears show well defined papillary masses, with a fronded appearance and central vascular cores. The blood vessels usually lack the characteristic serpiginous outline seen in smears of normal plexus tissue and are harder to identify. They are often more prominent in toluidine blue stained preparations because of the contrasting green colour of the erythrocytes in their lumina. The tumour tissue is generally much more cellular than normal choroid plexus, with several layers of tumour cells surrounding the papillary structures. Around the margins, the cells are typically arranged as a regular layer of columnar epithelium, with basally-orientated nuclei and well-defined apical cytoplasmic surfaces. Cilia are not usually present, but may be seen occasionally in congenital and infantile examples. In some tumours, there is also a tendency for the tissue to smear out into epithelial sheets, looking rather like cross-cut epithelium in tissue sections. This phenomenon may be seen either within larger papillary structures or in separately smeared islands of tumour tissue which lack central blood vessels. Such islands of tissue are again likely to have an organized layer of columnar cells around their margins and may sometimes show rosette-like organization. Individual tumour cell cytology is best seen where the tumour cells are thinly smeared into small clusters. The nuclei are small, round and very uniform in appearance, with pale, finely stippled chromatin and one or more small, ill-defined nucleoli. The perinuclear cytoplasm is discreet and does not form processes. In contrast to ependymoma smears, a fibrillar background stroma is entirely lacking.

Where tumours are smeared more thickly into larger masses of tissue, the fronded pattern may be lost and replaced by a coarser, lobulated outline. Central blood vessels can be quite invisible in such circumstances, but even in the thicker areas of tissue it is often possible to discern an infolded papillary pattern, which may be superimposed on a background of cells arranged in epithelial sheets. In addition, some stretches of typical columnar epithelial organization can usually be found around the margins, where the tissue is more thinly spread. Both calcospherites and old blood pigment are commonly present in smears of choroid plexus papillomas, especially in the central areas of larger tissue fragments.

Frozen sections

In frozen sections, the features of choroid plexus papillomas are again very distinctive and unlikely to cause a diagnostic problem in the right clinical circumstances. A typical, fronded, papillary architecture may predominate in some cases but perhaps rather unexpectedly, it is more usual to see a villous pattern. This can be reminiscent of cross-cut small intestinal mucosa, but with delicate, capillary-type blood vessels in the centre of most of the villous structures. Other examples may show a pattern of longitudinal folds, in which the relationship of the blood vessels to the epithelium is not at all obvious. The well-organized, regular epithelial cells vary from one to several layers in thickness and have very uniform small, rounded nuclei. The marginal epithelial layer is usually columnar in appearance with a smooth, flattened apical surface, in contrast to the 'cobblestone' pattern associated with normal choroid

plexus tissue. Rather uncommonly, the tumour cells show pronounced oncocytic change, a helpful indicator of choroid plexus origin. Goblet-cell secretory change in the epithelial cells is also a possibility, but this is excessively rare and should arouse suspicion of a metastatic or teratoid lesion. As in smear preparations, calcification and haemosiderin pigment are frequently present, and frozen sections may also reveal areas of old fibrous scarring, fibrin deposition or even cholesterol granulomas.

9.1.4. GRADING AND MALIGNANCY

Choroid plexus papillomas are biologically benign lesions and there is no real evidence for a spectrum of malignancy linking them with overt carcinomas (see below). In consequence, a true carcinoma of the choroid plexus or other malignant tumour such as a teratoma or metastasis should be considered if intra-operative preparations show evidence of vascular proliferation, necrosis or significant cytological pleomorphism. Even the isolated finding of mitotic figures should alert suspicion that the lesion may not be a simple papilloma but a well-differentiated carcinoma. This is an important observation to make intra-operatively, since choroid plexus carcinomas not only carry a much poorer prognosis, but may be diffusely infiltrating brain tissue and therefore less amenable to total resection.

9.1.5. DIFFERENTIAL DIAGNOSIS

The differential diagnosis of choroid plexus papillomas theoretically includes any intraventricular tumour, but in practice the possibilities are usually limited by clinical details, including the very young age of presentation, the presence of communicating hydrocephalus, strong radiological contrast enhancement and profuse haemorrhage on surgical manipulation. Once confronted with intra-

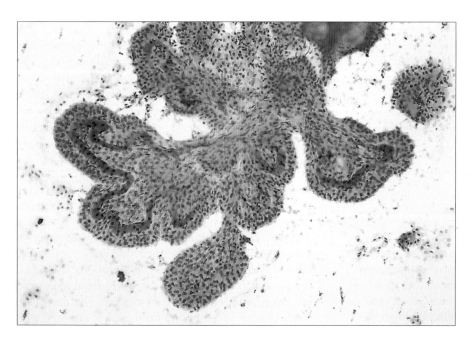

Figure 9.1

Normal choroid plexus tissue. If a ventricle is penetrated, fragments of choroid plexus can be inadvertently incorporated into a non-diagnostic biopsy and mistaken for papilloma. In smear preparations, normal choroid plexus forms very uniform papillary fronds, with a delicate, serpiginous pattern of central blood vessels. The epithelial layer may appear more than one cell deep due to the thickness of tissue smeared, but it is lower and more regular than the epithelium in most cases of papilloma. Smear preparation, toluidine blue, ×110.

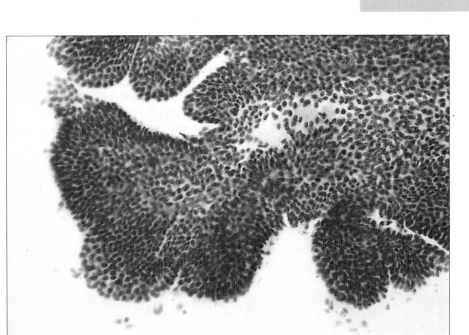

Figure 9.2
Choroid plexus papilloma. Female aged 14 years, fourth ventricle. The papillary masses of very uniform epithelial tissue bear a strong resemblance to those seen in smears of normal choroid plexus. The smeared tissue usually appears much more cellular, however, with an epithelial layer which is many cells deep. Central blood vessels tend to be less prominent in papilloma smears, and are most easily seen in toluidine blue stained preparations because of the greenish colour of erythrocytes. Smear preparation, toluidine blue, ×175.

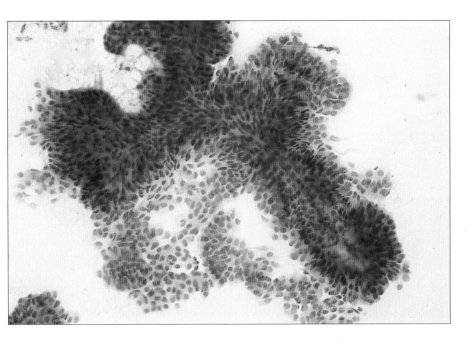

Figure 9.3
Choroid plexus papilloma. Male aged 40 years, recurrent lesion of the fourth ventricle. The appearances are similar to those of the case shown in Fig. 9.2. There is again an obvious papillary architecture, although the central blood vessels are more difficult to see. The epithelial layer is thinner and less well organized in this example, with cells smearing out into epithelial islands around the margins. Smear preparation, haematoxylin eosin, ×175.

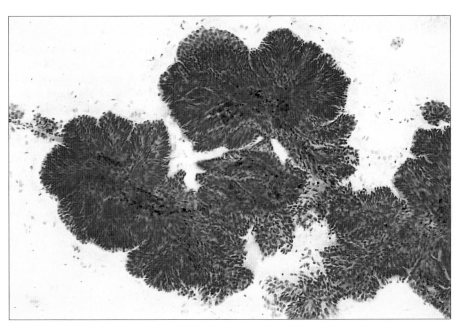

Figure 9.4
Choroid plexus papilloma. Male aged 24 years, partly ossified tumour of the fourth ventricle. The tumour has smeared rather thickly into large masses of tissue with a coarse, lobulated outline. The papillary nature of the lesion remains apparent despite this, with epithelial palisading of peripheral cells and blood vessels buried in more central areas. Smear preparation, toluidine blue, ×110.

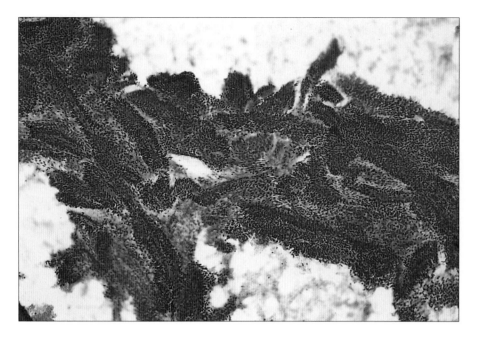

Figure 9.5
Choroid plexus papilloma. Male aged 20 years, fourth ventricle. This tumour was again quite tough and smeared mostly into large, thick clumps which lack the typical fronded appearance of papillomas. The blood vessels are hard to pick out, but viewed at this low magnification there is an infolded papillary pattern superimposed onto sheets of regular epithelial tissue. Smear preparation, toluidine blue, ×90.

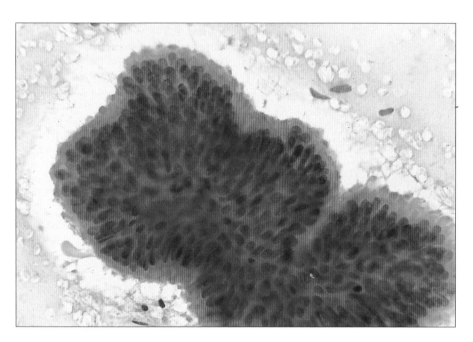

Figure 9.6
Choroid plexus papilloma. Same case as Fig. 9.4. The epithelial tissue forming the papillary structures is usually many cells thick, but the nuclei are very uniform and there is no evidence of maturation towards the margins. The surface shows a regular layer of columnar cells with basally orientated nuclei and a well-defined apical zone of cytoplasm. Cilia are not usually present except in some cases presenting in early infancy. Smear preparation, haematoxylin eosin, ×350.

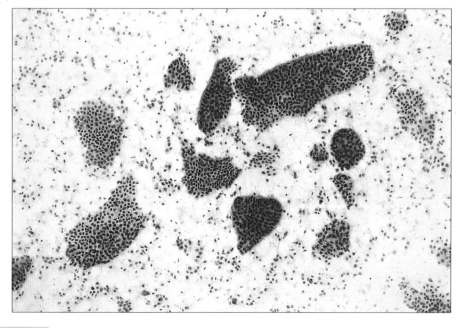

Figure 9.7
Choroid plexus papilloma. Female aged 71 years, fourth ventricle. In some papillomas the tissue smears out from the papillary areas into sheets of epithelial cells, which may form separate islands like those seen here. At higher magnification, a regular surface layer of columnar epithelium like that shown in Fig. 9.6 can usually be found around the margins of these islands. Smear preparation, toluidine blue, ×110.

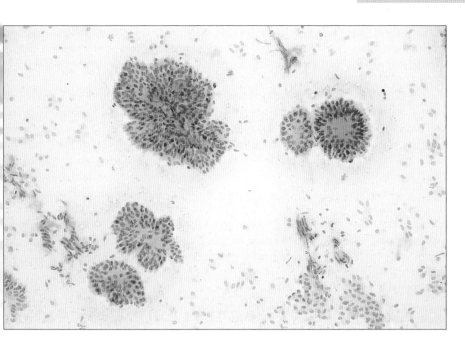

Figure 9.8
Choroid plexus papilloma. Same case as Fig. 9.4. In addition to a typical papillary fragment, this field shows small epithelial islands with a rosette-like pattern. These rosettes show no association with vessels and have presumably been avulsed from larger papillary structures by the smearing technique. Individual cells smeared out in the background are also present. Smear preparation, haematoxylin eosin, ×110.

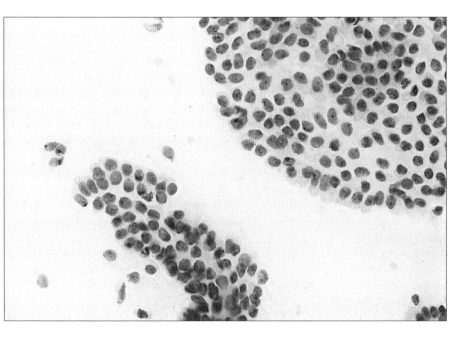

Figure 9.9
Choroid plexus papilloma. Same case as Fig. 9.2. The cytological features of individual tumour cells is best seen where the tissue is thinly smeared into small separate fragments of epithelium. Tumour cell nuclei are small, round and very uniform in appearance with finely stippled chromatin. A nucleolus is not usually present. The cytoplasmic borders are very ill-defined except along the apical surfaces, where at least some stretches with a columnar arrangement and basally-orientated nuclei are normally visible. Smear preparation, toluidine blue, ×350.

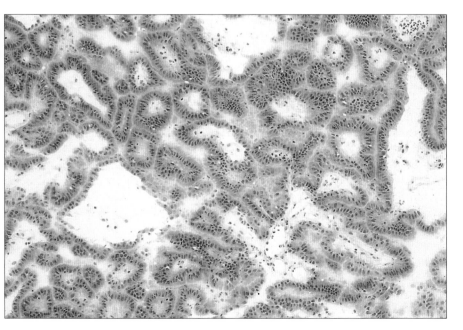

Figure 9.10
Choroid plexus papilloma. Same case as Fig. 9.4. Frozen sections most commonly show a villous arrangement like this, reminiscent of cross-cut intestinal mucosa. A pattern of longitudinal folds or obvious papillary fronding may also be encountered. The fibrovascular stroma consists of sparse collagen and delicate, thin-walled vessels. The overlying epithelium is always very regular but varies greatly in thickness. The apical surface is usually flat and lacks the typical 'cobblestone' appearance seen in sections of normal choroid plexus tissue. Frozen section, haematoxylin eosin, ×110.

operative smears or frozen sections, it is not difficult to exclude obviously malignant childhood tumours like medulloblastomas and teratomas, since papillomas are always pathologically benign lesions. In older age groups, however, it is important to remember that **well-differentiated metastatic adenocarcinomas** can look very like choroid plexus papillomas in both smears and frozen sections. Confusion is most likely to arise in patients with an unsuspected primary systemic tumour and a solitary metastasis growing within the choroid plexus. Evidence of mucin production and goblet cells make a primary choroid plexus tumour most unlikely and the presence of true acini or tubules virtually excludes the diagnosis. Any cytological features of malignancy should likewise arouse suspicion of a metastasis, remembering that primary carcinomas of the choroid plexus are very uncommon in adulthood.

In any age group, **ependymoma** is a most important intra-operative differential diagnosis of choroid plexus papilloma. Ependymomas usually lack the intense radiological contrast enhancement of papillomas and they tend to be less haemorrhagic when manipulated during surgery. However, in smears and frozen sections the two lesions display a similar papillary architecture which can confuse an unwary pathologist. In smear preparations, the papillary fronds of choroid plexus papillomas tend to have a much more regular, organized appearance than those of most ependymomas, and there is a complete absence of gliofibrillary stroma even at the edges of the papillary masses. Instead of individual cells smearing out from the tissue margins with fine cytoplasmic processes, the cells of choroid plexus papillomas tend to form a surface layer of columnar-type epithelium, usually with basal orientation of nuclei. The tumour cell nuclei are smaller and blander than those of most ependymomas with less obvious nucleoli, and there is often a distinct tendency for the cells to form discreet epithelial clumps separate from the main papillary masses. In frozen sections, the distinction between choroid plexus papillomas and ependymomas is likely to be even more obvious, the epithelial organization of papillomas contrasting with the characteristic glial background and perivascular pseudorosettes of ependymomas. **Papillary ependymomas** constitute a potential trap, but these will generally show malignant features and have at least some areas of more typical ependymomatous growth pattern.

A rather different problem involves the inadvertent incorporation of **normal choroid plexus tissue** into a non-diagnostic biopsy. This may occur if the ventricle is unwittingly penetrated during attempted biopsy of a deep-seated intrinsic lesion. A mixture of reactive brain and choroid plexus tissue usually results, and the latter needs to be recognized for what it is. The tissue is tougher and smears less easily than that of most papillomas, but still gives the impression of more uniform papillary fronding, with a delicate, serpiginous outline to the central blood vessels. Perhaps more specifically, the apical surface epithelium of normal choroid plexus shows a highly characteristic 'cobblestone' appearance in both smears and frozen sections, which contrasts with the smooth columnar surface layer of the papillary structures in papillomas.

Finally, where smear preparations produce a prominent pattern of epithelial sheets without obvious papillary organization, the outside possibility of a **craniopharyngioma** or a **dermoid/epidermoid cyst** of the third or fourth ventricle needs to be excluded. Such lesions are very unlikely to be confused either radiologically or surgically with a choroid plexus tumour and usually smear very poorly, but they can yield similar sheets of regular epithelial tissue. Frozen sections are likely to be necessary in these circumstances and should leave no doubt about the matter.

9.2. CHOROID PLEXUS CARCINOMA

9.2.1. CLINICAL AND RADIOLOGICAL FEATURES

Carcinomas of the choroid plexus are almost exclusively tumours of early infancy. They are less common in later childhood than their benign counterparts and virtually never occur in adult life. The overwhelming majority of cases arise in one or other lateral ventricle, but many examples will also cross the midline to occupy the opposite ventricular cavity, or invade deep hemispheric white matter. The tumours have a pronounced tendency to disseminate in the CSF pathways and in some instances there can be multiple spinal and cranial seedlings by the time of presentation. There is typically a short clinical history and rapid downhill course. Signs and symptoms mostly relate to acute hydrocephalus, but focal deficits such as hemiparesis are found in about one third of cases.

The radiological characteristics of choroid plexus carcinomas are similar to those of benign papillomas. They are hyperdense in CT scans, iso- or hypodense with T1-weighted MR and hyperdense with T2 weighting. There is always bright signal enhancement following administration of intravenous contrast media. Clues to the malignant nature of the lesion include heterogeneity of signal due to cysts or focal necrosis and an absence of calcification. The carcinomas also tend to be less well circumscribed than papillomas, frequently showing extraventricular extension with reactive signal changes in the adjacent hemispheric white matter. Hydrocephalus is apparent radiologically in about two thirds of cases and is nearly always of obstructive type, in contrast to the communicating hydrocephalus associated with most benign papillomas of the lateral ventricle.

9.2.2. SURGICAL FINDINGS

Choroid plexus carcinomas are mostly very large tumours by the time of surgery and they are extremely haemorrhagic when manipulated. The tumour tissue is friable and reddish in colour, and the surface tends to be less obviously fronded than that of benign papillomas. There is a very varied appearance on cut section, which frequently reveals cysts, old blood pigmentation and large areas of central necrosis. Grittiness due to calcification is uncommon. Many examples deeply infiltrate brain adjacent to the expanded ventricular cavity, and here the surgeon may have difficulty finding a clear plane of dissection. Another sinister surgical finding is the presence of satellite nodules dotted around the ventricular lining away from the main tumour bulk.

9.2.3. INTRA-OPERATIVE PATHOLOGY

Smear cytology

The tissue is usually soft enough to make good smear preparations, which can show a wide range of cytological appearances depending on the degree of differentiation of the tumour. At one end of the spectrum, the features are similar to those of a benign papilloma, with well organized papillary structures, central vascular cores and cells arranged in clearly epithelial layers or sheets. In such cases, the only clue to the malignant nature of the tumour may be the presence of readily identifiable mitotic figures, which are not normally seen in benign papillomas. More clearly malignant lesions will show progressively less organized papillary architecture, with increasing degrees of cytological pleomorphism and proliferation of blood vessels. The latter feature can be quite marked, with florid capillary budding like that seen in smears of glioblastomas. Necrotic tumour tissue may also be apparent in some cases and there are frequently small, cohesive clumps of clearly malignant epithelial tumour cells which smear out separately from the larger papillary masses. The overall effect can be cytologically indistinguishable from smears of metastatic carcinoma in an adult, excepting that the young age of the patient usually precludes this diagnosis. A choroid plexus origin may also be suggested by the presence of a regular columnar epithelial layer around the margins of larger papillary formations, even in smears from quite cellular, pleomorphic tumours. The most anaplastic lesions, however, can lose any semblance of papillary or epithelial organization, with very marked cytological atypia and no real hint of a choroid plexus origin. In such cases, clinical details such as patient age, the haemorrhagic nature of the tumour and its predominantly intraventricular location all need to be taken into account in reaching a sensible conclusion at the time of surgery.

Frozen sections

The appearance of cryostat sections will again vary considerably with the extent of tumour differentiation. Well differentiated lesions with an obvious papillary or villous pattern can be distinguished from papillomas by the presence of mitoses, necrosis and other features of malignancy. In the more anaplastic tumours, evidence of papillary organization can sometimes be more apparent in frozen sections than in smear preparations, with fibrovascular cores surrounded by an epithelial mantle of tumour. A regular surface layer of columnar cells with a smooth apical surface is also a useful feature if present, but cannot be relied on in very poorly differentiated cases. Exceptionally, a gradation of anaplastic tumour with more obvious choroid plexus tissue may be encountered, and such a fortunate observation will obviously help clinch the diagnosis. A more constant feature is the presence of very exuberant vascular proliferation, sometimes in the pattern of multiple, glomeruloid lumina cuffed by anaplastic tumour cells. As in benign papillomas, evidence of haemorrhage, fibrin deposition and fibrous scarring are all common, if rather non-specific features.

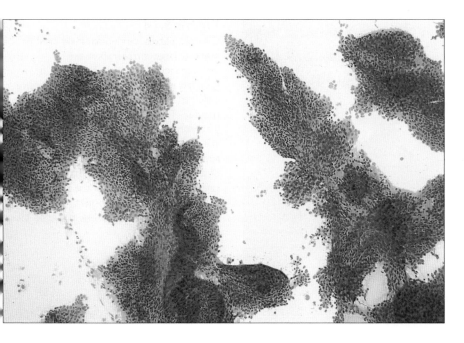

Figure 9.11

Choroid plexus carcinoma. Male aged 3 years, lateral ventricle tumour deeply infiltrating cerebral white matter. The smear shows ill-defined papillary masses merging with irregular sheets of epithelial tissue. Vascular cores are not visible and the appearances are rather disorganized compared with most benign papillomas. Mitotic figures were found at higher magnification. Smear preparation, haematoxylin eosin, ×90.

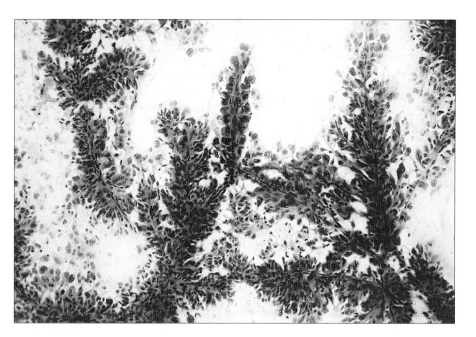

Figure 9.12
Choroid plexus carcinoma. Male aged 9 years, trigone region tumour. There is an obvious papillary architecture with numerous branching blood vessels. The tumour cells show very marked pleomorphism and cytological atypia, but attempts at epithelial layering are still apparent in some places. The cells also have a cohesive, epithelial quality, despite being smeared out individually at the margins of the papillary structures. Smear preparation, toluidine blue, ×110.

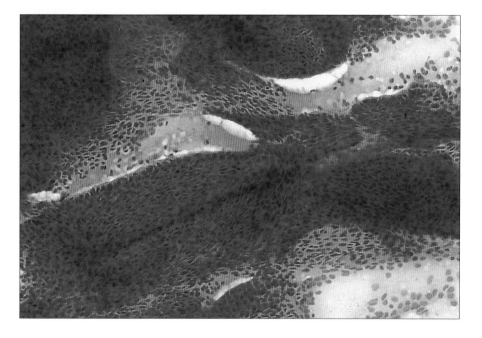

Figure 9.13
Choroid plexus carcinoma. Same case as Fig. 9.11. In this area the tumour is forming twisted and folded sheets of a clearly epithelial nature. There is no hint of papillary architecture, but in places the cells are arranged in organized epithelial layers with well-defined apical cytoplasmic borders. Smear preparation, haematoxylin eosin, ×175.

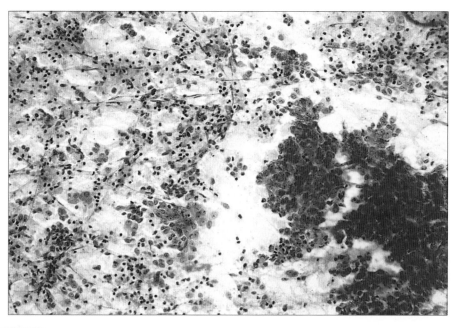

Figure 9.14
Choroid plexus carcinoma. Male aged 6 months, large intracerebral and intraventricular tumour. The tissue is grouped into irregular clumps of cohesive cells set in a background of necrotic tumour. There is considerable pleomorphism and numerous mitotic figures are visible at higher magnification. The appearances are indistinguishable from those of a poorly differentiated metastatic carcinoma, but the age of the patient helped to suggest the correct diagnosis in this case. Smear preparation, toluidine blue, ×175.

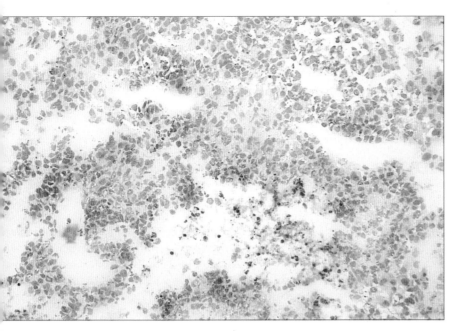

Figure 9.15
Choroid plexus carcinoma. Male aged 2 months, fourth ventricular tumour. The appearance of frozen sections varies widely depending on the degree of tumour differentiation. Poorly differentiated tumours like this one lack obvious choroid plexus features and simply show irregular sheets of clearly malignant epithelial tissue. There are no papillary structures or obvious epithelial surface layers. Many choroid plexus carcinomas are richly vascular, and the tumour here shows numerous sinusoidal vascular channels. The appearances are not specific, however, and at the intra-operative diagnosis relied heavily on knowledge of the clinical, radiological and surgical findings. Frozen section, haematoxylin eosin, ×175.

9.2.4. DIFFERENTIAL DIAGNOSIS

In early infancy the most important differential diagnosis is that of **malignant teratoma**, either as a primary lesion or a metastasis to the choroid plexus from an undisclosed systemic site. The presence of other germline elements is obviously a helpful feature in this context, but they may not always be apparent in smear preparations. Even using frozen sections, a poorly differentiated, predominantly epithelial teratoma can be difficult to entirely exclude. In general, high or intermediate grade teratomas are less likely to show the exuberant vascular proliferation typically associated with choroid plexus carcinomas, but this is obviously not a very specific feature. In the final event, suspicion that the tumour is teratoid rather than of choroid plexus origin is most likely to be aroused if it is in an unlikely site for a choroid plexus carcinoma, such as the suprasellar/third ventricle region or midline posterior fossa. A **medulloepithelioma** is a much rarer possibility, but also needs to be considered in infants presenting with a relatively circumscribed, cytologically malignant intraventricular tumour. These lesions can show evidence of a papillary architecture in smears or frozen sections, but the epithelial layer has a distinctive, quite orderly, pseudostratified arrangement. Many cases also show areas of overt neuroglial differentiation, which is

never seen in choroid plexus tumours. A frozen section is likely to be necessary if there is any suspicion of this diagnosis using smear preparations. The only kind of **ependymoma** likely to be confused with choroid plexus carcinoma intra-operatively is the malignant papillary variety. Despite their papillary architecture, however, these lesions will usually show obvious evidence of a glial stromal component in both smears and frozen sections.

In adults, the intra-operative diagnosis of choroid plexus carcinoma should only be made with extreme caution, in view of its rarity in this age group and the obvious trap of a **metastatic adenocarcinoma** with an undisclosed primary systemic site. Metastasis to the choroid plexus is not uncommon, although the lesions are usually smaller than most choroid plexus carcinomas at presentation. If there is radiological evidence of multiple tumours, this clearly argues in favour of metastatic disease, although it must be remembered that some choroid plexus carcinomas can present after seeding into the CSF pathways has already occurred. Any hint of acini, goblet cells or mucin production in the smears or frozen sections is again a strong indicator of a metastatic lesion, mucous secretion being an extremely rare phenomenon in choroid plexus tumours.

NEURONAL TUMOURS

10.1. GANGLIOCYTOMA AND GANGLIOGLIOMA

These uncommon tumours have a mature neuronal or ganglionic element which may occur either in a relatively pure form or in association with a glial element. If present there is a frequently considerable difficulty in determining whether the glial component is neoplastic or reactive and consequently gangliocytoma and ganglioglioma are often considered together under the term **ganglion cell tumour**.

10.1.1. CLINICAL AND RADIOLOGICAL FEATURES

Ganglion cell tumours present predominantly in children or young adults. They may occur at any site in the CNS but most are supratentorial and the temporal lobe is the most common location. Ganglion cell tumours usually present with a long-standing history of seizures. This is an indication that these tumours generally have very limited growth potential and as they are often small and well-circumscribed, surgical excision is likely to be curative. Malignant forms are very rare and in these it is generally the glial component which proliferates (**anaplastic or malignant ganglioglioma**). Ganglion cell tumours may be solid or cystic. In cystic examples there may be a mural tumour nodule. There may be radiological evidence of calcification and enhancement with contrast.

10.1.2. SURGICAL FINDINGS

Ganglion cell tumours are generally small, firm, well-circumscribed and grey in colour. There may be a cystic component and calcification is common. These tumours may be encountered in elective surgery for intractable epilepsy and may be excised as part of a therapeutic temporal lobectomy.

10.1.3. INTRA-OPERATIVE PATHOLOGY

Criteria for the diagnosis of a ganglion cell tumour include the presence of cells exhibiting mature ganglionic or neuronal differentiation and recognition that the cells are neoplastic. Intra-operatively both of these points present a challenge and considerable care should be exercised before offering a firm diagnosis. In

general terms criteria for the recognition of neoplasia include: demonstration that the cells are clearly heterotopic, i.e. that they are within white matter or abnormally large neurons are present in the superficial cerebral cortex; abnormality of the architectural arrangement of the cells with grouping in clusters or random orientation of the cells in contrast to the usual parallel arrays of neurons in the laminae of the cerebral cortex; atypical or bizarre cell morphology and binucleation or multinucleation.

Smear cytology

Ganglion cell tumours are frequently tough in texture and they may not be easy to smear. The cells have a tendency to be arranged in large clusters, often arranged around blood vessels which may be prominent. The appearances on smear preparations are highly variable. The tumour may be composed predominantly of large mature ganglion cells with large vesiculated nuclei, prominent nucleoli and abundant cytoplasm. Binucleate or multinucleate cells may be identified and the cell processes may appear morphologically abnormal. In tumours with a predominant ganglion cell component the background resembles neuropil. If a glial component predominates the background comprises the coarser processes of the glial cells. Often the smear contains a chaotic mixture of ganglion cells, pilocytic astrocytes and small round cells. If small round cells are present these may represent neuroblasts, lymphocytes, which are commonly encountered in ganglion cell tumours, or a glial component. If a glial component is present it is usually astrocytic in nature. Granular bodies and Rosenthal fibres may be encountered giving reassurance to the impression of a low grade lesion. Mitotic figures are not found. The ganglionic component may be inconspicuous and pass unnoticed in smears, or be interpreted as residual pre-existing neurons in an infiltrating astrocytic tumour. The tumour may be too tough to make satisfactory smears and it may be necessary to prepare frozen sections.

Frozen sections

The cytological features described above will be encountered. In addition, some of the architectural features which are helpful in making the diagnosis of a ganglion cell tumour and which are not available in smear preparations may be seen in frozen sections. As outlined above these include demonstration that the ganglion cells are heterotopic in location, clustering of the cells, abnormalities in orientation of the cells and multinucleation.

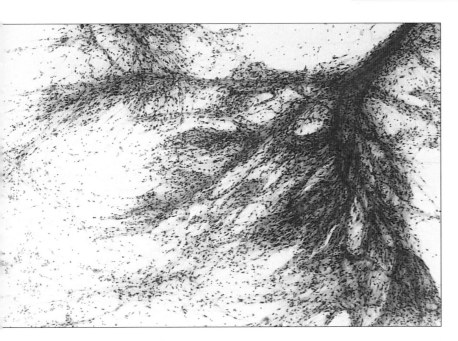

Figure 10.1

Ganglioglioma. Male aged 12 years, temporal lobe. The low power view resembles that of an astrocytic tumour with the cells clustered around blood vessels. The margins of the clusters appear irregular as a consequence of the coarse fibrillar nature of the tumour. This example was tough and so when smeared it gives the appearance of being quite a densely cellular tumour. Some gangliogliomas are too tough to smear and frozen sections are required. Smear preparation, toluidine blue, ×175.

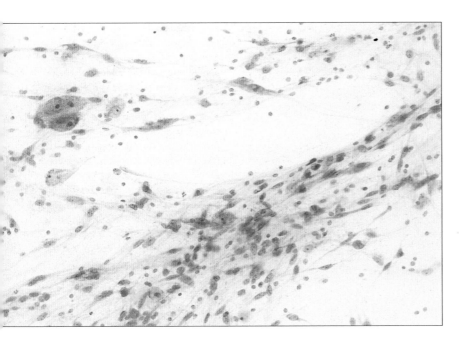

Figure 10.2

Ganglioglioma. Male aged 12 years. A higher power view of the same case illustrated in Fig. 10.1 shows a rather chaotic mixture of cell types. Included in this field are spindle-shaped cells with elongated nuclei and bipolar processes resembling the cells of a pilocytic astrocytoma; small round cells which could be glial cells, neuroblasts or lymphocytes; and a large binucleate ganglion cell with large rounded pale-staining nuclei and prominent nucleoli (top left). The presence of binucleate cells distinguishes them from incorporated pre-existing neurons and clinches the diagnosis of a ganglion cell tumour. Smear preparation, toluidine blue, ×700.

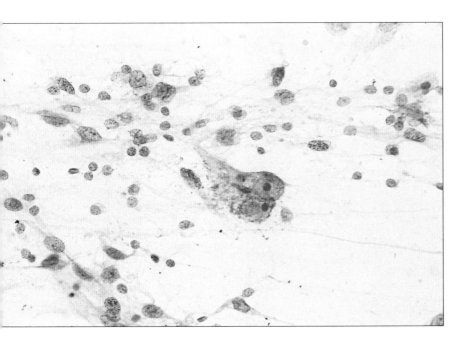

Figure 10.3

Ganglioglioma. Male aged 12 years. Another view of the same tumour illustrated in Figs 10.1 and 10.2 at a slightly higher power emphasizing the variation in morphology of the cells. In this example there were numerous binucleate ganglion cells and there was no doubt as to the correct diagnosis. However, if the ganglionic component is inconspicuous, and particularly if there is a prominent coarse fibrillar background, the tumour may be interpreted as being astrocytic in nature. Smear preparation, toluidine blue, ×1400.

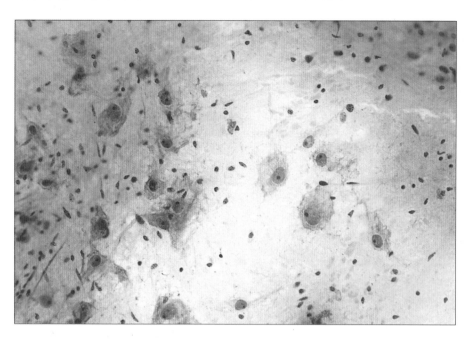

Figure 10.4
Gangliocytoma. Female aged 16 years, temporal lobe. Although there are no binucleate ganglion cells, this tumour contains numerous large ganglion cells with abnormal morphology, leaving little doubt as to the diagnosis. This is a relatively pure gangliocytoma in which the background is composed of blue-staining very fine fibrillar material resembling neuropil. This is in contrast to the coarser processes in the ganglioglioma illustrated above in Figs 10.1–10.3. In addition to the ganglion cells there are other cells most of which have small round nuclei. Smear preparation, toluidine blue, ×700.

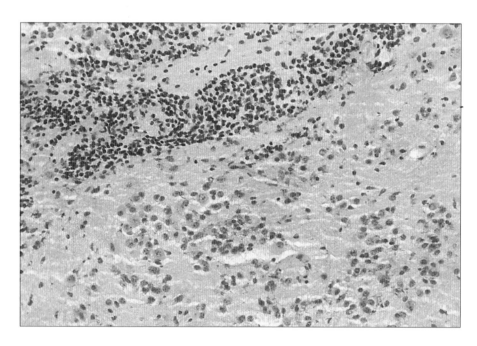

Figure 10.5
Gangliocytoma. Female aged 23 years, frontal lobe. Frozen sections allow appreciation of the abnormal clustering of ganglion cells (seen at the bottom and to the right) which is a common feature of ganglion cell tumours. The margin of a large cluster is illustrated here. Smear preparations do not readily show this feature which is diagnostically helpful if the ganglion cells are not multinucleated or morphologically bizarre. This tumour also contains a substantial population of small round cells which were identified as neuroblasts on paraffin histology. Frozen section, haematoxylin eosin, ×700.

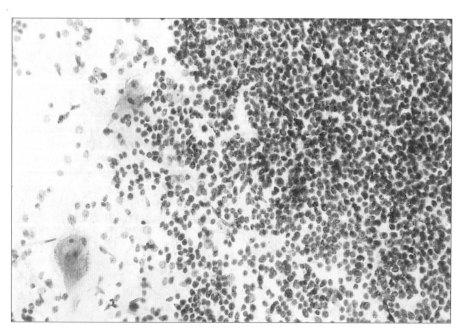

Figure 10.6
Anaplastic ganglion cell tumour. Female aged 16 years, temporal lobe. Ganglion cell tumours are usually of low grade. If there is evidence of significant proliferative activity it is most commonly identified in the glial component of the tumour. The tumour illustrated here contained a large population of mitotically active neuroblasts among which were scattered ganglion cells which were clearly morphologically abnormal and not representing incorporated pre-existing neurons. Arguably this could be interpreted as a neuroblastoma with ganglionic differentiation. Smear preparation, toluidine blue, ×700.

10.1.4. DIFFERENTIAL DIAGNOSIS

The most important differential diagnoses include other lesions which present with a long history of seizures in the young. Awareness of the typical anatomical location of the relevant tumours is helpful: **pleomorphic xanthoastrocytoma** usually occurs superficially in the cerebral hemispheres whereas, in contrast, **subependymal giant cell astrocytoma** occurs in the wall of a ventricular cavity. In both of these entities the tumour cells typically have bizarre morphology with large vesiculated nuclei, prominent nucleoli and abundant cytoplasm – and they may therefore appear very similar to the cells of a ganglion cell tumour. Indeed, the cells of these neoplasms may show mixed neuronal/glial features when paraffin sections are available for immunohistochemistry. A helpful point is that subependymal giant cell astrocytoma usually occurs in the clinical setting of tuberous sclerosis.

Dysembryoplastic neuroepithelial tumour may have many features in common with a ganglion cell tumour, including presentation with intractable seizures in a young patient, a location in the temporal lobe and the participation of abnormal neurons. Distinction between ganglion cell tumour and dysembryoplastic neuroepithelial tumour is likely to require paraffin histology to appreciate the specific features required for diagnosis of the latter entity (see below).

There is a wide spectrum of lesions that contain cells having neuronal and/or glial features which are **developmental abnormalities** rather than neoplasms and these include: clusters of heterotopic neurons in white matter, cortical dysplasia, cortical tubers in tuberous sclerosis, and lesions of variable appearance which may occur in the context of neurofibromatosis.

Diffusely infiltrating glial tumours have a tendency to contain **entrapped residual neurons** and awareness that this happens is necessary to avoid overdiagnosis of ganglion cell tumours. In this situation the neurons are morphologically normal. Conversely, underdiagnosis may occur if a ganglioglioma has a prominent glial component; the ganglionic element may be overlooked and the lesion interpreted as a pure glial tumour.

The appearance on smear preparations or frozen sections of large bizarre and pleomorphic cells may prompt confusion with **glioblastoma**.

Three further very rare entities warrant separate mention. Although a definite diagnosis is unlikely to be achieved intra-operatively it is necessary to be aware of these entities.

Dysplastic gangliocytoma of cerebellum (Lhermitte-Duclos) is a very rare tumour-like lesion of the cerebellum in which there is focal thickening of the cerebellar folia. Microscopically the abnormality bears some architectural resemblance to the cerebellar cortex and includes large bizarre neurons resembling Purkinje cells. This lesion has a low growth potential.

Desmoplastic infantile ganglioglioma presents as large superficial cerebral mass in infancy. It is a mixed neuronal-glial tumour with a prominent connective tissue component and grows relatively slowly.

Very uncommonly **paraganglioma** may occur as a primary lesion of the filum terminale and is indistinguishable from paragangliomas occurring at other locations. In neuropathological practice extradural paragangliomas may also be encountered such as those arising in the glomus jugulare, the carotid body and the paraspinal sympathetic chain.

10.2. DYSEMBRYOPLASTIC NEUROEPITHELIAL TUMOUR

10.2.1. CLINICAL AND RADIOLOGICAL FEATURES

This is a relatively recently recognized entity which presents in childhood or early adult life with seizures and is usually therefore encountered in surgery for intractable epilepsy. Dysembryoplastic neuroepithelial tumours (DNT) occur in the supratentorial compartment and the temporal lobe is the most common site. On MR scans the intracortical and nodular characteristics of DNT may be apparent. There may be evidence of calcification and cyst formation. DNTs have little if any growth potential and it seems likely that surgical resection may be curative.

10.2.2. SURGICAL FINDINGS

The appearances are variable, but key features include an intracortical location and the formation of multiple nodules which may be apparent on macroscopic examination.

10.2.3. INTRA-OPERATIVE PATHOLOGY

It may not be appropriate to offer a firm diagnosis of DNT at the time of surgery. Even when the full extent and characteristics of the lesion are available for examination on paraffin histology there is still debate as to how broad is the spectrum of lesions which the term DNT encompasses. One of the key diagnostic features is the presence of multiple intracortical nodules. The nodules have appearances which vary and may resemble oligodendroglioma, astrocytoma or ganglion cell tumour. The lesion may be associated with dysplasia of the adjacent cortex. The importance of this entity is evolving to the extent that some argue it may be responsible for the majority of focal lesions in young patients presenting with intractable seizures due to a temporal lobe focus.

Smear cytology

Smear preparations, if made and depending on which component of the lesion is sampled, may show cells resembling those of oligodendroglioma, astrocytoma, ganglion cell tumour or relatively unremarkable central nervous tissue. Some of the smears we have encountered have been composed on low power examination of irregular clusters of cells with coarse fibrillar margins and prominent vessels. At higher power a chaotic mixture of ganglion cells, astrocyte-like cells, including cells with pilocytic morphology, and cells resembling oligodendrocytes have been apparent. Other smears have closely resembled oligodendroglioma or central neurocytoma with scattered ganglions cells included. Calcospherites may be present. Mitotic figures are not identified.

Frozen sections

Frozen sections have the potential to illuminate some of the important architectural features of the lesion, particularly the formation of nodules. With luck definite intracortical nodules of different cytological composition may be present. In addition to the different appearances described above the so-called 'specific glio-neuronal element' may be encountered. This is composed of cords of oligodendrocyte-like cells enclosing microcysts which contain ganglion cells. Calcospherites and Rosenthal fibres may be present both features pointing to a low grade lesion. The spectrum of cytological appearances seen in the surgical specimen from any one patient may be confusing. It may be wise to indicate to the neurosurgeons that they are dealing with a low grade intrinsic lesion, with definite diagnosis to await examination of all of the features of the lesion on paraffin histology.

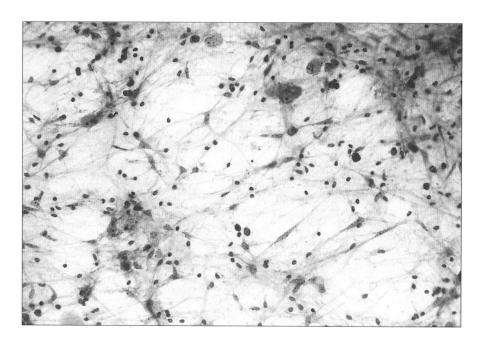

Figure 10.7
Dysembryoplastic neuroepithelial tumour. Male aged 24 years, temporal lobe. This field shows a mixture of cell types including ganglion cells, cells resembling pilocytic astrocytes and small round cells. The picture is very similar to that of the ganglioglioma illustrated in Fig. 10.2. However, a characteristic feature of dysembryoplastic neuroepithelial tumour is the variability of appearances in different parts of the lesion. With luck this variability may be represented within one smear preparation or in smears made from different sites with in the lesion. Smear preparation, toluidine blue, ×350.

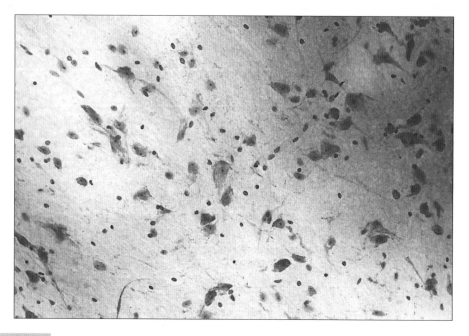

Figure 10.8
Dysembryoplastic neuroepithelial tumour. Male aged 24 years, temporal lobe. Another part of the same smear preparation illustrated in Fig. 10.7 but showing a very different appearance. In this field there are numerous large ganglion cells set in a fine fibrillar background resembling neuropil. The appearance is very similar to that of the gangliocytoma illustrated in Fig. 10.4. Smear preparation, toluidine blue, ×700.

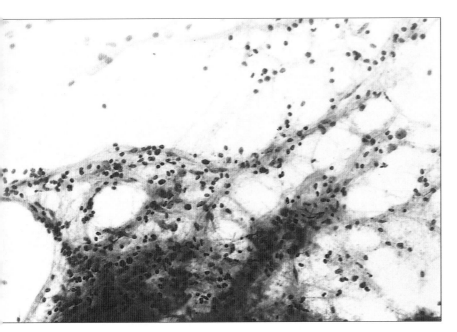

Figure 10.9
Dysembryoplastic neuroepithelial tumour. Male aged 24 years, temporal lobe. The same case as illustrated in the previous two figures but showing a very different appearance. In this smear small round oligodendroglioma-like cells are arranged in strands. This may well represent the smear appearance of the so-called 'specific glio-neuronal element' of dysembryoplastic neuroepithelial tumour. The appearance of this element in sections is illustrated in the following figure. Smear preparation, toluidine blue, ×700.

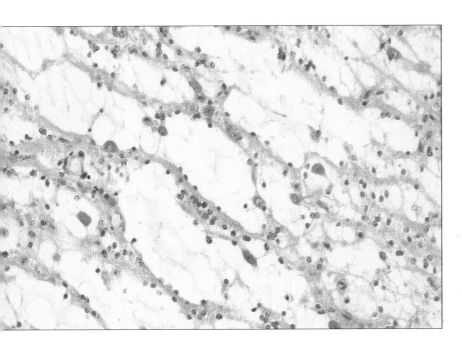

Figure 10.10
Dysembryoplastic neuroepithelial tumour. Male aged 18 years, temporal lobe. The 'specific glio-neuronal element' of dysembryoplastic neuroepithelial tumour in sections is composed of oligodendroglioma-like cells arranged in strands which enclose cystic spaces in which are individually arranged neurons. Paraffin section, haematoxylin eosin, ×700.

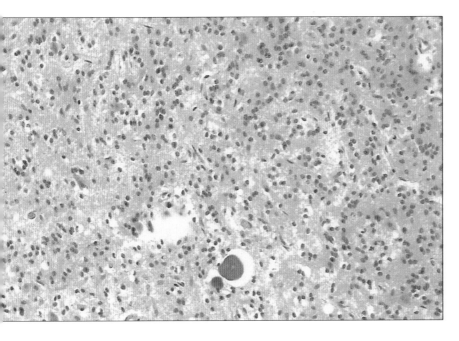

Figure 10.11
Dysembryoplastic neuroepithelial tumour. Female aged 27 years, temporal lobe. This frozen section has sampled a nodule composed of small round cells resembling those of an oligodendroglioma. A calcospherite is included at the bottom of the picture. Frozen section, haematoxylin eosin, ×700.

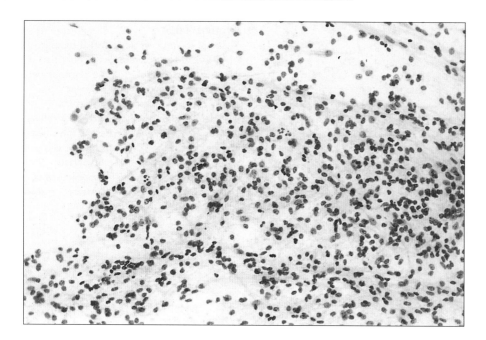

Figure 10.12
Dysembryoplastic neuroepithelial tumour. Female aged 27 years, temporal lobe. This figure shows the same tumour as illustrated in Fig. 10.11 and the area sampled has a corresponding oligodendroglioma-like appearance. Smear preparation, toluidine blue, ×700.

10.2.4. DIFFERENTIAL DIAGNOSIS

Oligodendroglioma is composed of cells which are morphologically similar, often involve cortical grey matter and occasionally may form nodular structures. The distinction between the two entities may require awaiting paraffin histology.

Parts of a DNT may resemble **ganglion cell tumour** with a mixture of cells showing ganglionic differentiation and glial differentiation.

The different lesions which may present with focal seizures in young patients have a wide variety of appearances with cells resembling neurons and/or glial cells and possibly cells with intermediate features. Definite characterization of these lesions is often challenging even when information is available from paraffin histology and immunohistochemistry – for example determining whether it is appropriate to categorize these as ganglion cell tumours, DNT or maldevelopmental lesions.

10.3. CENTRAL NEUROCYTOMA

10.3.1. CLINICAL AND RADIOLOGICAL FEATURES

Central neurocytoma arises characteristically within the ventricular system. Nearly all examples are located within the lateral ventricles and straddle the midline, being related to the septum pellucidum. The tumour is uncommon, most examples occurring in young adults. Central neurocytomas may be large tumours when they present with signs and symptoms of raised intracranial pressure, often in part due to obstruction of CSF flow.

On CT and MR scans the intraventricular and midline location of the tumour is apparent. The tumour may contain areas of calcification.

Central neurocytoma has been recognized only relatively recently as a distinct entity and as it is rare there is some uncertainty as to its behaviour. Available evidence suggests however that it has a relatively low growth potential and surgical resection may possibly result in cure.

10.3.2. SURGICAL FINDINGS

Central neurocytomas are large, well-circumscribed often lobulated tumours lying within the ventricular system with a point of attachment to the ventricular wall. The tumour may have a gritty texture because of calcification.

10.3.3. INTRA-OPERATIVE PATHOLOGY

Smear cytology

Central neurocytomas smear easily to produce sheets of separated cells with no tendency for cohesion. The tumour cells have uniform spherical nuclei with diffuse or finely granular chromatin, little apparent perinuclear cytoplasm and a background of fine fibrillar material resembling neuropil. In a few examples we have seen non-uniformity in the distribution of the nuclei in the smear preparations giving a hint of the anuclear zones described below. Occasionally we have seen a suggestion of perinuclear haloes, which may be a prominent feature on paraffin histology. Mitotic figures are absent or few. Small clusters of fine calibre multi-branching blood vessels, similar to those seen in oligodendroglioma, may be scattered throughout the smears. Calcospherites are often seen.

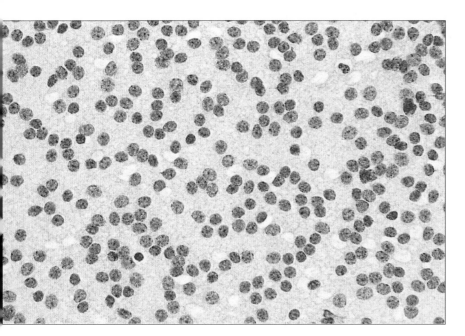

Figure 10.13
Central neurocytoma. Female aged 29 years, lateral ventricle. The cells of central neurocytoma smear out into a monotonous sheet with no suggestion of cell cohesion. The nuclei are round and uniform in size. The background is composed of fine fibrillar material resembling neuropil. Mitoses absent or few. Clusters of fine calibre blood vessels and occasional calcospherites may disturb the uniformity of the smear. Smear preparation, toluidine blue, ×1400.

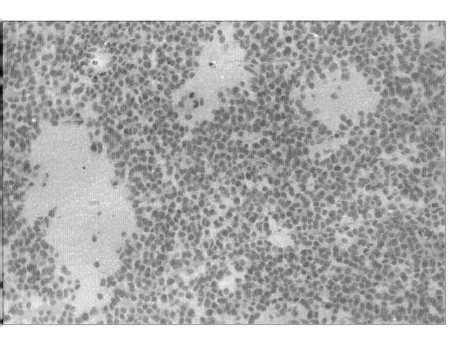

Figure 10.14
Central neurocytoma. Male aged 32 years, lateral ventricle. Sections show a moderately cellular tumour composed of cells with uniform round nuclei and no discernible cytoplasm with a fine fibrillar intervening matrix. If present the large areas of fibrillar material devoid of cell nuclei help to distinguish central neurocytoma from oligodendroglioma. Frozen section, haematoxylin eosin, ×700.

Frozen sections

The tumour is typically moderately cellular and is composed of sheets of cells with uniform round nuclei and indistinct cytoplasm. A useful diagnostic architectural feature if present, and which is not readily seen on smear preparations, is areas of eosinophilic fibrillar material without nuclei, somewhat resembling those seen in pineocytoma.

10.3.4. DIFFERENTIAL DIAGNOSIS

The principal differential diagnosis is **oligodendroglioma** which appears almost identical both on smear preparations and in frozen sections. The diagnosis of a central neurocytoma should only be offered when the intraventricular location of the tumour is

known and even then it is probably appropriate to offer it as a differential diagnosis together with oligodendroglioma. Indeed, even on paraffin histology, before the relatively recent recognition of central neurocytoma most of these tumours were labelled as oligodendroglioma. Morphologically the only helpful distinguishing feature is the presence of anuclear areas of fibrillar material which may be seen in frozen sections of central neurocytoma and are not present in oligodendroglioma. Definite distinction between these two tumours requires demonstration of neuronal differentiation by immunohistochemistry and/or electron microscopy.

Pituitary adenoma may have a very similar appearance, both on smear preparations and frozen sections, and as large adenomas may present as intraventricular masses there exists the potential for confusion. However pituitary adenomas usually occupy the third ventricle and are in continuity with an intrasellar component. These are important distinguishing features at the time of operation.

Cerebral neuroblastoma may present as a mass involving the ventricular system, but is generally intraparenchymal and is recognizable by its malignant cytological features (*see* Chapter 12).

It is necessary to have an awareness of **other intraventricular tumours** which include ependymoma, subependymoma, choroid plexus tumour, subependymal giant cell astrocytoma and, on occasion, meningioma and craniopharyngioma (*see* Chapter 5).

10.4. OLFACTORY NEUROBLASTOMA (AESTHESIONEUROBLASTOMA)

10.4.1. CLINICAL AND RADIOLOGICAL FEATURES

Olfactory neuroblastomas are thought to be derived from the neuroepithelial sensory cells of the olfactory mucosa and consequently arise in the nasal cavity in the region of the cribriform plate. They typically present with obstruction of the nasal cavity or epistaxis – symptoms which may have been present for a considerable time. There may be intracranial extension of the tumour beneath the frontal lobe presenting a somewhat dumb-bell shape on imaging. Olfactory neuroblastoma is a relatively slowly growing tumour but infiltration of local structures occurs and lymph node metastases have been described.

10.4.2. SURGICAL FINDINGS

The tumour forms polypoid masses and there is frequently involvement of the sinuses and bony structures forming the skull base.

10.4.3. INTRA-OPERATIVE PATHOLOGY

Smear preparations

Smears of olfactory neuroblastoma show the cells smearing out individually with a picture resembling that of central neurocytoma. The tumour cells have uniform round nuclei and mitotic figures, if present, are usually sparse.

Frozen sections

The tumour architecturally is formed from sheets of closely packed cells with uniform round nuclei and scanty cytoplasm. Occasionally small eosinophilic fibrillar areas between nuclei resembling Homer Wright rosettes may be seen.

10.4.4. DIFFERENTIAL DIAGNOSIS

Olfactory neuroblastoma is a rare tumour and the diagnosis should only be offered in the appropriate clinical setting. Other tumours which may appear similar and which can occur at this location include **metastatic carcinoma**, **neuroendocrine tumour** which may arise locally, and **pituitary adenoma**.

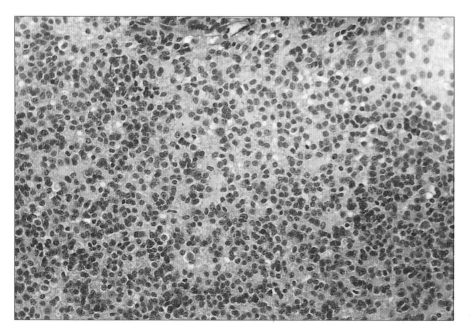

Figure 10.15
Olfactory neuroblastoma (aesthesioneuroblastoma). Male aged 55 years, skull base, midline. The cells have regular round nuclei and smear out uniformly in a fashion resembling that seen in central neurocytoma (Fig. 10.13) or medulloblastoma. The tumour is usually of relatively low grade and mitoses are few. The neuropil-like background of the smear again bears resemblance to that seen in tumours at other sites demonstrating neuronal differentiation. Smear preparation, toluidine blue, ×700.

ELEVEN

PINEAL TUMOURS

Although a wide range of CNS tumours can arise in the region of the pineal gland, the two most important categories of tumour are the pineal parenchymal tumours and germ cell tumours. These will be considered separately, since both categories contain a variety of neoplasms which may be encountered in clinical practice and, particularly since the increasingly widespread use of stereotaxy, hitherto inaccessible tumours are now sampled for intra-operative diagnosis. The classification of pineal germ cell tumours is based on the WHO classification for testicular germ cell tumours; see Table 11.1 for a summary of the classification of pineal neoplasms used in this chapter.

11.1 PINEAL GERM CELL TUMOURS

11.1.1. CLINICAL AND RADIOLOGICAL FEATURES

Most intracranial germ cell tumours arise in the midline, usually in the region of the pineal gland, but the suprasellar region is the second commonest site and occasional tumours may be laterally located in the thalamus or basal ganglia. Primary intracranial germ cell tumours are uncommon in Western countries (around 1% of all primary CNS neoplasms), but occur at a high incidence in Japan where they may represent up to 12% of all brain tumours. This increased frequency is largely accounted for by intracranial germinomas, but the underlying biological basis for this remarkable variation is uncertain. Most intracranial germinomas occur in males and present in the first two decades of life, with most patients being diagnosed between the ages of 10 and 20 years. In males, most germinomas are located in the pineal region whereas in females there is an increased incidence of tumours in the suprasellar region. Teratomas tend to occur in younger children (mean age 5 years).

The clinical features associated with these tumours depends upon the location of the tumour within the CNS. Tumours within the pineal region tend to cause obstructive hydrocephalus by compressing the third ventricular outflow. Headache is the commonest presenting feature which can be followed by nausea vomiting and papilloedema. Direct compression of the brain stem can result in disturbances of extraocular movements, classically known as Parinaud's syndrome with paralysis of upgaze or convergence, but other eye movement dysfunction may occur. Compression of the

Table 11.1
WHO classification of pineal neoplasms

Pineal parenchymal tumours	Pineocytoma (Grade II)
	Pineoblastoma (Grade IV)
	Mixed/transitional pineal tumours (Grade II–IV)
Germ cell tumours	Germinoma
	Embryonal carcinoma
	Yolk sac tumour (endodermal sinus tumour)
	Choriocarcinoma
	Teratoma: immature
	mature
	with malignant transformation
	Mixed germ cell tumours

superior cerebellar peduncles can cause ataxia, but this is an uncommon presenting feature. Germ cell tumours in the pineal region may cause endocrine abnormalities although this is uncommon and may result from the secondary effects of hydrocephalus or direct tumour invasion of the hypothalamus. Precautious puberty has been associated with pineal region tumours in males with ectopic β-HCG secretion from choriocarcinomas or mixed germ cell tumours with trophoblastic cells. Haemorrhage may rarely occur into a pineal germ cell tumour, resulting in pineal apoplexy. Tumours in the suprasellar region may present with diabetes insipidus and visual field effects with endocrine dysfunction occurring as a result of compression of the hypothalamus and pituitary gland. Hypothalamic compression may also result in behavioural disturbances, eating disorders and obesity.

11.1.2. RADIOLOGICAL FINDINGS

High resolution contrast enhanced MRI scans are the investigation of choice in patients with germ cell tumours, because of the superior delineation of tumour size, vascularity and relationship with adjacent structures. Germinomas are relatively isodense to normal white matter on T1-weighted images and may appear hyperintense on T2-weighted images. The tumours enhance homogeneously with gadolinium and tumour calcification can be detected on CT scans which show a slightly higher attenuation than normal grey matter. Teratomas in contrast are of heterogeneous composition and this is reflected in their neuroradiological features which show variable contrast enhancement and cystic change. Malignant teratomas may invade into surrounding structures, and haemorrhage can be detected in both these tumours and in choriocarcinoma.

11.1.3. SURGICAL FINDINGS

Germinomas are soft in consistency with a grey/pink colour, which often infiltrate adjacent structures and are poorly-defined at the tumour margin. Cystic change is uncommon, in contrast to teratomas which are well defined tumours of mixed composition frequently containing cysts. The surface is lobulated and well-differentiated neoplasms may contain a mixture of tissues including hair, bone, cartilage or teeth. Keratin may be produced by some tumours, which may give rise to a foreign body giant cell reaction causing the lesion to become markedly fibrotic and strongly adhesive to

the adjacent structures. The other forms of germ cell tumour are usually ill-defined lesions; choriocarcinomas in particular are characterized by haemorrhage.

11.1.4. INTRA-OPERATIVE PATHOLOGY

Smear cytology

Most germinomas are soft enough to make good smear preparations on which it is usually possible to arrive at a diagnosis. These tumours are histologically and cytologically identical to seminomas of the testis and dysgerminomas of the ovary and are characterized by the presence of two distinct cell types: large tumour cells and small lymphocytes (which are often perivascular). The large tumour cells tend to spread away from the blood vessels in a diffuse monolayer and appear polygonal or spheroidal with ill-defined cell boundaries,

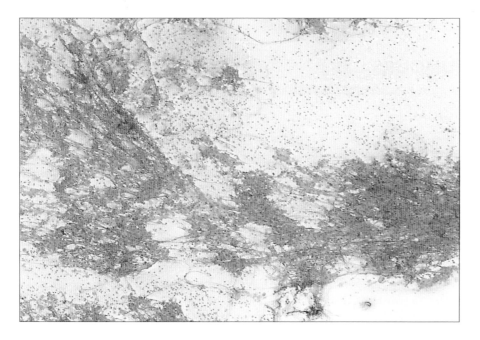

Figure 11.1
Germinoma. Male aged 14 years, pineal region. The large malignant cells in germinomas tend to form ill-defined aggregates around the numerous small capillary vessels within the tumour. No evidence of a gliofibrillary matrix is present. Smear preparation, haematoxylin eosin, ×70.

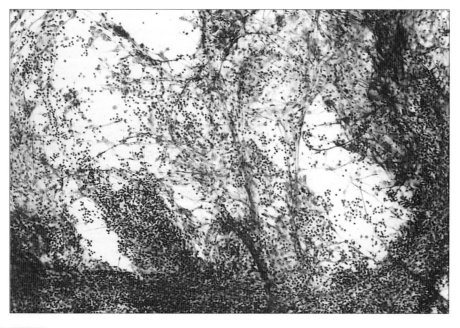

Figure 11.2
Germinoma. Female aged 12 years, pineal region. The reactive lymphocytes in germinomas contain small densely-staining rounded nuclei and form a variable admixture with the larger tumour cells. Smear preparation, toluidine blue, ×70.

containing a large rounded vesicular nucleus and a prominent nucleolus which is often central. Mitotic activity can be identified in this cell population, particularly in smear preparations. The tumour-associated lymphocytes tend to be aggregated around finely branching blood vessels but often in smear preparations can appear admixed within the tumour cell population. These cells are T-lymphocytes and are characterized by a small round densely-staining nucleus.

Teratomas contain variable admixtures of tissue which can include tissues of firm consistency on which it is impossible to perform smear examinations including cartilage, bone and teeth. In the softer areas of teratomas a variety of tissue can be encountered, ranging from primitive neuroectodermal tissue to mature benign or malignant epithelial tissues, keratin and hair. A diagnosis of teratoma is often better made on cryostat sections.

Choriocarcinomas are characterized by populations of large multinucleate giant cells which spread uniformly in smears away from the prominent vascular structures. The diagnosis of endodermal sinus tumour and embryonal cell carcinoma is better made in paraffin sections where immunocytochemistry for germ cell markers is often required for diagnosis.

Frozen sections

Typical germinomas can be identified in cryostat sections by the aggregates of large tumour cells containing abundant faintly eosinophilic cytoplasm around a vesicular nucleus and prominent nucleolus. These cells are aggregated in solid sheets and although occasional lymphocytes may be interspersed through these aggregates, most of the lymphocytes are present around the fine blood vessels within the tumour. Foci of calcification may occur and cause confusion with oligodendroglioma

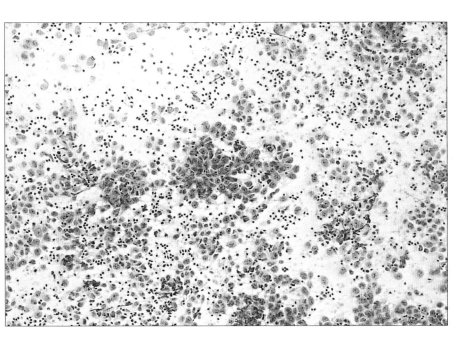

Figure 11.3
Germinoma. Male aged 12 years, pineal region. The irregular clusters of large tumour cells stand out in relief against the smaller reactive lymphocytes. Smear preparation, toluidine blue, ×140.

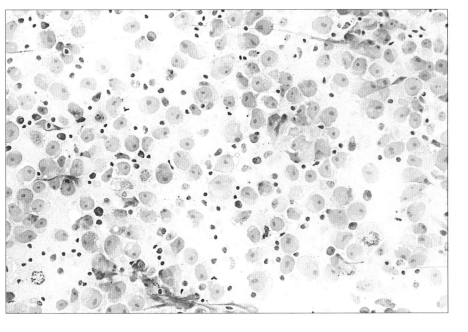

Figure 11.4
Germinoma. Male aged 12, pineal region. The pleomorphic nature of the large tumour cells is most readily appreciated in the monolayer region of the smear, where the large irregular nuclei with prominent nucleoli are identified. Occasional mitotic figures are present and an occasional neutrophil polymorph is present in addition to the reactive lymphocytes. Smear preparation, toluidine blue, ×700.

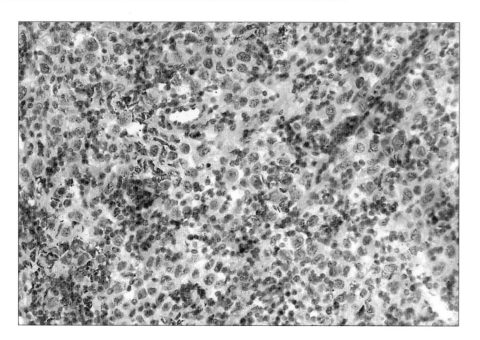

Figure 11.5
Germinoma. Male aged 14 years, pineal region. The irregular clusters of large tumour cells are clearly identifiable in cryostat sections where the prominent nucleolus and irregular nucleus are also clearly represented. The population of small reactive lymphocytes is clearly identifiable around blood vessels in this section. Cryostat section, haematoxylin eosin, ×350.

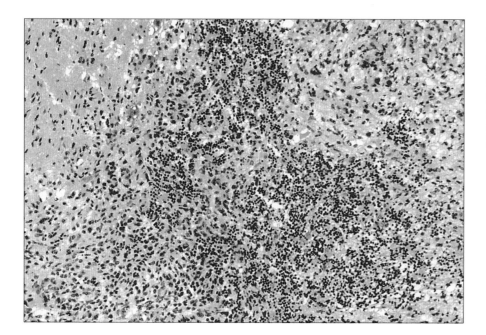

Figure 11.6
Germinoma. Male aged 13 years, pineal region. The reactive lymphocyte population is prominent in this tumour, and at the infiltrating edge can raise the suspicion of an inflammatory process. However, closer inspection reveals the characteristic large pleomorphic tumour cells. Cryostat section, haematoxylin eosin, ×140.

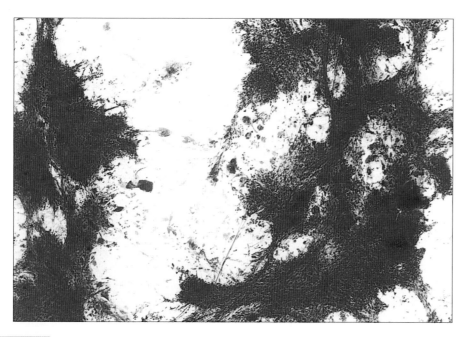

Figure 11.7
Malignant teratoma with choriocarcinoma. Male aged 4 years, pineal region. Malignant teratoma frequently contain a pleomorphic cell population, including large bizarre giant cells which are evident on low power examination. Smear preparation, toluidine blue, ×140.

although the neoplastic cells in germinomas are larger than the tumour cells of oligodendrogliomas.

Frozen sections of teratomas can exhibit a wide range of appearances depending on the individually varying tissue constituents, ranging from mature epithelial tissues of squamous or glandular type to epithelial carcinomas, cartilage, bone, hair, adipose tissue or malignant immature tissues including neuroblastic tissue and rhabdomyoblasts. Choriocarcinomas appear in frozen sections as tumours with bizarre multinucleate cells which are arranged in irregular aggregates around blood-filled vascular spaces. The entire tumour may be haemorrhagic, thus making interpretation difficult. The diagnosis of endodermal sinus tumour and embryonal carcinoma can be made on frozen sections if the typical histological structures are present, although immunocytochemistry is required to confirm the diagnosis.

11.1.5. GRADING AND MALIGNANCY

Although the WHO grading system for neuroepithelial tumours is not applicable to germ cell tumours, it is important to realize that this group of tumours exhibits a spectrum of malignancy. The only benign tumour in this group is the mature teratoma, which grows through expansion and cystic enlargement in a manner similar to epidermoid and dermoid cysts. Germinomas invade adjacent structures and may occasionally disseminate through the CSF pathway. All the other germ cell tumours are malignant and locally invasive. They have a high capacity to spread through the CSF pathway, and may metastasize outwith the CNS to other sites, the commonest of which are the lung and long bones. Mixed germ cell tumours are not uncommon; extensive histological sampling and immunocytochemical screening are required to assess adequately the presence of other germ cell tissues in apparently monomorphous tumours.

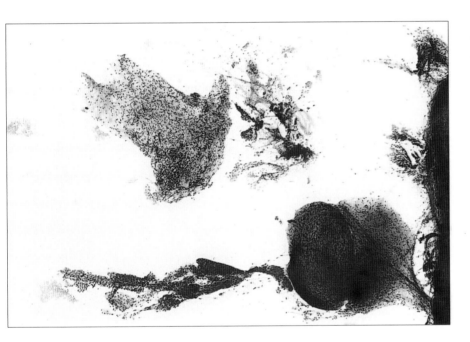

Figure 11.8
Teratoma with malignant transformation. A wide range of discernible cell types may occur in teratomas with malignant transformation, including glial tissue (centre) and malignant epithelial tissue. Smear preparation, haematoxylin eosin, ×70.

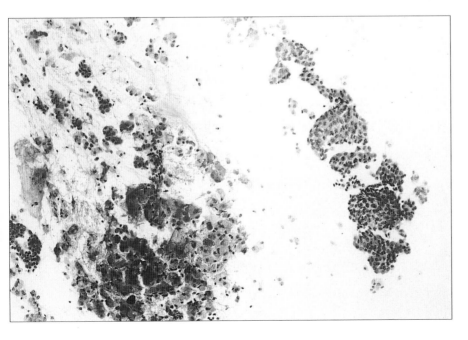

Figure 11.9
Teratoma with malignant transformation. Male aged 3 years, pineal region. In this tumour, two distinct epithelial cell populations are identified, corresponding to adenocarcinoma (left) and transitional cell carcinoma (right). Smear preparation, haematoxylin eosin, ×140.

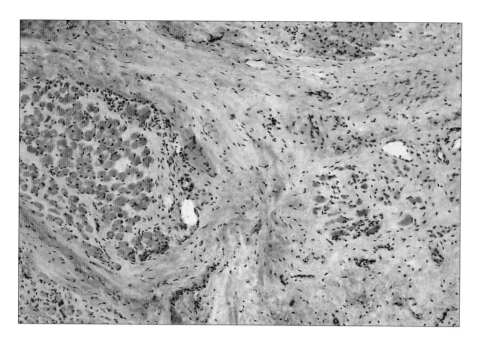

Figure 11.10
Mature teratoma. Male aged 6 years, pineal region. Mature teratomas are characterized by a haphazard arrangement of different tissue types, in this case including skeletal muscle, fibrous connective tissue, vascular endothelium and neural tissue. Cryostat section, haematoxylin eosin, ×140.

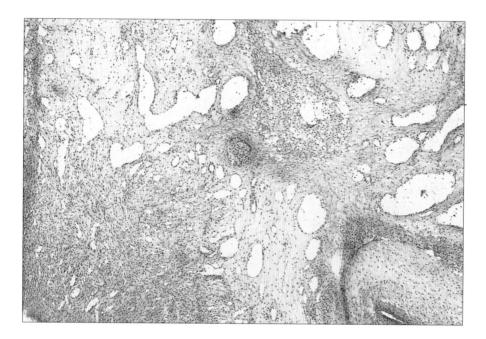

Figure 11.11
Immature teratoma. Male aged 2 years, pineal region. A wide variety of both mature and immature tissues, including immature neuroepithelial tissue (centre) and germ cell elements. Cryostat section, haematoxylin eosin, ×140.

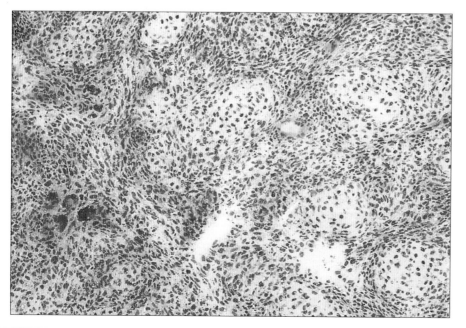

Figure 11.12
Immature teratoma. Male aged 5 years, pineal region. This malignant teratoma contains an immature germ cell component with large bizarre multinucleate cells; malignant cartilaginous tissue is present in small nodules within the tumour. Cryostat section, haematoxylin eosin, ×140.

11.1.6. DIFFERENTIAL DIAGNOSIS

Germinomas may be confused in smear and cryostat sections with **oligodendrogliomas**, although the neoplastic germ cells contain more abundant cytoplasm and have a larger nucleus with a prominent nucleolus. The finely branching vascular pattern and occasional foci of calcification in germinomas may add to the confusion, but their population of reactive T-lymphocytes is not usually found in oligodendrogliomas. Similar confusion may occur with a **central neurocytoma**, particularly if the tumour is located close to the third ventricle. However, the dual cell population characteristic of germinomas is not present in central neurocytomas, which additionally lack the prominent nucleolus and more abundant cytoplasm of the large germinoma tumour cells.

Germinomas may also be confused with malignant **lymphomas**, particularly if the population of reactive T-lymphocytes is prominent in the tissue examined. Malignant lymphoma cells usually have a more marked perivascular aggregation than the germinoma cells, and contain less abundant cytoplasm with a more widespread variety of nuclear morphologies and may often show necrosis, which is rare in germ cell tumours. The neoplastic cells in germinomas are often relatively uniform in their nuclear morphology in contrast to lymphomas.

Suprasellar germ cell tumours may be confused with **pituitary adenomas** or **pituitary carcinoma** if mitotic activity is pronounced within the neoplasm. The dual cell population characteristic of germinomas is not usually identified in pituitary neoplasms, which often exhibit a more marked range of nuclear pleomorphism (even in pituitary adenomas) than in germinomas. The germinoma tumour cells usually contain a larger quantity of cytoplasm than the cells in a pituitary tumour, and the vascular network in germinomas is less prominent and thick-walled than in pituitary tumours. Germinomas may also be confused with **metastatic carcinoma**, although this is relatively uncommon in the age range in which intracranial germinomas are encountered. Metastatic carcinomas characteristically appear in smear preparations as cohesive sheets of pleomorphic cells in contrast to the uniform monolayer of germinoma. Another potential confusion may arise with **malignant melanoma** (either primary or metastatic), in view of the prominent nucleoli and relatively abundant cytoplasm of the tumour cells in germinoma. However, malignant melanomas usually do not contain a prominent population of reactive T-lymphocytes and of course the presence of melanin pigmentation is extremely helpful in differential diagnosis.

Well-differentiated teratomas may be confused with **epidermoid or dermoid cysts** and this confusion may be impossible to resolve at the time of surgery. The same applies to teratomas in which well-differentiated carcinoma is a prominent component, since a distinction from **metastatic carcinoma** will not be possible until all the available tissue has been sampled and the presence of other types of tissue identified. Malignant teratomas in which immature tissues predominate can be confused with **pineoblastomas, supratentorial PNET** and **small cell glioblastomas**. Again, this confusion may be difficult to resolve until all the available tissue has been examined, although smears of small cell glioblastomas usually contain areas where a gliofibrillary matrix is present and typical astrocytic processes are present on at least some tumour cells around a markedly hyperplastic endothelium.

The other types of germ cell tumour are extremely rare and may be confused with metastatic deposits from other sites in the body. The bizarre giant cells of choriocarcinoma may be confused with those of **glioblastoma multiforme** or a **subependymal giant cell astrocytoma**, but adequate knowledge of the clinical and radiological findings will usually provide helpful information to clarify the diagnosis.

11.2. PINEAL PARENCHYMAL TUMOURS

11.2.1. CLINICAL AND RADIOLOGICAL FEATURES

These tumours arise from the parenchymal cells of the pineal gland and occur in two main categories (Table 11.1). The incidence of these tumours is uncertain, but they are extremely uncommon, accounting for around 0.5% of all cerebral neoplasms. Earlier studies have indicated that pineocytomas and pineoblastomas occur at an approximately equal incidence (30–40% of cases in each category) with the remainder of tumours showing a mixed composition. These tumours can occur in children and adults; pineoblastomas occur over a wide age range (1–65 years) with an average age of onset of around 18 years. Pineocytomas tend to occur in older patients with an average age of onset of around 40 years, ranging from 21–55 years, with a slight male predominance. The presenting clinical features for pineal parenchymal tumours are similar to those for germ cell tumours arising in the pineal gland. Pineoblastomas are particularly liable to invade adjacent structures and tend to present early with the signs and symptoms of hydrocephalus and raised intracranial pressure. Occasional cases of pineoblastoma occur in association with bilateral retinoblastoma (the so-called 'trilateral retinoblastoma'), usually in families with an inherited germline mutation in the retinoblastoma gene.

11.2.2. NEURORADIOLOGY

Pineal parenchymal tumours are hypodense or isointense on T1-weighted imaging and hyperintense on T2-weighted MRI scans. Pineocytomas tend to be well demarcated and homogeneous in appearance on MRI scans, with uniform enhancement and occasional small cystic structures. Calcification can be present usually scattered throughout the neoplasm (in contrast to germinomas where the tumour appears to engulf a calcified pineal gland). Pineoblastomas are ill-defined invasive neoplasms which are more heterogeneous in composition, frequently containing areas of necrosis and haemorrhage.

11.2.3. SURGICAL FINDINGS

Pineocytomas tend to be relatively well-defined tumours which occupy the pineal gland in an expansive manner, frequently causing compression of the third ventricle with less invasion of surrounding structures than pineoblastomas, which are malignant tumours and extensively invade local structures. Pineoblastomas may contain multiple areas of haemorrhage and necrosis, whereas pineocytomas are usually solid, occasionally with small cysts. Pineoblastomas may also invade into the CSF pathway and can metastasize to other sites in the CNS, although this usually occurs at a relatively late stage in the disease.

11.2.4. INTRA-OPERATIVE PATHOLOGY: PINEOCYTOMAS

Smear preparations

The neoplastic cells in pineocytomas tend to smear in aggregates rather than in a diffuse monolayer. The tumour cells are small and polygonal with a tendency to form 'pineocytomatous rosettes', which may be identified only with difficulty in smear preparations since they lack a relationship to blood vessels. The blood vessels in pineocytomas are fine capillary structures with an irregular branching pattern. The tumour cells are relatively regular in size and shape, although neuronal or glial differentiation can be identified, with a gliofibrillary matrix present in cases with predominant glial differentiation. Calcification can also be identified in smear preparations, but mitotic figures are usually inconspicuous and necrosis is absent.

Frozen sections

Pineocytomas usually exhibit a lobulated architecture, with evidence of neuronal differentiation and very occasional pineocytomatous rosettes which are unrelated to the delicate blood vessels within the tumour. A central zone of fibrillary matrix may occur within the rosettes, reminiscent of the normal structure of the pineal gland. Patchy calcification can also be identified in these tumours, although this is rarely extensive. Glial differentiation is occasionally apparent, with perivascular orientation of process-bearing tumour cells forming a gliofibrillary matrix. The tumour margins are usually clearly defined, with compression of adjacent structures rather than invasion.

Grading and malignancy

Pineocytomas are slow-growing neoplasms which are well circumscribed and seldom, if ever, metastasize through the CSF pathway. These correspond to Grade II tumours. Occasional pineal parenchymal neoplasms contain areas of both mature (pineocytoma) and immature (pineoblastoma) cells. In some of these cases the cytological features of the tumour cells may be intermediate between these categories, but in all instances the tumour should be graded according to the most malignant areas within the tissue submitted for examination.

Differential diagnosis

Although a wide range of tumours can arise in the region of the pineal gland, the main difficulties in differential diagnosis of pineal parenchymal tumours concern other neuroepithelial tumours which arise at this site. **Astrocytomas** can be distinguished from pineocytomas by their characteristic vascular endothelial hyperplasia and the gliofibrillary matrix with prominent cell processes in the perivascular regions. Rosette formation is not encountered in astrocytomas and calcification is less frequent than in pineocytomas. The presence of calcification might raise the possibility of an **oligodendroglioma**, although the characteristic finely branching capillary network and relatively uniform population of small rounded cells in these tumours should allow distinction from pineocytoma. Rosette formation is not encountered in oligodendrogliomas, although cyst formation is relatively common. **Ependymomas** may also be distinguished from pineocytomas by the presence of a gliofibrillary matrix and the characteristic perivascular orientation of the cells in smear preparations. In cryostat sections, the presence of ependymal pseudorosettes and canaliculi might lead to confusion with the rosette structures occasionally present in pineocytomas; the close relationship of ependymal pseudorosettes to blood vessels and the characteristic nuclear features of ependymomas should allow a clear distinction to be made. Non-neoplastic **glial cysts** may arise in the pineal gland, and are sometimes associated with haemorrhage. The neuroradiological features of these lesions are usually characteristic, but the presence of dense gliotic tissue without appreciable nuclear pleomorphism should allow distinction from a pineocytoma.

Pineocytomas may also be confused with other tumours exhibiting neuronal differentiation including the **central neurocytoma** and the **ganglioneuroma**. In both cases, the presence of rosettes is helpful in the diagnosis of pineocytoma. The cells of the central neurocytoma are relatively small and rounded without the elongated cell processes seen in pineocytoma. The presence of calcification in central neurocytomas can cause additional confusion, but the vascular pattern of these tumours with a finely branching capillary network will allow distinction from pineocytoma. Ganglionic differentiation is exceptional in pineal tumours, and should allow a clear distinction from a ganglioneuroma.

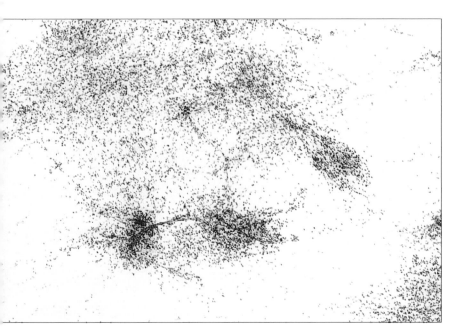

Figure 11.13
Pineocytoma. Male aged 22 years, pineal region. Vascular endothelial hyperplasia is not a prominent feature of pineocytomas; the neoplastic cells tend to aggregate around the delicate capillary network in irregular clusters. Smear preparation, toluidine blue, ×70.

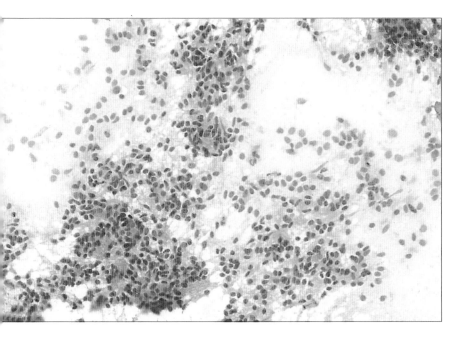

Figure 11.14
Pineocytoma. Female aged 28 years, pineal region. The neoplastic cells tend to spread away from the thin walled capillaries in irregular clusters and eventually form a monolayer of relatively uniform cells with a variable quantity of eosinophilic cytoplasm. The cytoplasmic component may raise suspicions of a gliofibrillary matrix, but this is not a uniform feature in pineocytoma. Smear preparation, haematoxylin eosin, ×140.

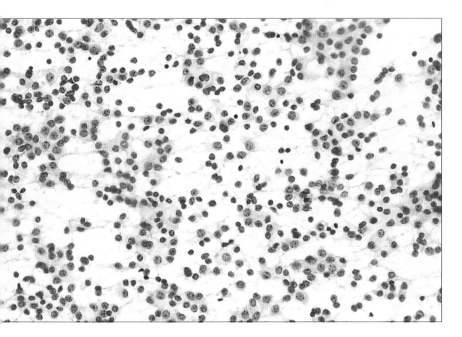

Figure 11.15
Pineocytoma. Male aged 36 years, pineal region. The neoplastic cells in pineocytoma usually show only a mild degree of nuclear pleomorphism with little evidence of mitotic activity. The cells tend to aggregate in small clusters and occasional rosette-like structures are identified (centre right). Smear preparation, toluidine blue, ×350.

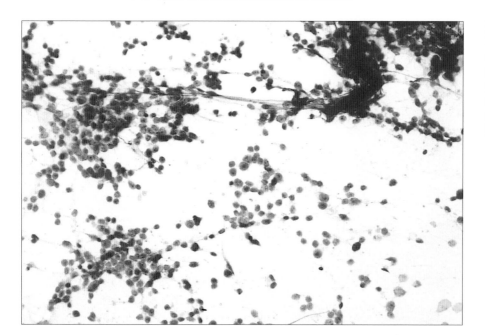

Figure 11.16
Pineocytoma. Male aged 24 years, pineal region. Occasional rosette-like structures (centre) are identified in the monolayer away from blood vessels, being composed of small uniform cells with rounded finely stippled nuclei. Smear preparation, toluidine blue, ×350.

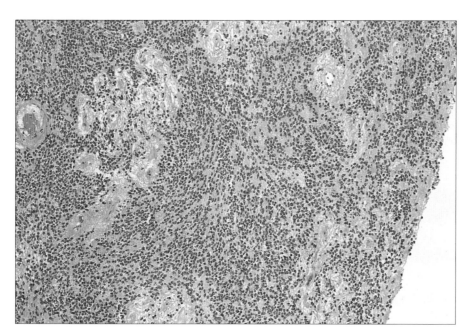

Figure 11.17
Pineocytoma. Female aged 27 years, pineal region. On low power examination, pineocytomas are composed of small uniform cells arranged in clusters of varying size within a fine fibrillary stroma, which may resemble an ependymoma. However, canalicular structures and ependymal rosettes are absent. Cryostat section, haematoxylin eosin, ×140.

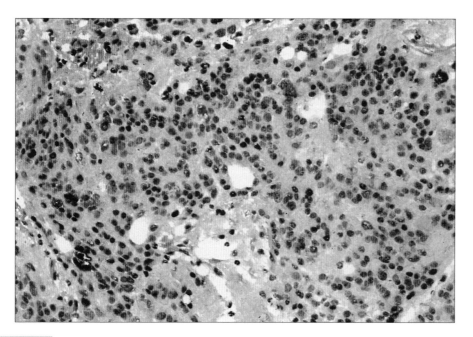

Figure 11.18
Pineocytoma. Male aged 32 years, pineal region. The relatively uniform tumour cells of pineocytomas are aggregated in irregular clusters, and occasionally form rosettes or tubular structures (centre). Mitotic activity is not usually present in these neoplasms. Cryostat section, haematoxylin eosin, ×350.

Pineocytomas are usually easily distinguished from **meningiomas**, although the presence of calcification in psammoma bodies might cause initial diagnostic confusion. The characteristic nuclear and cytological features of meningiomas, with their characteristic arachnoidal morphology, relatively abundant cytoplasm and ill-defined cell membranes, allow a clear distinction from pineocytoma. Rosette formation does not occur in any of the histological subtypes of meningioma. Pineocytomas can be distinguished from **germ cell tumours** by the presence of the characteristic rosette structures in cryostat sections, although in smear preparations a careful distinction from **germinoma** needs to be made in view of the calcification which can occur in both lesions. The large tumour cells in germinomas have more abundant cytoplasm and a larger rounded nucleus and a more prominent nucleolus than is encountered in pineocytoma cells. The presence of perivascular lymphocytes in germinomas is a further aid in differentiating these lesions from pineocytomas. The other forms of germ cell tumours are usually easily distinguished from pineocytomas in both smear preparations and cryostat sections.

11.2.5. INTRA-OPERATIVE PATHOLOGY: PINEOBLASTOMAS

Smear preparations

Pineoblastomas exhibit the cytological features of malignant embryonal tumours, and are characterized by numerous small irregular cells which smear away from the numerous thickened capillary-like blood vessels in a diffuse monolayer. The cells possess scanty cytoplasm and contain an elongated or carrot-shaped nucleus. Occasional pineoblastic rosettes may be identified in smear preparations, but are more readily identifiable in cryostat sections. Mitotic figures are easily detected and necrosis is present in many cases.

Frozen sections

Pineoblastomas appear as small cell embryonal tumours which in cryostat may contain multiple foci of necrosis and haemorrhage. Nuclear pleomorphism and mitotic activity is usually evident and occasional pineoblastic rosettes may be present. Although photoreceptor differentiation can be identified in paraffin sections, this is not usually readily appreciated in cryostat sections; most of the tumour cells contain scanty cytoplasm with an elongated nucleus. The tumour margin is ill-defined and invasion of adjacent structures may be detected.

Grading and malignancy

Pineoblastomas are malignant tumours which infiltrate extensively and are well known for their capacity to spread through the CSF pathway. These tumours correspond to Grade IV.

Differential diagnosis

The differential diagnosis of pineoblastoma includes other malignant **embryonal tumours**, particularly the **ependymoblastoma** which can arise in the third ventricle. The neoplastic cells of both these embryonal tumours are similar in smear preparations, and the presence of ependymoblastic tubules can be confused with pineoblastic rosettes in cryostat sections. Immunocytochemistry and electron microscopy may be required to finally differentiate between these lesions, although such a distinction at the time of surgery is not usually of major clinical significance. Metastatic deposits of **medulloblastoma** can be confused with pineoblastoma, although the clinical history in such cases would clearly be helpful in establishing the diagnosis. Pineoblastomas can be distinguished from **cerebral neuroblastomas** by their higher cellularity, scanty cytoplasm and absence of ganglionic or neuronal differentiation in most cases. However, a distinction between these entities may also be impossible at the time of intra-operative diagnosis and additional immunocytochemical and ultrastructural investigations may be required on fixed material. Pineoblastomas can be distinguished from **small cell glioblastomas** by their relative lack of vascular endothelial hyperplasia and the presence of rosette formation, which is extremely uncommon in glioblastomas. Small cell glioblastomas in general exhibit a wider range of nuclear morphology than pineoblastomas, and careful examination will usually reveal occasional multinucleate cells and, in most cases, evidence of astrocytic differentiation with a gliofibrillary matrix. In adults, pineoblastomas can be distinguished from **metastatic small cell anaplastic carcinomas** by their tendency to form monolayers in smear preparations, in contrast to carcinomas in which the cells characteristically aggregate in clusters. Rosette formation is uncommon in metastatic small cell anaplastic carcinoma, in which the cells are generally larger and contain more abundant cytoplasm in both cryostat sections and smear preparations than in pineoblastomas. Pineoblastomas can be confused with malignant **germ cell tumours**, particularly **immature teratomas** in which primitive neuroepithelial tissue is present. A final distinction will depend upon extensive histological sampling of the tissue submitted for examination, which is usually best done on paraffin sections, in order to establish the presence of other tissue types within the teratoma. Rosette formation may be encountered in malignant neuroepithelial tissue in immature teratomas and its presence cannot be relied upon solely for differentiation from pineoblastoma. Pineoblastomas are unlikely to be confused with other types of germ cell tumours arising in the region of the pineal gland on account of their distinctive cytological and architectural features.

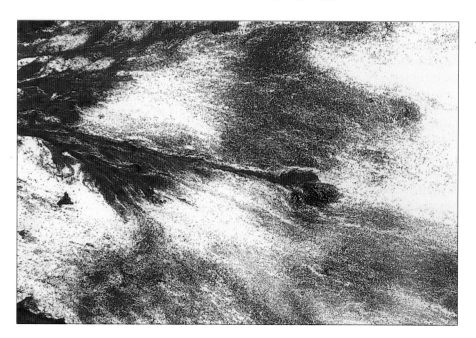

Figure 11.19
Pineoblastoma. Male aged 7 years, pineal region. Vascular endothelial hyperplasia is frequently a prominent feature in these tumours, with dense aggregates of small darkly staining cells which spread away from the vessels in a monolayer. Smear preparation, toluidine blue, ×70.

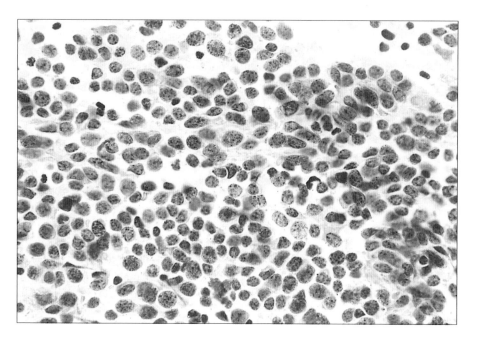

Figure 11.20
Pineoblastoma. Male aged 3 years, pineal region. In the monolayer, the tumour cells exhibit the features of an embryonal tumour, with pleomorphic nuclei, scanty cytoplasm and occasional cellular aggregates. Pineoblastic rosettes are difficult to identify in smear preparation. Smear preparation, toluidine blue, ×350.

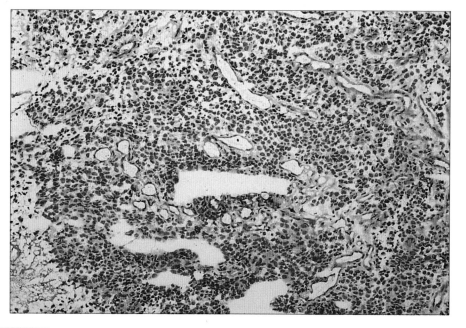

Figure 11.21
Pineoblastoma. Female aged 6 years, pineal region. Occasional pineoblastomas contain cyst-like spaces, with prominent vascular channels in the adjacent tumour parenchyma. The cell density is much higher than in pineocytomas, with a correspondingly wide range of nuclear pleomorphism. Cryostat section, haematoxylin eosin, ×140.

T W E L V E
PRIMITIVE NEUROECTODERMAL TUMOURS

12.1. CLINICAL AND RADIOLOGICAL FEATURES

The term 'primitive neuroectodermal tumour' (PNET) encompasses a number of malignant embryonal tumours arising in the central nervous system which exhibit a capacity for divergent differentiation, including astrocytic, neuronal, ependymal, rhabdoid, lipomatous and melanotic differentiation. These tumours tend to occur most frequently in childhood, the commonest example of which is the cerebellar medulloblastoma. The histogenesis of this group of tumours is uncertain, but the PNET concept is useful in denoting tumours which share a number of biological and clinical features, and are related to the more distinct categories of embryonal tumours, including the ependymoblastoma, pineoblastoma and cerebral neuroblastoma.

Medulloblastomas are the second most frequent brain tumour to occur in children (after the pilocytic astrocytoma) and constitute around 25% of all paediatric brain tumours. They occur with a peak incidence at 3–8 years but a significant sub-group, approximately 20%, occur beyond the age of 20 years. Occasional congenital cases have been reported and medulloblastomas are one of the commoner tumours occurring within the first year of life. There is a preferential occurrence in males, and occasional cases occur in families, particularly those with p53 germline mutations (Li-Fraumeni syndrome), or the Gorlin syndrome (*see* Chapter 5).

Presenting features in children with medulloblastomas are often non-specific, including irritability, lethargy and loss of appetite. These are usually followed by the signs and symptoms of raised intracranial pressure including headache, nausea and vomiting which are often worse in the mornings. Intracranial hypertension usually occurs as a consequence of obstructive hydrocephalus as the tumour compresses or invades the cerebral aqueduct or fourth ventricle. At a later stage, gaze palsy may occur with neck stiffness and cerebellar abnormalities including ataxia and nystagmus. Most medulloblastomas in children arise in the region of the vermis, but in adults an origin in the cerebral hemispheres is more common and this can produce a lateral cerebellar syndrome including unilateral dysdiadochokinesia and intention tremor. Medulloblastomas can metastasize through the CSF pathway, and occasionally patients may present with signs and symptoms relating to metastatic deposits,

e.g. around lumbar spinal nerve roots, or in the frontal lobes, although this is uncommon.

Supratentorial primitive neuroectodermal tumours occur more frequently in children than in adults, although these are rare tumours and probably account for no more than 5% of all PNET. The tumours tend to arise in the cerebral hemispheres and present with signs and symptoms of raised intracranial pressure and localizing neurological deficit. Meningeal invasion and CSF spread may produce signs and symptoms of obstructive hydrocephalus at a relatively later stage in the natural history of the tumour than the obstructive hydrocephalus caused by medulloblastomas.

12.2. NEURORADIOLOGY

Many patients with cerebellar medulloblastomas suffer from obstructive hydrocephalus, which is readily demonstrable on CT and MRI studies. On CT scans, medulloblastomas usually occur as a hyperdense mass with uniform contrast enhancement although occasionally areas of haemorrhage and cystic change can be identified. An origin in the cerebellar vermis in children is the most common, whereas in adults the tumours tend to arise in the cerebellar hemisphere. On MRI scans the T1-weighted images demonstrate a hypodense mass with compression or invasion of the fourth ventricle. Calcification is infrequent in medulloblastomas. Peritumeral oedema is often present and is readily identified on contrast-enhanced MRI scans. Metastatic deposits often exhibit sparse contrast enhancement, and myelography with CT scans has until recently been the most precise method of investigating spinal metastases. MRI scans also have a role to play in the detection of tumour recurrence, both locally in the posterior fossa and at other sites. Very rarely, medulloblastomas have metastasized outwith the CNS (usually in long bones) following surgery; these can be detected on a standard skeletal survey.

12.3. SURGICAL FINDINGS

Medulloblastomas usually occur as lobulated pink tumours which are usually highly vascular and may appear encapsulated. Occasional tumours invade the subarachnoid space and can appear as a white plaque of tumour over the surface of the cerebellum, but invasion into the ventricular system is more common.

Cystic degeneration and necrosis are unusual, but large lesions may compress the brainstem and result in haemorrhage in the surrounding tissues.

Supratentorial PNET usually occur as ill-defined infiltrative lesions involving the cerebral cortex and surrounding white matter, often associated with extensive oedema. Haemorrhage and necrosis have been described in these tumours, which may mimic anaplastic astrocytomas or glioblastomas at the time of surgery and on neuroradiological studies.

12.4. INTRA-OPERATIVE PATHOLOGY

Smear cytology

Most medulloblastomas are soft enough to make good smear preparations, upon which a diagnosis can be made. Typically, the smear preparations consist of large numbers of densely packed cells with oval or carrot-shaped nuclei which may occasionally exhibit nuclear moulding. The cells tend to spread in a monolayer widely from the blood vessels, which may vary from small capillary-like structures to large vessels with hyperplastic endothelium. Mitotic figures are readily identified in smear preparations and occasional tumours contain foci of necrosis. Neuroblastic rosettes can be identified occasionally in smear preparations; these usually resemble the Homer-Wright rosettes identified on paraffin histology. The nuclear chromatin in medulloblastomas is usually finely granular and best appreciated in toluidine blue stained sections. On haematoxylin and eosin stained smears, a variable quantity of cytoplasm is present in the tumour cells and occasional cells may exhibit neuronal differentiation, to assume a ganglionic appearance, or astrocytic differentiation with occasional astrocytic processes or a patchy gliofibrillary

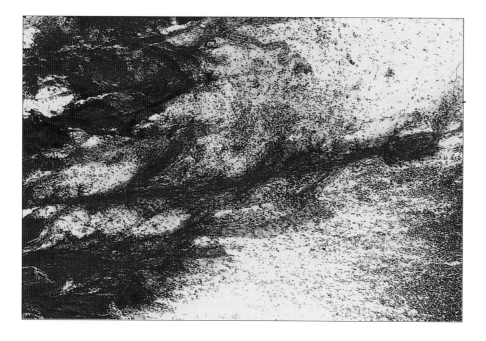

Figure 12.1
Medulloblastoma. Male aged 3 years, cerebellar vermis tumour. A dense vascular endothelial component is present in most tumours, from which the neoplastic cells spread in an irregular monolayer. Smear preparation, toluidine blue, ×35.

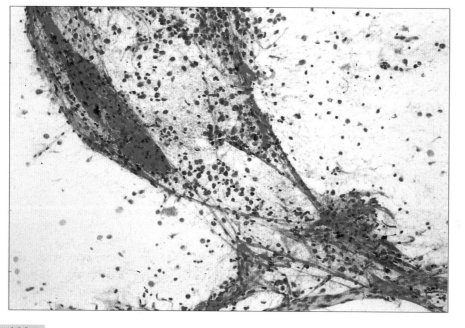

Figure 12.2
Medulloblastoma. Male aged 9 years, cerebellar vermis tumour. Capillary endothelial hyperplasia is variable, but there is no gliofibrillary matrix around the capillaries, in contrast to ependymomas and astrocytomas. Smear preparation, haematoxylin eosin, ×70.

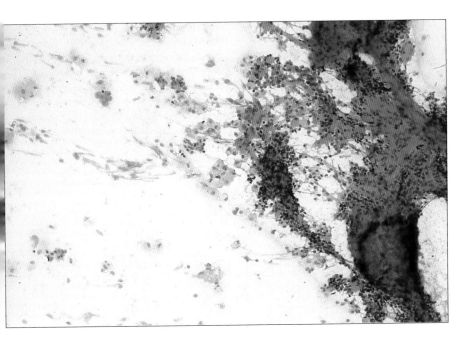

Figure 12.3
Medulloblastoma. Male aged 4 years, cerebellar vermis tumour. Necrosis and infarction are not uncommon in medulloblastomas, and can produce cellular reactions within the tumour tissue, including the presence of large 'foamy' macrophages with uniform nuclei (centre). Smear preparation, haematoxylin eosin, ×70.

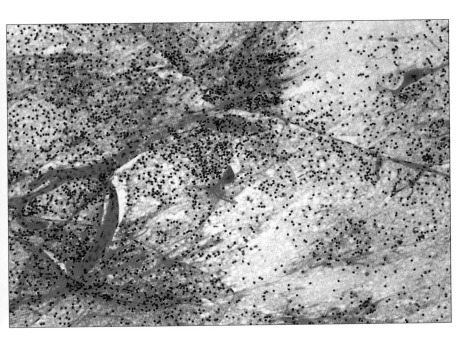

Figure 12.4
Medulloblastoma. Female aged 6 years, left cerebellar hemisphere tumour. Cerebellar cortical invasion is common, and biopsy specimens frequently include cerebellar neurones, within which large Purkinje cells (centre and right) are conspicuous by their size and eosinophilic cytoplasm. Smear preparation, haematoxylin eosin, ×140.

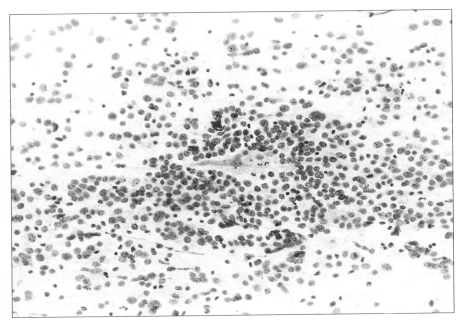

Figure 12.5
Medulloblastoma. Male aged 4 years, cerebellar vermis tumour. The neoplastic cell nuclei are often elongated or carrot-shaped, but a wide range of nuclear morphology is not uncommon. The nuclei tend to 'mould' to the shape of the adjacent tumour cells; aggregation around normal cerebellar neurones (Purkinje cell – centre) is a common finding in cases with extensive local invasion. Smear preparation, toluidine blue, ×350.

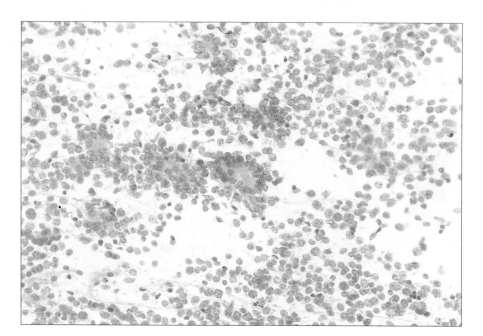

Figure 12.6

Medulloblastoma. Female aged 8 years, cerebellar vermis tumour. The neoplastic cells frequently aggregate in irregular clusters within a monolayer away from blood vessels. Occasional rosettes (centre) may be present in tumours with neuronal differentiation. Smear preparation, haematoxylin eosin, ×350.

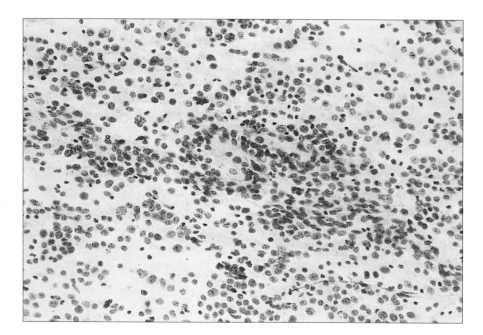

Figure 12.7

Medulloblastoma. Male aged 1 year, cerebellar vermis tumour. Tumours in young infants show similar cytological features to those in older children, and contain small pleomorphic tumour cells with scanty cytoplasm. Nuclear moulding is also present, along with a rosette-like structure (centre). Smear preparation, toluidine blue, ×700.

matrix. The latter, however, are uncommon. Neuronal differentiation may be more evident in cerebellar hemispheric tumours in adults (desmoplastic medulloblastomas) but even in these tumours the small primitive neuroectodermal tumour cell population is readily identifiable in smear preparations. Occasional rare variants of medulloblastoma can exhibit ependymal differentiation which can be detected in smear preparations, although the embryonal tumour cell component is also present. Exceptionally, tumours containing melanotic cells, adipocytes or rhabdomyoblasts have been described, but as in other variants of this tumour, the embryonal cell population is readily identifiable within the other cellular components.

One of the commonest difficulties encountered in examining smear preparations in patients with medulloblastomas is potential confusion of small cerebellar granular neurones for medulloblastoma cells (*see*

Chapter 5). Since medulloblastomas frequently invade the cerebellar cortex, it is not surprising that intraoperative biopsy samples may occasionally include fragments of cortical tissue. Cerebellar granular neurones are small cells with very scanty cytoplasm and the uniformly rounded nuclei. In smear preparations, they are often admixed with occasional Purkinje cells which can be readily distinguished by their large cell body, extensive cytoplasm and large nucleus with a prominent nucleolus (*see* Chapter 3). In contrast, medulloblastoma cells have larger nuclei than granular neurones with an elongated or carrot shape, a more variable chromatin pattern and dense packing with nuclear moulding and frequent mitotic activity.

Smear preparations of supratentorial primitive neuroectodermal tumours usually exhibit similar appearances to those of cerebellar medulloblastomas. Since confusion of granular neurones with tumour cells is not a

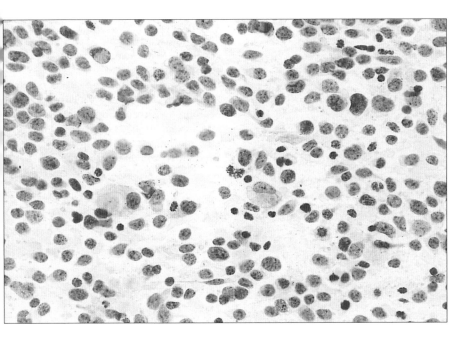

Figure 12.8
Medulloblastoma. Male aged 25 years, left cerebellar hemisphere tumour. Tumours in the cerebellar hemispheres in adults commonly show evidence of neuronal differentiation, with large neoplastic cells containing abundant cytoplasm and a large nucleus with a prominent nucleolus (centre). Smear preparation, toluidine blue, ×700.

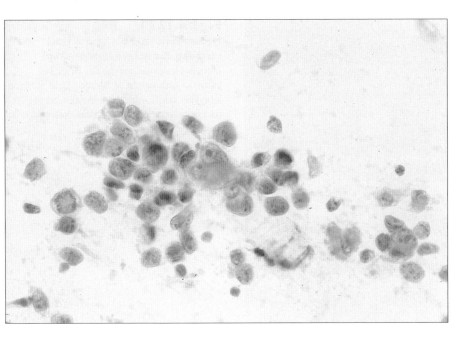

Figure 12.9
Medulloblastoma. Male aged 39 years, right cerebellar hemisphere tumour. A spectrum of neuronal differentiation can be detected in adult hemispheric tumours, ranging from small primitive neuroectodermal cells to large cells with abundant eosinophilic cytoplasm and a prominent nucleolus within a large nucleus, which may appear bilobed (centre). Smear preparation, haematoxylin eosin, ×1400.

difficulty in supratentorial tumours, a diagnosis of neoplasia is often straightforward, although confusion may arise between metastatic small cell anaplastic carcinoma or small cell glioblastoma and supratentorial PNET. Other specific categories of PNET which occur in the supratentorial region (ependymoblastoma and pineoblastoma) obviously come under the differential diagnosis of supratentorial PNET and are described more fully in Chapters 8 and 11 respectively. The diagnosis of these particular entities depends on full clinical and neuroradiological details; distinction of these entities from a supratentorial PNET may not be possible on cytological grounds alone.

Frozen sections

Medulloblastomas appear in cryostat sections as highly cellular tumours with hyperchromatic nuclei which are densely packed and often exhibit nuclear moulding.

Mitotic figures are frequent and occasional small areas of necrosis may be present. The tumour cells infiltrate into the surrounding tissues and can usually be distinguished from cerebellar granular neurones on their nuclear morphology. Neuroblastic rosettes may be present in cryostat sections, but the most frequently encountered tumour architecture is solid irregular sheets of densely packed tumour cells around an irregular vascular network.

Tumours exhibiting neuronal differentiation, particularly the hemispheric desmoplastic medulloblastomas in adults, may contain larger cells with more abundant pale eosinophilic cytoplasm which are grouped in irregular clusters, sometimes surrounded by smaller embryonal tumour cells. Mitotic figures are usually less evident in the islands of larger cells. Occasional medulloblastomas are highly vascular and contain thick-walled blood vessels with hyperplastic endothelium,

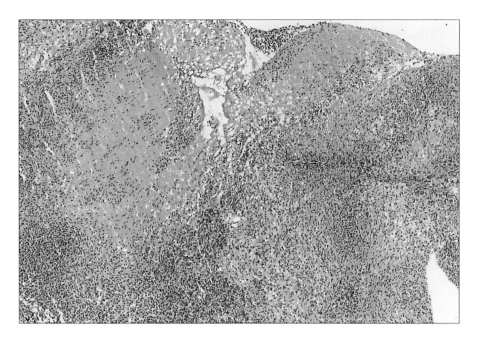

Figure 12.10
Medulloblastoma. Female aged 5 years, cerebellar vermis tumour. Cerebellar cortical invasion is readily detected in cryostat sections, with solid sheets of small dark-staining primitive cells infiltrating the neuropil. Invasion of the subarachnoid space may also be identified (top), and should raise the suspicion of CSF metastases. Cryostat section, haematoxylin eosin, ×70.

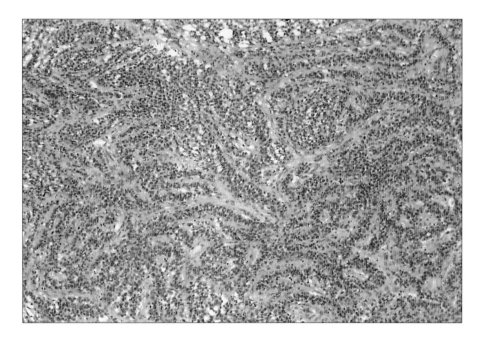

Figure 12.11
Medulloblastoma. Male aged 7 years, right cerebellar hemisphere tumour. Some medulloblastomas exhibit an organoid pattern, with bands of tumour cells forming irregular cords which invade the cerebellar parenchyma. Cryostat section, haematoxylin eosin, ×140.

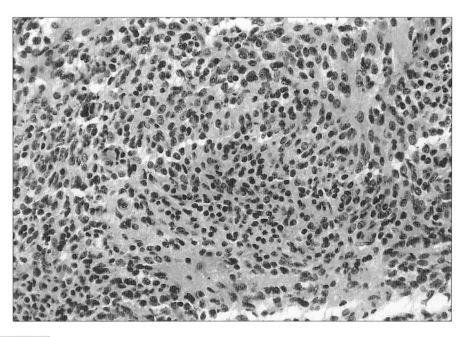

Figure 12.12
Medulloblastoma. Male aged 34 years, left cerebellar hemisphere tumour. Neuronal differentiation in medulloblastomas in adults often occurs in 'nodules' or 'islands', within which the tumour cells are irregularly dispersed and contain a variable quantity of eosinophilic cytoplasm. Cryostat section, haematoxylin eosin, ×350.

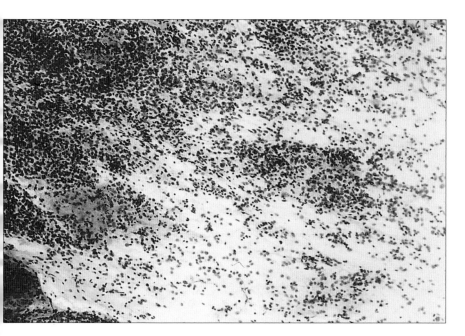

Figure 12.13
Cerebral PNET. Male aged 38 years, right temporal tumour. The neoplastic cells tend to spread away from blood vessels in irregular clusters within a monolayer, resembling an astrocytic glioma at low magnification. Smear preparation, toluidine blue, ×70.

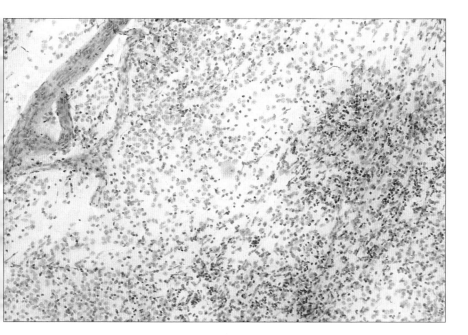

Figure 12.14
Cerebral PNET. Male aged 14 years, left frontal tumour. The neoplastic cells and vascular endothelium extensively infiltrate the adjacent brain, entrapping cortical neurones (centre). Smear preparation, haematoxylin eosin, ×70.

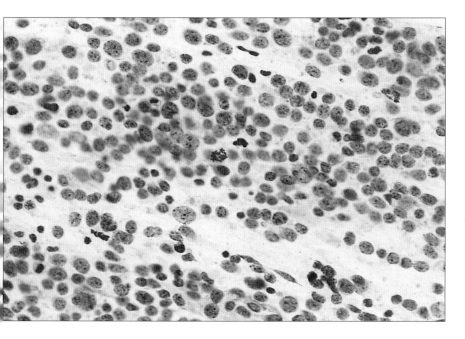

Figure 12.15
Cerebral PNET. Female aged 17 years, left parietal tumour. The neoplastic cells show marked nuclear pleomorphism, with nuclear moulding within some of the cellular aggregates and occasional mitotic figures. Smear preparation, toluidine blue, ×350.

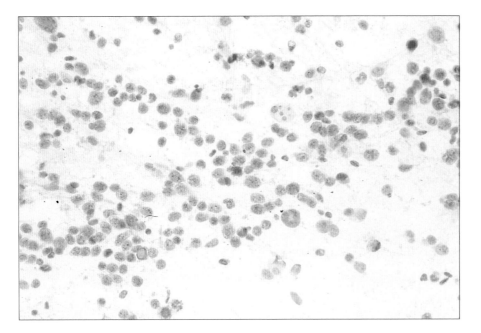

Figure 12.16
Cerebral PNET. Male aged 24 years, right parietal lobe. The neoplastic cells contain a small quantity of eosinophilic cytoplasm, but show marked nuclear pleomorphism, with occasional bilobed nuclei. No gliofibrillary matrix is present, allowing distinction from an astrocytic glioma. Smear preparation, haematoxylin eosin, ×350.

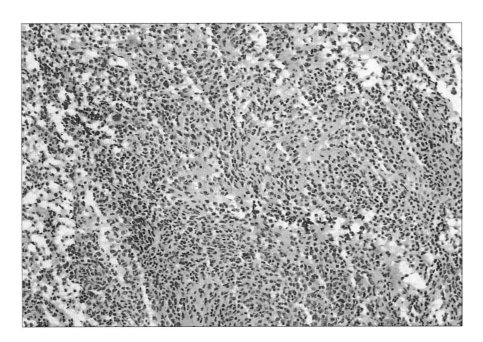

Figure 12.17
Cerebral PNET. Male aged 19, left temporal lobe. Sheets of tumour cells form a solid mass of tumour, with occasional small groups of cells containing more abundant eosinophilic cytoplasm which should not be confused with a gliofibrillary matrix. Marked nuclear pleomorphism is also evident. Cryostat section, haematoxylin eosin, ×70.

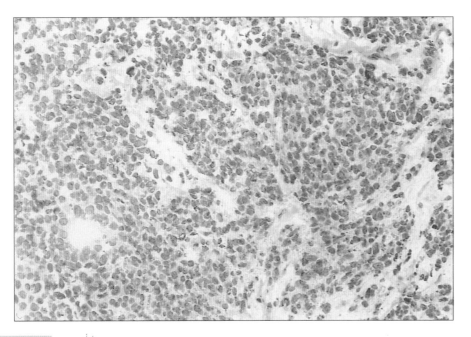

Figure 12.18
Cerebral PNET. Female aged 24 years, left frontal lobe. In some tumours, the neoplastic cells are grouped into well-demarcated clusters, with an intervening fibrillary stroma. A poorly-formed tubular structure (left) suggests ependymal differentiation, but subsequent immunocytochemical studies found predominant neuronal differentiation. Cryostat section, haematoxylin eosin, ×140.

sometimes surrounded by dense aggregates of tumour cells. These tumours may also exhibit haemorrhage and necrosis, which might cause confusion with a glioblastoma multiforme. The rare variants of medulloblastomas containing melanotic cells, rhabdomyoblasts or lipidized cells may be recognized in frozen sections but these tumours are extremely rare and are therefore infrequently encountered in routine diagnostic practice.

Cryostat sections of supratentorial PNET show similar appearances to medulloblastomas, and show irregular solid sheets of small malignant cells with scanty cytoplasm; extensive neuronal differentiation (as in the desmoplastic medulloblastoma) is usually not identifiable. Necrosis and haemorrhage can occur in supratentorial PNET and may lead to confusion with glioblastoma. However, multinucleate tumour cells, marked vascular endothelial hyperplasia and widespread astrocytic differentiation are infrequent in supratentorial PNET, in contrast to glioblastoma. Tumour cell rosettes are usually less apparent in PNET than in medulloblastomas.

12.5. GRADING AND MALIGNANCY

All PNET are highly malignant tumours which are capable of widespread local infiltration, invasion of the subarachnoid space and may metastasize through the CSF pathway to the spinal canal or other sites within the CNS. The diagnosis of metastatic PNET can be made on smear preparations and cryostat sections, and an intra-operative diagnosis may be required for re-exploration of a recurrent cerebellar medulloblastoma. In these instances, the same diagnostic criteria apply although the context in which the neoplastic cells are identified will obviously vary according to the site of metastatic disease.

12.6. DIFFERENTIAL DIAGNOSIS

The clinical and radiological diagnosis of cerebellar medulloblastomas include other tumours occurring in the posterior fossa in childhood, particularly **pilocytic astrocytomas**, **ependymomas** and **choroid plexus tumours**. **Pilocytic astrocytomas** are readily distinguishable from medulloblastomas on smear preparations and cryostat sections on account of their obvious astrocytic differentiation, low cellularity, gliofibrillary matrix and lack of mitotic activity. Medulloblastomas usually smear out in a diffuse monolayer, unlike **ependymomas**, which show an obvious gliofibrillary stroma and form cohesive clumps of tissue with perivascular palisades. Frozen section preparations are useful in the demonstration of ependymal perivascular pseudo-rosettes or tubular rosettes, which are not encountered in medulloblastomas. Medulloblastomas are generally more cellular than ependymomas both in smears and cryostat sections, although **anaplastic ependymomas** may cause confusion on account of their high cellularity, mitotic activity and focal necrosis. Close inspection of smears

for the nuclear features of these tumours, the relationship of the tumour cells to blood vessels and the presence of a gliofibrillary stroma will aid in the differential diagnosis. **Choroid plexus papillomas** are similarly distinguishable from medulloblastomas in smear and cryostat preparations on account of their obvious papillary architecture and epithelial cytological features, but diagnostic difficulties may be encountered with the rarer **choroid plexus carcinomas** of childhood, particularly the **anaplastic carcinomas** which tend to occur in the posterior fossa in young males. In these tumours, the neoplastic cells are usually larger than in medulloblastomas, and exhibit a cellular cohesion in smear preparations which indicates their epithelial origin. However, mitotic activity and necrosis may occur in choroid plexus carcinomas and these tumours may also invade the cerebellar cortex. The nuclei in these tumours are usually large and rounded with a prominent nucleolus, in contrast to medulloblastomas.

Medulloblastomas arising in the cerebellar hemisphere in adults may be confused with **metastatic small cell anaplastic carcinoma**. Although the nuclear features of these tumours are superficially similar, small cell anaplastic carcinomas usually contain a more obvious nucleolus within the nucleus and the cells tend to smear in aggregates rather than in a diffuse monolayer. Supratentorial PNET in adults may also be distinguished from metastatic small cell anaplastic carcinoma by these features. Supratentorial PNET can be distinguished from **small cell glioblastomas** by the abundant vascular endothelial proliferation, the characteristic perivascular orientation of tumour cells and the presence of a gliofibrillary matrix and cell processes in the glioblastoma. Small cell glioblastomas will occasionally contain multinucleate cells which are unusual in PNET, whereas neuroblastic rosettes are infrequently encountered in glioblastomas.

In adults, medulloblastomas and supratentorial PNET also need to be distinguished from primary **CNS lymphoma** and **metastatic lymphoma**. In smear preparations although lymphoma cells usually spread out in a monolayer, the extreme nuclear pleomorphism present in medulloblastomas is not usually encountered and carrot-shaped nuclei are uncommon. Medulloblastomas lack the marked perivascular orientation of malignant lymphoma, and a lymphocytic infiltrate around tumour vessels is uncommon in medulloblastomas. Cerebellar and cerebral PNET can be distinguished from **oligodendrogliomas** by their extreme nuclear pleomorphism, the lack of perivascular orientation, the absence of calcification and their irregular vascular network. **Astroblastomas** may be differentiated from medulloblastomas and supratentorial PNET by their tendency to form perivascular palisades and relatively uniform cytology with prominent gliofibrillary stroma and broad cytoplasmic processes around the prominent blood vessel walls.

The factors enabling a distinction between cerebellar medulloblastoma cells and **normal granular layer** neurones of the cerebellum are described above. Distinction of supratentorial PNET from other specific embryonal tumours particularly the **ependymoblastoma** and **pineoblastoma** may prove impossible at intra-operative diagnosis, and in practical terms this is unlikely to influence the immediate clinical management of the patient. Other rare tumours occurring in children which might potentially be confused with medulloblastoma include the **medulloepithelioma**, an extremely rare tumour which tends to occur in children under the age of 5 years in the cerebral hemispheres or cerebellum. Medulloepitheliomas are composed of cells which are larger than those usually encountered in medulloblastomas, with more abundant eosinophilic cytoplasm and a marked tendency to form extensive tubules and rosettes. Other tumours which occur more frequently within the cerebral hemispheres are the **cerebral neuroblastoma** and **ganglioneuroblastoma**, which may be distinguished from medulloblastomas and supratentorial PNET by the presence of a more uniform population of small neoplastic cells with poorly defined cytoplasm and round to ovoid nuclei. Ganglionic differentiation can be identified in these tumours and neuroblastic rosettes may occasionally be detected. Immunocytochemistry on paraffin sections will be required for a confident diagnosis of cerebral neuroblastoma and, as in other subtypes of embryonal tumours, an immediate distinction between this neoplasm and supratentorial PNET is unlikely to influence the immediate clinical management of the patient. Medulloblastomas and supratentorial PNET can be distinguished from **olfactory neuroblastoma** on clinical grounds according to the site of origin and the predominant neuroblastic and neuronal differentiation, which can include neuroblastic and neurosensory rosettes.

Atypical teratoid-rhabdoid tumours are extremely uncommon tumours occurring in children under the age of 6 years which predominantly involve the cerebellum. These unusual lesions exhibit a diversity of differentiation including neuronal, ependymal, mesenchymal and epithelial cells. The clinical manifestations are similar to those of medulloblastoma, although multiple areas of necrosis and cystic degeneration are more likely to be encountered on MRI scans. The phenotypic diversity in these tumours will allow a distinction from medulloblastomas and other malignant tumours arising in the posterior fossa, although immunocytochemistry on paraffin sections is required for the diagnosis of this uncommon entity.

THIRTEEN

TUMOURS OF CRANIAL AND SPINAL NERVE SHEATHS

13.1. SCHWANNOMA

13.1.1. CLINICAL AND RADIOLOGICAL FEATURES

The vast majority of sporadic intracranial Schwannomas are cerebellopontine angle tumours arising from the vestibular part of the eighth cranial nerve. They present with increasing frequency in older age groups, most commonly with unilateral deafness. Larger examples may also cause ataxia and other disturbances of cerebellar function. Very rarely, solitary Schwannomas may also arise from the roots of the trigeminal or lower cranial nerves, presenting as mass lesions in the middle fossa or foramen magnum region. In the spine, sporadic Schwannomas may arise at any level, although they are slightly more common in the lumbar region. They usually cause signs and symptoms of nerve root or spinal cord compression appropriate to the level of the tumour. Back pain is also a feature, especially with lesions in the lumbosacral region. Large, dumb-bell tumours can sometimes present as mediastinal or abdominal retroperitoneal masses.

Schwannomas are also a common manifestation of neurofibromatosis of either main type, and may be the earliest recognized feature of the syndrome. They tend to present earlier in life than sporadic Schwannomas, often in young adulthood. In NF II, intracranial examples most commonly arise from the eighth nerve and are usually bilateral. The initial signs and symptoms are frequently unilateral, however, since the tumour on one side is often much more advanced. Intracranial Schwannomas arising from other cranial nerves can also occur in NF II, and even if solitary must be regarded as suspicious of the syndrome. Spinal root Schwannomas may be a feature of NF I or NF II. They frequently arise at multiple levels, although many of the smaller ones may be asymptomatic at the time of presentation. In NF I, Schwannomas can also arise within the parenchyma of the brain or spinal cord, apparently unrelated to cranial or spinal nerve roots. These lesions again tend to present in younger age groups, usually with the clinical features of a meningioma or intrinsic spinal cord tumour.

Radiologically, MR scanning is the investigation of choice for both posterior fossa and spinal Schwannomas, these sites being much less easily imaged using CT scans. The tumours are iso- or hypo-intense to brain/cord in T1-weighted images and usually non-homogeneously hyper-intense with T2 weighting. Cystic change may be apparent in larger tumours and there is usually diffuse enhancement after administration of contrast media. A majority of eighth nerve Schwannomas will show radiological evidence of widening of the internal acoustic meatus, an important distinguishing feature from meningiomas of the cerebellopontine angle. Scans of larger spinal root Schwannomas may again demonstrate expansion of the corresponding bony meatus. This is particularly true of dumb-bell lesions, where there can be evidence of quite marked local bone erosion.

13.1.2. SURGICAL FINDINGS

Schwannomas are tough, well-circumscribed masses which are usually bounded by a thick fibrous capsule. The nerve root of origin, and sometimes neighbouring ones, are stretched over the tumour mass and may be partly embedded in the capsule. With larger tumours, these roots are frequently so attenuated as to be unrecognizable to the naked eye. The tumour tissue has a firm rubbery texture with a greyish, whorled appearance on cut section. Softer, bright yellow areas are often seen, especially in eighth nerve tumours. Cystic degeneration and evidence of old haemorrhage may also be apparent at the time of surgery. Cerebellopontine angle Schwannomas are approximately spherical in shape and can deeply indent the neighbouring brainstem or cerebellum. They frequently have a cone-like extension into the internal auditory meatus. Spinal Schwannomas practically always arise from sensory roots and thus tend to be posteriorly situated. Smaller examples are often sausage-shaped, especially those in the lumbosacral canal, and are usually entirely intradural. A proportion, however, extend far enough laterally to have an extradural component. The largest tumours protrude right out through the expanded meatus in a dumb-bell fashion, and may be predominantly paraspinal in extent.

13.1.3. INTRA-OPERATIVE PATHOLOGY

Smear cytology

Schwannomas are usually quite tough tumours, but it is possible to make diagnostic smear preparations from most cranial and spinal root examples if a little care is exercised. The main difficulty is avoiding squash artefact whilst at the same time exerting enough pressure to create a sufficiently thin film of tissue. It is the fasciculated Antoni A tissue which gives Schwannomas their diagnostic appearance in smears, the cords of spindle cells becoming separated and entwined about each other by the smearing process. The result has been described as resembling twisted rope and is best appreciated at quite low magnification. Closer examination confirms that the twisted structures are sheaves of closely packed spindle cells with axial orientation. They should not be confused with blood vessels, which are not a conspicuous feature in most Schwannoma smears. The tumour cell nuclei in these sheaves of tissue may be ovoid or very elongate and cigar-shaped, but always with rounded ends. They usually have uniform, stippled chromatin without a prominent nucleolus. Bipolar cytoplasmic processes may be apparent in some cases, but individual cell cytoplasm is often indistinct, giving the impression of a coarsely fibrillar background stroma. This is very cohesive, even at the margins of the twisted fascicles, and may be weakly metachromatic in toluidine blue stained preparations. Although Antoni A tissue provides the most useful information in Schwannoma smears, a variable amount of looser Antoni B tissue is often present and a gradation between the two appearances should also be expected in some cases. This is particularly the case with eighth nerve tumours and so-called 'ancient' spinal root lesions. Where loose and degenerate Antoni B tissue predominates, a careful search may be necessary to identify areas of the smear which show the characteristic twisted rope pattern, and the importance of using a low magnification lens for this cannot be over-emphasized. The looser tissue smears out more thinly, with stellate or bipolar cells set in a coarsely fibrillar background. Variable traces of a twisted fascicular architecture may be apparent, but this is often entirely lost. The cells have large and irregular nuclei with pale chromatin and sometimes a distinct nucleolus. There is frequently quite a marked degree of cytological pleomorphism, but this is of a degenerate nature and mitoses are not seen unless there is malignant change (see below). In some tumours the looser, more degenerate tissue appears markedly hypercellular due to the presence of numerous small lymphocytes, scattered in a 'pepper and salt' fashion across the smear. The lipidized cells sometimes seen in paraffin sections of Schwannomas are only rarely identified in smears, but haemosiderin pigment is often a prominent and helpful feature.

Frozen sections will demonstrate the tumour architecture of well preserved Schwannomas, especially the characteristic biphasic pattern of Antoni A and B type tissue. In tumours which have proved too tough to make satisfactory smear preparations, there is likely to be a predominance of densely fasciculated type A tissue, and there is rarely a problem making the diagnosis from cryostat sections. Rhythmic nuclear palisades and Verocay bodies may be visible in this type of tumour,

although such features are rarely appreciated in smear preparations. The situation is rather less straightforward with degenerate tumours, especially those of the eighth nerve, where interpretation of smear preparations has proved difficult and there is little or no recognizable fascicular architecture in the cryostat sections. Hypercellularity due to lymphocytic infiltration and tumour cell pleomorphism may again be prominent features in the frozen sections and can easily mislead the unwary into suspicion of malignancy. Useful histological features in these lesions include the presence of abundant haemosiderin pigment, typical hyaline vascular degeneration, xanthomatous areas, and large cystic spaces lined by flattened tumour tissue.

13.2. NEUROFIBROMA

13.2.1. CLINICAL FEATURES

Neurofibromas of the craniospinal axis are virtually unknown except in the context of neurofibromatosis, and even an apparently solitary lesion is highly suspicious of this disorder. They are very rare in the cranial cavity and unlike Schwannomas show no predilection for the eighth nerve. In the spine, they usually occur at multiple levels and are much more likely to be encountered in cases of NF I than NF II. The clinical presentation is like that of spinal root Schwannomas and may include solitary root symptoms, evidence of cord compression and back pain. There are frequently cutaneous stigmata of NF I. Radiologically, spinal root neurofibromas have very similar signal characteristics to Schwannomas and it is often not possible to distinguish between them, even when MR scans are used. Neurofibromas are perhaps more likely to be multiple and bilateral by the time of presentation and widespread expansion of nerve root foramina is often a prominent radiological feature.

13.2.2. SURGICAL FINDINGS

Like Schwannomas, spinal neurofibromas almost always arise from sensory roots and therefore tend to be sited posteriorly in the spinal canal. Smaller examples take the form of fusiform expansions of the roots, which often extend out into the bony foramina to involve the dorsal root ganglia. The margins of the expanded area are ill-defined and it can be difficult for the surgeon to ascertain the full lateral extent of the tumour. There is typically a stringy, rather mucoid consistency on cut section, blending imperceptibly with the firmer, whitish tissue of the adjacent unaffected nerve root. In contrast to Schwannomas, the parent nerve root is entirely engulfed by the tumour and inevitably must be sacrificed during surgical excision. Large neurofibromas assume a dumbbell distribution similar to giant spinal Schwannomas, with a variable paraspinal component. There is often considerable bony erosion in these circumstances and the

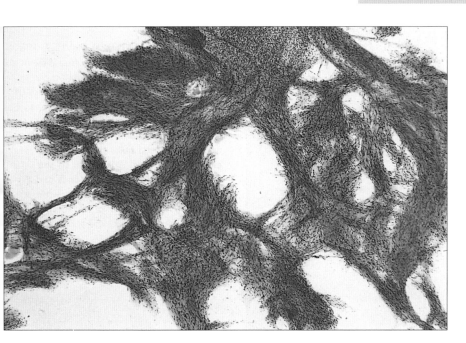

Figure 13.1

Schwannoma. Female aged 37 years with a solitary intradural nodule in the mid thoracic region. Fascicles of tumour cells from the dense Antoni A areas of tumour become separated and intertwined about each other by the smearing process. This results in a highly characteristic appearance, sometimes described as resembling twisted rope. It is most easily recognized at quite low magnifications. Smear preparation, toluidine blue, ×35.

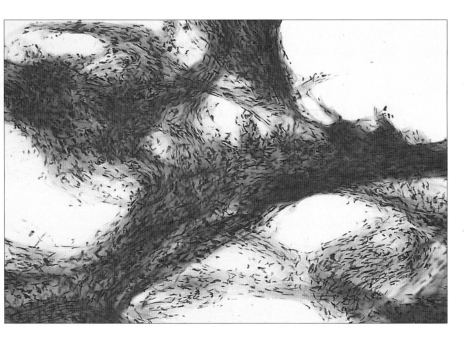

Figure 13.2

Schwannoma. Male aged 51 years presenting with unilateral deafness and a cerebellopontine angle tumour. The interlacing fascicles of smeared Antoni A tissue consist of tightly packed, elongate tumour cells. Smear preparations are often quite thick because of the toughness of the tissue, and at higher magnifications it may be necessary to rack the focus up and down to appreciate the fascicular architecture. Smear preparation, toluidine blue, ×110.

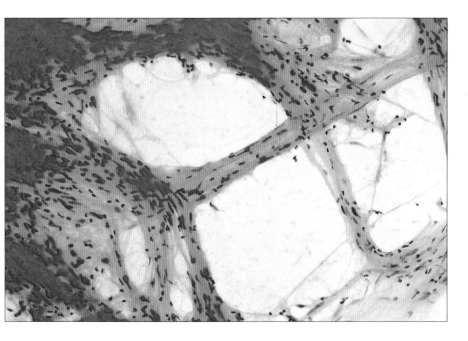

Figure 13.3

Schwannoma. Male aged 25 years with neurofibromatosis type 2 and bilateral eighth nerve root tumours. The twisted rope pattern is again clearly seen. Antoni A tissue is very cohesive, and there is little tendency for the cells or background stroma to dissociate at the edges of the cord-like fascicles. These structures should not be confused with blood vessels, which are not a prominent feature of Schwannoma smears. Smear preparation, haematoxylin eosin, ×175.

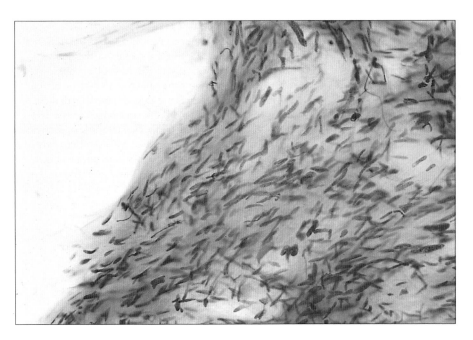

Figure 13.4

Schwannoma. Same case as Fig. 13.2. The cells of Antoni A tissue are often difficult to see in smears because of the cohesive nature of the tumour and the thickness of the fascicles. Individual cell cytoplasm is usually indistinct and there is a dense fibrillar background stroma. The tumour cell nuclei tend to be quite narrow and elongate, with axial orientation to the fascicles. They have rounded ends and a homogeneous chromatin pattern without obvious nucleoli. Smear preparation, toluidine blue, ×220.

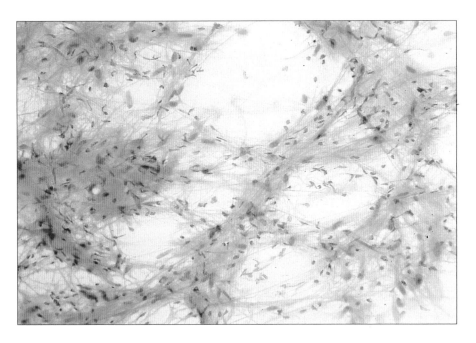

Figure 13.5

Schwannoma. Unilateral cerebellopontine angle tumour in a male aged 76 years. Gradations between Antoni A tissue and very loose, degenerate tumour are common, especially in eighth nerve Schwannomas. The tumour sampled here shows the vestiges of twisted interlacing fascicles, but it is much more loosely smeared than typical Antoni A tissue. Many of the tumour cells have spread out individually and have a stellate appearance with coarse cytoplasmic processes. Smear preparation, haematoxylin eosin, ×175.

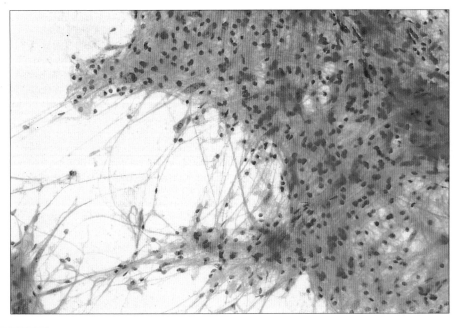

Figure 13.6

Schwannoma. Same case as Fig. 13.5. Degenerate tumour tissue, including that from Antoni B areas, tends to smear in a more diffuse fashion without evidence of fascicular architecture. Individual tumour cells dissociate easily from the margins of larger clumps of tissue and often show considerable pleomorphism. As in this case, lymphocytic infiltration may give an overall impression of hypercellularity. Smear preparation, haematoxylin eosin, ×220.

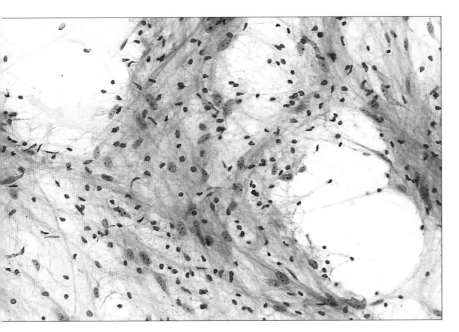

Figure 13.7
Schwannoma. Female aged 63 years. Histologically degenerate tumour from the lumbosacral spinal canal. The tumour cells have large, irregular nuclei with pale chromatin and occasional nucleoli. Many have a stellate or bipolar appearance with coarse cytoplasmic processes. The fibrillary background stroma is mildly metachromatic and numerous small lymphocyte nuclei are scattered across the smear. Smear preparation, toluidine blue, ×220.

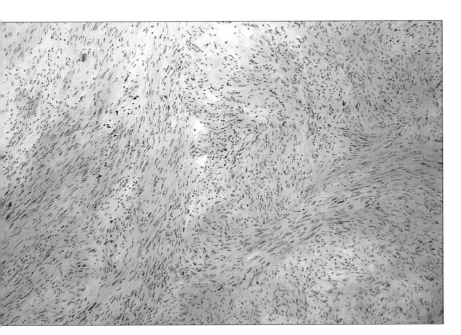

Figure 13.8
Schwannoma. Male aged 27 years with neurofibromatosis type 1 and multiple spinal lesions. In well-preserved Schwannomas, frozen sections will show this typical pattern of tightly interweaving fascicles of spindle cells, sometimes alternating with looser areas of Antoni B tissue. In some cases nuclear palisades and Verocay bodies may also be present, but these are less often encountered than in Schwannomas of peripheral nerves. Frozen section, haematoxylin eosin, ×90.

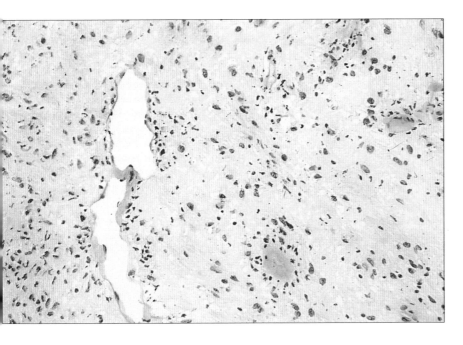

Figure 13.9
Schwannoma. Male aged 47 years with a solitary nodule in the lumbosacral canal. Degenerate tumour tissue lacks the fascicular architecture of Schwannomas and can be difficult to interpret in a small sample. The tissue is often quite sparsely cellular, although a prominent lymphocytic infiltrate may be present in some cases. The tumour cells occasionally show considerable nuclear pleomorphism, but this is a degenerative feature and does not indicate malignancy. The blood vessels seen here show the characteristic hyaline change of Schwannoma vessels. Frozen section, haematoxylin eosin, ×175.

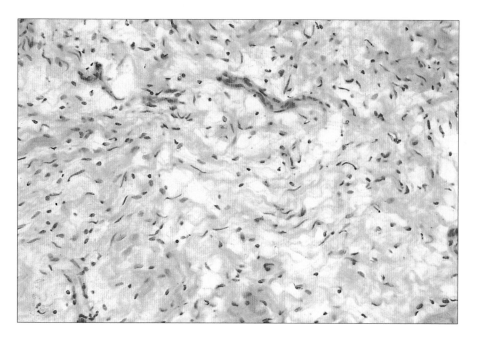

Figure 13.10
Neurofibroma. Paraspinal dumb-bell lesion in a male aged 13 years with presumptive neurofibromatosis. Frozen sections typically show tissue with a loose, rather myxoid appearance and quite widely spaced, undulating bundles of collagen. The cells vary widely in appearance, but many have elongated and slightly twisted nuclei with pointed ends. Bipolar cytoplasmic processes merge with the collagenous stroma. The blood vessels do not usually show the hyaline change typical of Schwannomas. Frozen section, haematoxylin eosin, ×220.

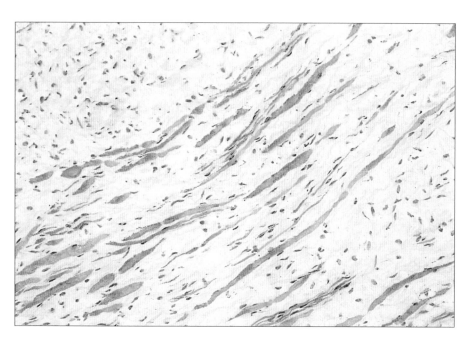

Figure 13.11
Neurofibroma. Male aged 51 years with a solitary fusiform lesion of the T1 posterior root. In smaller tumours, and near the ends of larger ones, myelinated nerve root fibres may be found dispersed within the tumour tissue. This is a helpful diagnostic feature which clearly distinguishes neurofibromas from Schwannomas and other compact tumours such as meningiomas. Frozen section, haematoxylin eosin, ×175.

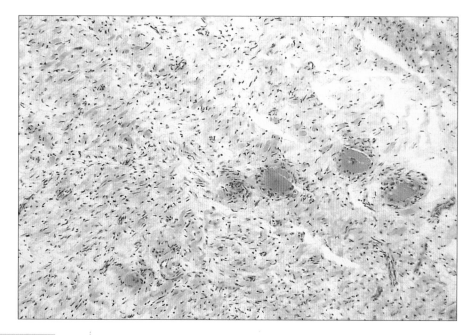

Figure 13.12
Neurofibroma. Same case as Fig. 13.10. In lesions which extend far enough laterally into the bony meatus it is not uncommon to find dorsal root ganglion cells embedded in the tumour tissue. These are easily recognized by their large size and encircling ring of capsule cells. The diagnostic implications are the same as for dispersed myelinated root fibres (see Fig. 13.11). Frozen section, haematoxylin eosin, ×110.

relationship of tumour to nerve root may no longer be apparent by the time of surgery.

13.2.3. INTRA-OPERATIVE PATHOLOGY

Most spinal neurofibromas are very difficult to smear, producing thick preparations which lack specific diagnostic features. In particular, they tend not to show the twisted rope pattern characteristic of Schwannomas. Frozen sections typically show loose, myxoid tissue with a greatly expanded extracellular space. The tumour cells give the appearance of a non-homogeneous population, but many have very thin, elongate nuclei, sometimes with pointed ends and a slightly folded or twisted outline. There is usually a loose background of undulating collagen fibres. Individual cell processes are attenuate and bipolar, merging with the stromal collagen. The tumour cells may be grouped into fascicles, but these are rarely compact and tend to run in the same direction, in contrast to the dense, interweaving pattern of Schwannoma Antoni A tissue. In some cases, dorsal root ganglion cells and widely separated myelinated root fibres may be found dispersed within the tumour tissue. Both are very helpful diagnostic features when present, emphasizing the diffuse nature of the tumour growth and helping with the distinction of neurofibromas from compact tumours such as Schwannomas and meningiomas.

13.3. MALIGNANCY IN NERVE SHEATH TUMOURS

True malignancy is exceptionally rare in craniospinal nerve sheath tumours unless neurofibromatosis is present. It is particularly unlikely to be encountered in cranial root lesions and does not occur in the relatively common sporadic eighth nerve Schwannomas. In practice, malignancy is most likely to be encountered in large spinal Schwannomas or neurofibromas in patients with either NF I or NF II. They may be primarily sarcomatous lesions or benign ones which have undergone focal malignant change. Subclassification of these lesions is not usually possible or necessary at the time of making an intra-operative diagnosis, and use of the generic term 'malignant peripheral sheath tumour' is recommended at this stage. The smear and frozen section appearances are usually indistinguishable from those of other types of sarcoma, and in many cases a nerve sheath origin will only be suggested by the radiological and surgical information available. There is typically a spindle-cell morphology, with frequent mitoses and markedly increased cellularity. Focal necrosis is also a useful indicator of malignancy, although care must be taken not to confuse this with the degenerative changes seen in some benign Schwannomas. A similar word of caution applies to nuclear pleomorphism, which can be very striking in some older Schwannomas. In general, malignant nerve sheath tumours are more likely to have a rather monotonous

cytological appearance, and a variety of sheet-like, storiform or herringbone growth patterns may be apparent in frozen sections.

In addition to overtly sarcomatous lesions, there is an important group of Schwannomas which show evidence of **rapid growth** whilst falling short of overt malignancy. Such tumours are again more likely in the context of neurofibromatosis and are sometimes referred to as the 'cellular variant' of Schwannoma. Their identification intra-operatively may alter surgical management, since they are much more likely than typical Schwannomas to recur locally if not completely excised. Smears and frozen sections continue to show recognizable architectural features of a Schwannoma, particularly the twisted rope pattern in smears, but there is an overall increase in cellularity, with little or no loose Antoni B tissue. Tumour cell nuclei are often noticeably larger and rounder than usual and mitotic figures easily found. Even occasional mitoses should alert suspicion of rapid growth in a Schwannoma, especially if there is clinical evidence of neurofibromatosis.

13.4. DIFFERENTIAL DIAGNOSIS

In the cerebellopontine angle, the most important differential diagnosis lies between an eighth nerve Schwannoma and either a meningioma or a metastasis. Whilst most typical **meningiomas** may be easily identified by their cell whorls and vesicular nuclei, those of fibroblastic pattern can be difficult to distinguish from cellular Schwannomas, and an intra-operative opinion may have to rely heavily on clinical information. In contrast to most Schwannomas, cerebellopontine angle meningiomas tend not to present with deafness as an early symptom and are most unlikely to show either radiological or surgical evidence of tumour involving the internal auditory meatus. In addition, they often show radiological evidence of dural spread (the so-called 'dural tail'), and an obvious dural attachment may be apparent at surgery. A **solitary metastasis** of the angle may be more difficult to distinguish from a Schwannoma pre-operatively in some cases, but is unlikely to present much difficulty to the pathologist, whether smears or frozen sections are used. The same applies to a predominantly solid **haemangioblastoma** sited in the cerebellopontine angle, although this will require frozen sections and is likely to have been recognized surgically on account of its intense vascularity. Cerebellopontine angle epidermoid cysts constitute a theoretical differential diagnosis, but are usually easily identified by their distinctive radiological and macroscopic features

Schwannomas of the trigeminal root may again present clinically as meningiomas, in this instance of middle fossa or sphenoid ridge origin. Those of the lower cranial nerve roots can mimic a variety of other **skull base tumours**, including paragangliomas, chordomas

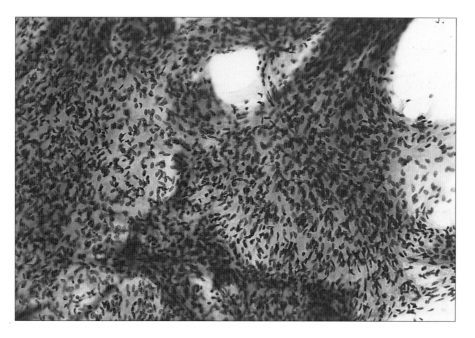

Figure 13.13
Schwannoma with evidence of rapid growth. Male aged 50 years with type I neurofibromatosis and a cervical intradural mass. Although this smear shows evidence of twisted, interlacing fascicles, it is markedly hypercellular. The nuclei are monotonous but rounder than usual, and mitotic figures were easily found at higher magnification. Typical histological features of Schwannomas were seen in the paraffin sections, but the tumour again appeared markedly hypercellular with numerous mitoses and no looser Antoni B areas. Smear preparation, toluidine blue, ×175.

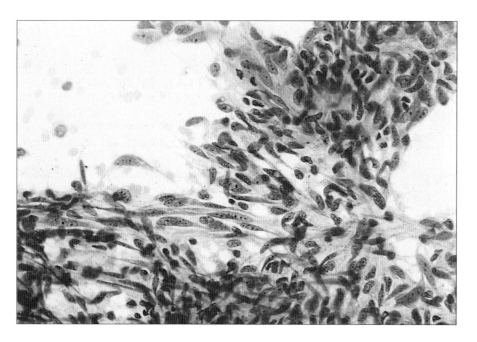

Figure 13.14
Malignant peripheral nerve sheath tumour. Large dumb-bell tumour in a male aged 32 years with type I neurofibromatosis. This smear shows frankly sarcomatous features, with large, pleomorphic spindle cells and a high mitotic rate. A twisted, fascicular architecture is not apparent and a nerve sheath origin was only suggested by the surgical relationship of the tumour to the nerve root. Smear preparation, toluidine blue, ×350.

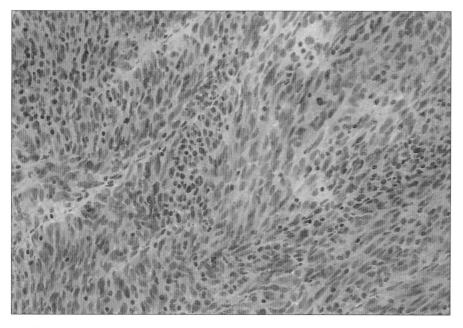

Figure 13.15
Malignant peripheral nerve sheath tumour. Same case as Fig. 13.14. The intra-operative frozen section again shows features of a sarcoma. There is a monotonous, predominantly sheet-like growth pattern with a vague impression of some cross-cut fascicles. The tumour cells have large, elongate nuclei and indistinct cytoplasm. Mitotic figures were easily found at higher magnification. Frozen section, haematoxylin eosin, ×220.

and primary bone or cartilaginous lesions. Radiological and surgical findings may be less helpful in this area and the tissue is frequently too tough to smear, except perhaps in the case of a chordoma. In the majority of cases, however, these lesions can be easily distinguished from a Schwannoma using intra-operative frozen sections.

In the spinal canal, posterior root **Schwannomas and neurofibromas** can be indistinguishable from each other on both radiological and surgical grounds, especially in the case of large, dumb-bell lesions. With some smaller tumours, the surgeon may be able to save the parent nerve root if the lesion is known to be a Schwannoma, but in practice the root can often be safely sacrificed without producing further clinical deficit, regardless of the type of nerve sheath tumour being excised. Using frozen sections, useful distinguishing features of neurofibromas include the myxoid stroma, loosely undulating architecture and very elongate cell nuclei with pointed ends. Diffusely enmeshed myelinated fibres or dorsal root ganglion cells are also extremely helpful in confirming that the lesion is a neurofibroma rather than a Schwannoma. **Meningiomas** of the spinal canal are most often of transitional type, with easily recognizable cell whorls and arachnoidal nuclei. They also frequently contain psammoma bodies. As with cerebellopontine angle lesions, however, the possibility of a fibroblastic meningioma needs to be kept in mind. Unlike nerve sheath tumours, meningiomas are not associated with expanded root foramina and do not usually assume a dumb-bell distribution. Occasionally, however, they may occur at multiple levels. Predominantly extramedullary **haemangioblastomas** can be closely associated with a spinal posterior root exit zone, and frozen sections may be necessary to exclude a small, entirely intradural Schwannoma. In the lumbosacral canal, extramedullary **metastases, paragangliomas** and **myxopapillary ependymomas** may all present as discreet nodules similar to small cauda equina nerve sheath tumours, but again should be easily distinguishable on the basis of their intra-operative pathology.

FOURTEEN
MENINGEAL TUMOURS

14.1. MENINGIOMA

14.1:1. CLINICAL AND RADIOLOGICAL FEATURES

Meningiomas are benign tumours which nearly always have a dural attachment. Clinical presentation is with the signs and symptoms of a mass lesion, namely focal neurological deficits, raised intracranial pressure or seizures. Radiologically meningiomas typically occur as well-circumscribed spherical masses expanding from the inner aspect of the dura and indenting the underlying brain. They usually enhance with contrast and, if angiography is performed, are seen to be fed from the external carotid artery. Calcification of the tumour may be apparent on CT scan. Rarely the tumour forms a widespread thickening of the dura known as **meningioma en plaque**. A relatively common feature is hyperostosis of the overlying cranial bone which may be accompanied by infiltration of the skull by tumour and extracranial soft tissues may also be involved. Indeed, on occasions meningioma may present as an extracranial soft tissue swelling or with bony deformity as a consequence of hyperostosis.

Meningiomas have a predilection for particular sites within the cranial cavity, including attachment to the dura overlying the convexities of the cerebral hemispheres, the falx cerebri and the sphenoid ridge. Other recognized sites include the olfactory grooves, the sellar region, the optic nerve sheath and the posterior fossa where meningiomas may present as cerebellopontine angle tumours. Uncommonly meningiomas may arise within the ventricular system, usually with an attachment to the choroid plexus. Special mention should be made of meningiomas arising within the spinal canal which present typically with spinal cord compression. Meningiomas occur most commonly in middle age and more frequently in women than in men. Neurofibromatosis provides a genetic predisposition to meningiomas. The most important environmental precipitating factor to have been identified is previous local irradiation.

Meningiomas are essentially benign tumours in the sense that they have a relatively low rate of cell proliferation, are well-circumscribed and do not metastasize. They would therefore be expected not to recur if completely excised. Experience shows however that a significant proportion do recur and this presumably is due to incomplete excision. As might be predicted the relatively accessible convexity tumours and spinal

meningiomas recur relatively infrequently, whereas less accessible tumours such as those arising from the skull base recur relatively more frequently. Recurrence is more likely if there is involvement of bone by the tumour. Recurrence of meningiomas remains unpredictable however and additional factors of relevance include the rate of cell proliferation and the demarcation at the interface between tumour and underlying brain.

14.1.2. SURGICAL FINDINGS

The combination of the relatively characteristic appearances of meningioma on imaging and the appearance at operation mean that the surgeon is rarely in doubt that a tumour is a meningioma. The identifying features of a typical meningioma are a smooth surfaced spherical or lobulated mass, an attachment to the inner aspect of the dura and expansion inwards to indent but not infiltrate the underlying brain. Meningiomas are red-brown or grey-brown in colour and the texture varies from soft to firm. Fibrous meningiomas are particularly tough and many meningiomas are gritty in texture as a consequence of calcification. If adjacent dura is involved by tumour this may be thickened – meningioma en plaque represents an extreme example of this phenomenon with dural thickening in the absence of a mass lesion. Extensive involvement of dura and bone, especially at the skull base, may cause considerable surgical difficulty. Spinal meningiomas are intradural, extramedullary masses and are frequently intensely calcified.

14.1.3. INTRA-OPERATIVE PATHOLOGY

Smear preparations

Most meningiomas are soft enough to be smeared satisfactorily. Even the relatively tough fibrous (fibroblastic) tumours can usually be smeared, although some are so rubbery as to require frozen sections. In most tumours the cells smear into clumps which vary in size, have irregular margins, and are unrelated to blood vessels unlike those of astrocytic tumours. Meningiomas are presumed to be derived from the meningothelial or arachnoidal cells of the arachnoid granulations and a large proportion of meningiomas reflect this origin in their cytological appearance. The nuclei are oval in shape with diffuse chromatin and indistinct or small nucleoli. Often intranuclear vacuoles (pseudo-inclusions) are identifiable and although not specific for meningioma (they may be found in melanoma for example), identification of these is reassuring. The nuclei are usually uniform although some examples show marked pleomorphism without sinister connotation. The cytoplasm of the cells is generally indistinct.

Although the majority of meningiomas are instantly recognizable as such, both the cytological and histological appearances of meningiomas can be remarkably varied. Commonly encountered variants include **meningothelial (syncytial) meningioma** in which typical meningothelial cells are arranged in sheets or lobules and **transitional (mixed) meningioma** in which there may be pronounced formation of cell whorls and lobules. Psammoma bodies are often identifiable in transitional meningiomas as spherical structures, unstained by toluidine blue in which the concentric laminations are visible. In **psammomatous meningioma**, which almost invariably occurs in the spinal canal, psammoma bodies may be so numerous that few tumour cells are identifiable in the intervening spaces. The cells of a **fibrous (fibroblastic) meningioma** are spindle shaped, usually lacking specific meningothelial features, and are arranged into ill-defined fascicles, giving an appearance closely resembling that seen in a Schwannoma. In practice these subdivisions are somewhat artificial as any one tumour may show a mixture of different histological patterns.

Many other patterns of differentiation may occur. Although generally they appear as typical meningiomas from a clinical and radiological point of view, these other variants may be less readily identifiable as meningiomas from the pathological point of view and can pose a diagnostic challenge even when paraffin histology is available. Fortunately these variants are encountered relatively infrequently. In examples which are proving difficult to identify on smear preparations because of absence of the characteristic meningothelial

nuclear morphology it is worth spending a considerable time looking for whorls because, if found, even one will provide reassurance that meningioma is the correct diagnosis.

Frozen sections

In frozen sections, in addition to the cytological features described above, the architectural patterns of the various forms of meningioma may be seen. These include the sheet-like arrangement of cells in meningotheliomatous (syncytial) meningioma; the whorls, lobules and psammoma bodies of transitional (mixed) meningioma; the elongated cells, abundant collagen and often fascicular architecture of the fibrous (fibroblastic) meningioma. Psammomatous meningiomas may be so densely calcified as to prove impossible to section.

14.1.4. RECURRENT MENINGIOMAS

Meningiomas which recur usually appear cytologically benign both in the first and subsequent operations. Comparison of smears or frozen sections with specimens from previous operations will help to determine whether or not there has been a fundamental change in the tumour cytology. Meningiomas with an attachment to the falx cerebri may evade the superior sagittal sinus even if they are cytologically benign. Although in this situation tumour cells may be identified within the venous channels distant metastases are almost unknown. The likelihood of recurrence of a meningioma depends to a large extent on the completeness of surgical excision. Tumours of the skull base, and particularly those involving bone, are more likely to recur. However, most tumours in which there is involvement of dura and infiltration of bone, and even those involving extracranial soft tissues, appear cytologically benign.

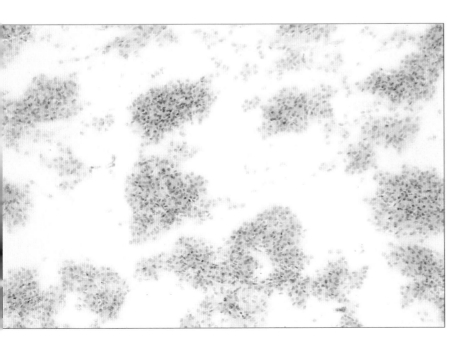

Figure 14.1
Meningotheliomatous meningioma. Male aged 55 years, convexity tumour. This relatively soft meningioma has smeared readily into clusters which have irregular margins and, unlike those of an astrocytic tumour, are unrelated to blood vessels. Smear preparation, haematoxylin eosin, ×350.

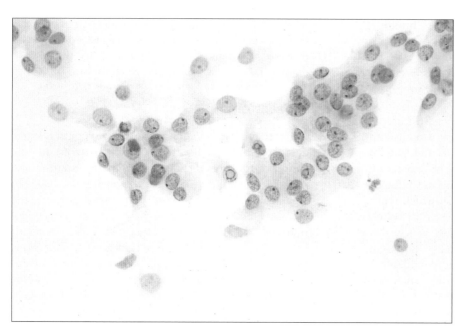

Figure 14.2
Meningotheliomatous meningioma. Female aged 42 years, falcine mass. A high power view shows the characteristic appearance of the nuclei resembling those of cells of arachnoidal granulations. The nuclei are uniform and ovoid or round with diffuse chromatin and small or indistinct nucleoli. Intranuclear vacuoles (pseudo-inclusions), such as seen in the cell in the centre of the field, are frequently found in meningiomas. The cytoplasm of meningioma cells is usually indistinct with ill-defined boundaries. Smear preparation, toluidine blue, ×1400.

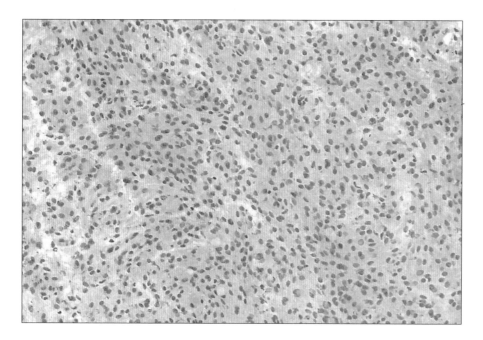

Figure 14.3
Meningotheliomatous meningioma. Female aged 45 years, parafalcine mass. In sections of meningotheliomatous meningiomas the cells are regular and are arranged in patternless sheets with no or few whorls or psammoma bodies. Frozen section, haematoxylin eosin, ×700.

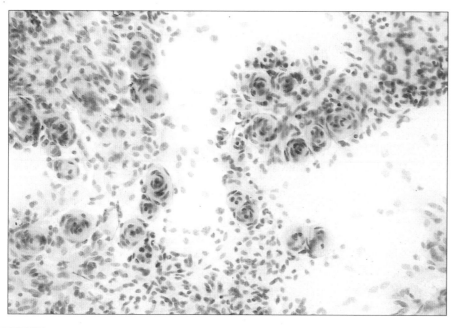

Figure 14.4
Transitional meningioma. Male aged 69 years, sphenoid ridge tumour. The cells of a transitional pattern meningioma generally smear readily into clusters with irregular margins. Whorls are easily identified in this tumour scattered amongst cells which are uniform in shape and size. Smear preparation, toluidine blue, ×700.

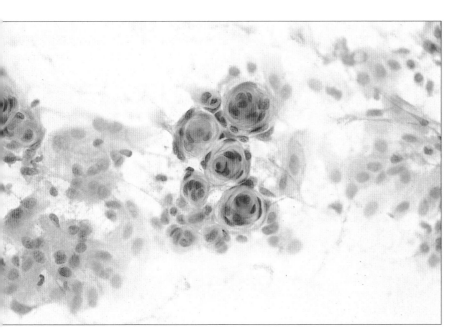

Figure 14.5
Transitional meningioma. Male aged 64 years, convexity tumour. A high power view of whorls shows the concentric arrangement of the tumour cells with prominent flattening of the cells forming the outer layers. Smear preparation, haematoxylin eosin, ×1400.

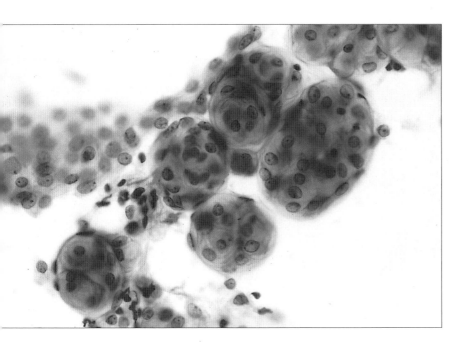

Figure 14.6
Transitional meningioma. Female aged 54 years, sphenoid ridge tumour. This tumour contains lobules which are larger than those in the previous figure and exhibit relatively little in the way of concentric whorling or flattening of the cells. The arachnoidal morphology of the nuclei is readily apparent. Smear preparation, toluidine blue, ×1400.

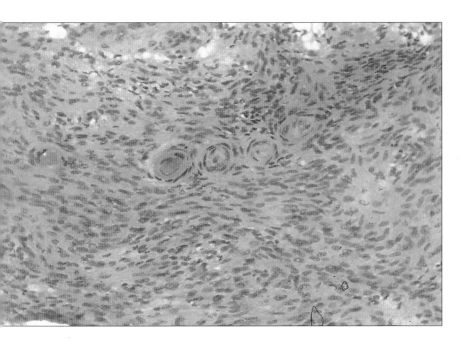

Figure 14.7
Transitional meningioma. Female aged 69 years, cerebellopontine angle mass. In sections sheets of uniform arachnoidal cells are interrupted by whorls which are rather ill-defined and relatively sparse in this example. A whorl to the left of centre is showing central calcification. Frozen section, haematoxylin eosin, ×700.

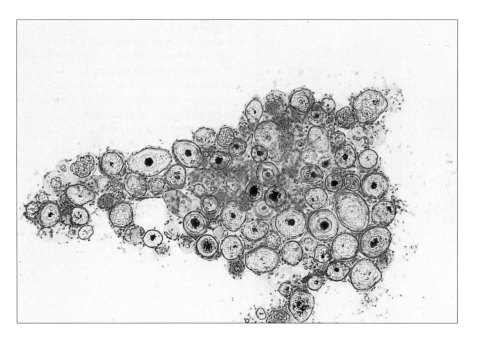

Figure 14.8
Psammomatous meningioma. Female aged 53 years, spinal intradural, extramedullary mass. This tumour is composed largely of psammoma bodies with relatively few arachnoidal cells arranged in the intervening spaces. Psammoma bodies do not take up the toluidine blue stain and appear as unstained spherical structures against the stained tumour cells. The microscope condenser has been left out to emphasize the slightly refractile quality of psammoma bodies. Smear preparation, toluidine blue, ×350.

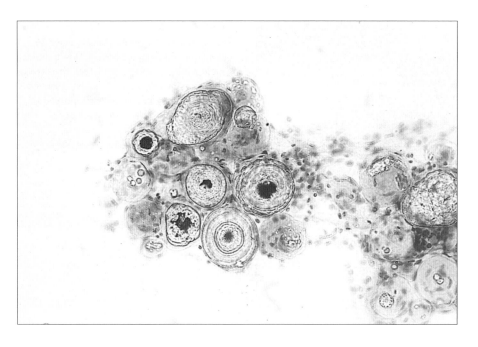

Figure 14.9
Psammomatous meningioma. The same tumour as illustrated in Fig. 14.8. Again the microscope condenser has been left out to emphasize the refractile quality of psammoma bodies and to demonstrate the concentric laminations which resemble tree rings. The majority of psammomatous meningiomas occur in the spinal canal. Smear preparation, toluidine blue, ×700.

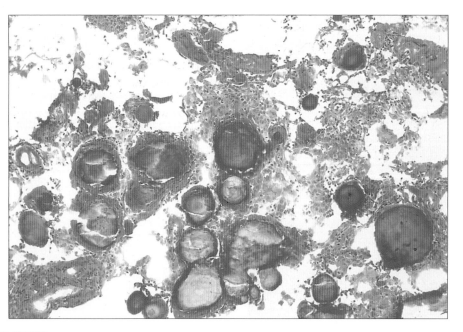

Figure 14.10
Psammomatous meningioma. Female aged 57 years, spinal intradural, extramedullary mass. It may be difficult to prepare frozen sections from meningiomas which contain numerous psammoma bodies. Several psammoma bodies in this field have cracked during sectioning. Psammoma bodies are intensely eosinophilic. The concentric rings are not as apparent as in smear preparations. Frozen section, haematoxylin eosin, ×350.

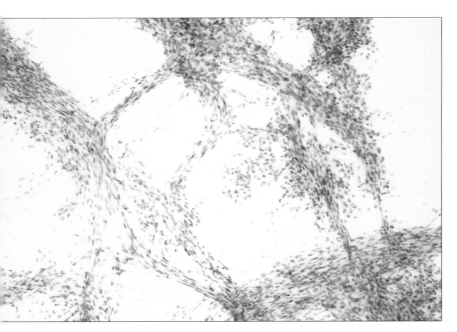

Figure 14.11

Fibrous meningioma. Male aged 62 years, convexity tumour. Fibrous meningiomas are tough and may be difficult to smear. When satisfactory smears can be made they show a low power appearance which is strikingly different to that of meningotheliomatous or transitional meningiomas. The tumour cells are arranged in fascicles which interweave and overlie each other. The low power view strongly resembles that of Schwannoma and in sites where both tumours occur, such as the cerebellopontine angle, it may not be possible to distinguish between them intra-operatively. Smear preparation, toluidine blue, ×350.

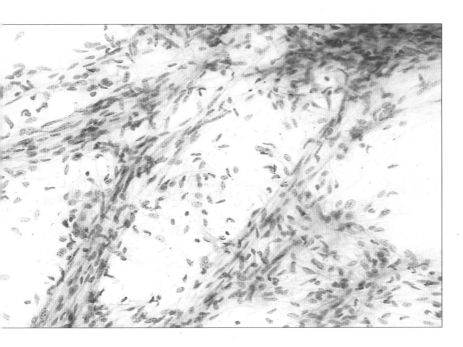

Figure 14.12

Fibrous meningioma. A higher power view of the same tumour illustrated in Fig. 14.11. The cells forming the fascicles are spindle-shaped and their elongated nuclei bear no resemblance to the arachnoidal nuclei of other forms of meningioma. As with the low power pattern, the high power view resembles that of Schwannoma. Smear preparation, toluidine blue, ×700.

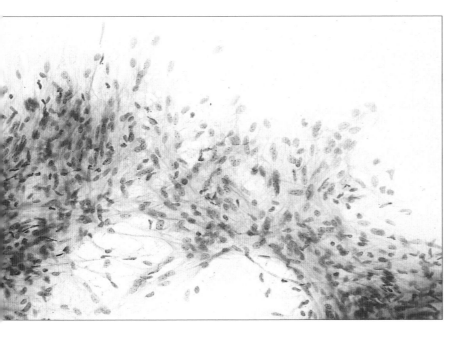

Figure 14.13

Fibrous meningioma. The same tumour as illustrated in the previous two figures. In this part of the smear the fascicular arrangement is not so prominent. Instead, the ill-defined margin of the cell clusters formed by wisps of collagen is reminiscent of an astrocytic tumour. Because fibrous meningiomas lack arachnoidal cytological features and generally lack whorls or psammoma bodies confident designation of the tumour as a meningioma intra-operatively may be problematic. Smear preparation, toluidine blue, ×700.

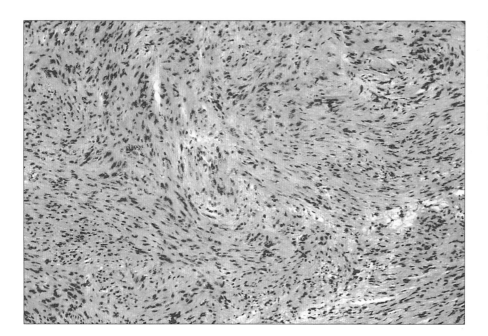

Figure 14.14
Fibrous meningioma. Female aged 64 years, olfactory groove tumour. Sections show cells with elongated nuclei arranged in ill-defined fascicles. As with smears the lack of specific meningothelial features may lead to uncertainty as to the correct diagnosis. Frozen section, haematoxylin eosin, ×350.

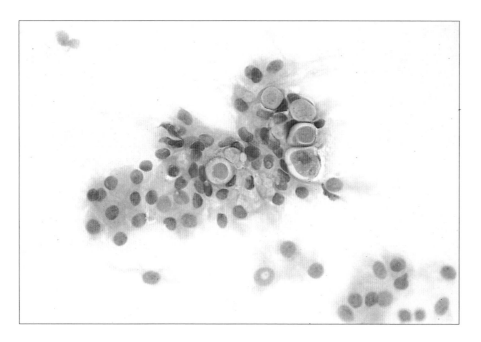

Figure 14.15
Secretory meningioma. Female aged 48 years, parafalcine tumour. The many patterns of differentiation that occur in meningiomas may present a substantial challenge for intra-operative diagnosis. This example is a secretory meningioma identified by the presence of pseudo-psammoma bodies which are small homogeneous spherical structures seen to be eosinophilic in this illustration. This particular variant is readily identifiable as a meningioma because the tumour cells have arachnoidal morphology. Note the intranuclear pseudo-inclusion at the bottom centre of the field. Smear preparation, haematoxylin eosin, ×1400.

14.1.5. DIFFERENTIAL DIAGNOSIS

Metastatic carcinoma may mimic meningioma radiologically and at operation by forming a well-circumscribed mass with a dural attachment. The benign cytology of meningioma usually readily distinguishes it from carcinoma and is especially apparent in smear preparations. Cerebellopontine angle and to a lesser degree spinal meningiomas may be confused with **Schwannoma**. It may be particularly difficult to determine whether a spindle-celled tumour forming fascicles in the cerebellopontine angle is a fibrous meningioma or a Schwannoma. Indeed it may not be possible to make the distinction with certainty either on smear preparations or frozen sections and it may be possible to be no more specific than to categorize the tumour as a benign mesenchymal tumour at the time of operation. In such a situation a discussion with the surgeon about the precise location of the tumour in the poste-

rior fossa, the presence or absence of a dural attachment and the relationship of the tumour to the eighth cranial nerve may be helpful pointers towards the correct diagnosis. Enlargement of the internal auditory meatus usually occurs with Schwannoma but rarely with meningioma. Frozen sections may reveal the biphasic compact cellular (Antoni A) and sparsely cellular (Antoni B) architectural patterns of a Schwannoma.

The cytoplasmic processes and nuclear characteristics of **glial tumours** usually readily distinguish these from meningiomas even in the potentially misleading situation where there is infiltration of the leptomeninges by glial tumour cells. However, fibrous meningioma, in particular, may lack arachnoidal features and the collagen fibres may resemble glial cytoplasmic processes. It should be noted that meningothelial cells, which may be arranged in small lobules or whorls, and occasional

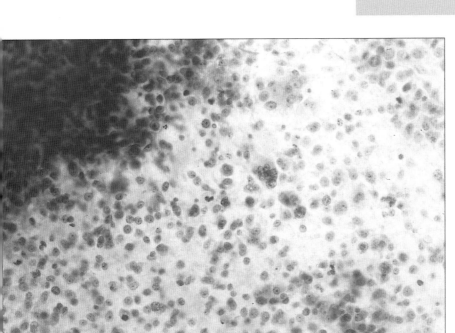

Figure 14.16
Malignant meningioma. Male aged 68 years, convexity tumour. This poorly differentiated recurrent tumour is difficult to identify as of meningeal origin. The cells lack arachnoidal morphology and there are no whorls or psammoma bodies. The thick mass of cells in the top left of the field shows the cells retain some of their tendency for cohesion, however many of the cells in this field show no such tendency. The tumour cells are pleomorphic and mitoses were readily identified. Smear preparation, toluidine blue, ×700.

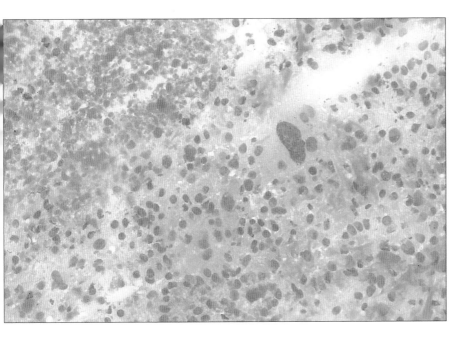

Figure 14.17
Malignant meningioma. Female aged 57 years, sphenoid ridge tumour. Frozen sections show a pleomorphic poorly differentiated tumour with necrosis in the top left of the field. Frozen sections allow the potential to examine the interface between tumour and brain which may reveal tumour infiltration in a malignant meningioma. Frozen section, haematoxylin eosin, ×700.

psammoma bodies, are normally present in the leptomeninges. These normal elements may therefore occasionally be seen in any tumour involving the meninges. The presence of normal or reactive meningeal elements in a superficial tumour should not cause confusion if the size of the tumour biopsy is adequate but may be problematic in a very small specimen.

Haemangiopericytoma is not a meningothelial tumour (see below) and is distinguished from meningioma by the absence of meningothelial cytological features, the absence of cell lobules, whorls and psammoma bodies. Haemangiopericytomas tend to be rather more densely cellular and to contain mitotic figures. If frozen sections are made the characteristic and diagnostically usefully 'stag horn' pattern of vascular channels within the tumour may be seen.

14.2. ATYPICAL/ANAPLASTIC (MALIGNANT) MENINGIOMA

There is undoubtedly a relatively small proportion of meningiomas which grow rapidly although there is no clear consensus as to what constitutes malignancy in a meningioma. The histological features which define atypical or malignant meningioma include poor differentiation, a high nuclear/cytoplasmic ratio and tumour necrosis. An important point in this context is that meningiomas are embolized prior to surgery in many neurosurgical centres and the process of embolization may result in multifocal tumour necrosis indistinguishable from that which may be present in unembolized rapidly growing tumours. A further important feature of malignant meningioma is infiltration of the brain surface beneath the tumour. This occurs almost exclusively in rapidly growing meningiomas and recurrence is almost inevitable. Malignant meningiomas almost never metastasize either cerebrospinally or sytemically.

14.2.1. DIFFERENTIAL DIAGNOSIS

Atypical or malignant meningiomas are distinguished from **benign meningioma** by the histological and cytological features described above. In tumours with evidence of rapid cell proliferation it may be wise to postpone definite characterization of the grade of the tumour until examination of paraffin sections allows assessment of the interface between tumour and brain.

Other malignant tumours which may have a meningeal attachment include metastatic carcinoma, malignant melanoma and sarcoma. In tumours with no definite evidence of meningothelial differentiation, or other form of differentiation, it may be necessary to postpone a definite diagnosis until the results of immunohistochemistry are available.

14.3. HAEMANGIOPERICYTOMA

14.3.1. CLINICAL AND RADIOLOGICAL FEATURES

Haemangiopericytomas occur as well-circumscribed tumours usually with a meningeal attachment. They occur most frequently within the cranial cavity. The importance of their recognition and distinction from meningioma is that they resemble in their biological behaviour haemangiopericytomas occurring elsewhere in the body i.e. they are frankly malignant tumours with the potential to metastasize both craniospinally and systemically.

14.3.2. SURGICAL FINDINGS

Haemangiopericytomas resemble meningiomas in that they have a meningeal attachment and appear well-circumscribed. Less commonly there may be infiltration of surrounding structures. These tumours are highly vascular and may bleed considerably during surgery.

14.3.3. INTRA-OPERATIVE PATHOLOGY

Smear preparations

Haemangiopericytomas tend to be rather tough and smear into highly cellular thick and irregular clusters of cells with relatively uniform round or oval, plump nuclei. In some examples the nuclei may have an angulated profile. Nucleoli are often prominent and this is relatively uncommon in tumours of meningothelial cells. Evidence of meningothelial differentiation in the form of lobules, whorls and psammoma bodies is absent. Mitotic activity may be identifiable. If the vascular nature of the tumour is not apparent it is a challenge to successfully distinguish haemangiopericytoma from meningioma intra-operatively when the clinical, radiological and operative findings are likely to suggest meningioma.

Frozen sections

There is probably a better chance of correctly identifying haemangiopericytoma on frozen sections than on smear preparations because, if present in the sections examined, the typical 'stag horn' shaped branching vascular channels which are so characteristic of this tumour may be seen. The tumour cells have uniform plump nuclei and are arranged in patternless sheets.

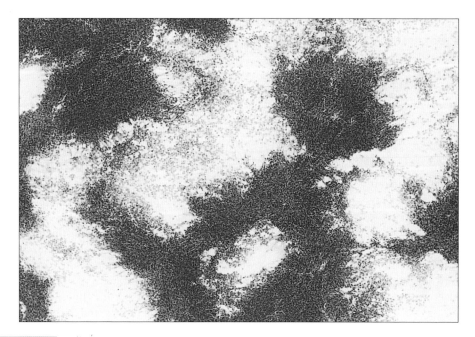

Figure 14.18
Haemangiopericytoma. Male aged 56 years, skull base tumour. Haemangiopericytomas tend to be tough and smear into thick irregular clumps, giving the impression of a highly cellular tumour. Smear preparation, toluidine blue, ×175.

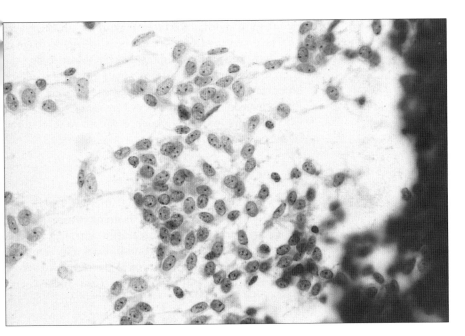

Figure 14.19
Haemangiopericytoma. Female aged 64 years, posterior fossa tumour. The cells have large ovoid or angular nuclei with scanty cytoplasm and do not have arachnoidal features. Nucleoli may be prominent. Mitotic figures may be identified. The characteristic vascular pattern of the tumour is not appreciated in smears making it difficult to achieve the correct diagnosis. Smear preparation, toluidine blue, ×1400.

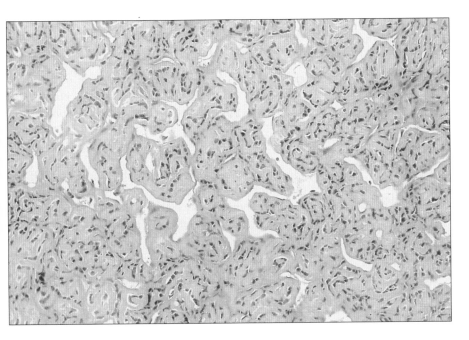

Figure 14.20
Haemangiopericytoma. Male aged 72 years, convexity mass. In frozen sections the diagnosis is readily made by identification of the characteristic 'stag horn'-shaped vascular channels. The nuclei are large and may have an angulated profile. This example contains abundant collagen which is separating the tumour cells and haemangiopericytomas often appear more densely cellular than this. Frozen section, haematoxylin eosin, ×700.

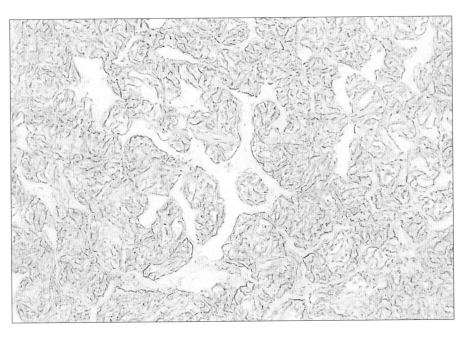

Figure 14.21
Haemangiopericytoma. The same tumour as illustrated in Fig. 14.20. If the time is taken to stain for reticulin, identification of the dense reticulin meshwork characteristic of this tumour adds certainty to the diagnosis. Frozen section, reticulin, ×700.

14.3.4. Differential diagnosis

The principal differential diagnosis is meningioma, particularly in its atypical or malignant form. A major identifying feature of haemangiopericytoma is the characteristic branching pattern of the vascular channels which may be seen on frozen sections but not on smear preparations. Recognition that a rapidly growing tumour attached to the meninges is a haemangiopericytoma may not be necessary intra-operatively as the knowledge is unlikely to influence the operative procedure. It is however obviously important that the correct diagnosis is achieved on subsequent examination of paraffin histology.

14.4. HAEMANGIOBLASTOMA (CAPILLARY HAEMANGIOBLASTOMA)

14.4.1. Clinical and radiological features

Haemangioblastomas occur most commonly in the cerebellum and less frequently in the brainstem and spinal cord. Cerebral examples of this tumour are rare. Haemangioblastomas frequently take the form of a fluid-filled cyst with a contrast enhancing mural nodule of tumour. Although not invariably haemangioblastomas often have a leptomeningeal attachment and it is for this reason that they are categorized as meningeal tumours in the WHO classification. The tumours may be multiple. Haemangioblastomas may occur sporadically or in patients with other features of von Hippel-Lindau disease which include cysts of the liver, pancreas and kidney, retinal haemangioblastomas and renal cell tumours. Most examples of haemangioblastoma occur in middle age. Those presenting earlier in life are more likely to be a manifestation of von Hippel-Lindau disease. A proportion of patients have polycythaemia resulting from secretion of erythropoietin by the tumour.

14.4.2. Surgical findings

As mentioned above haemangioblastomas are characteristically, although not invariably, associated with the presence of a smooth-walled cyst containing clear fluid. The tumour itself usually takes the form of a firm, dark red and vascular nodule in the wall of the cyst.

14.4.3. Intra-operative pathology

Smear preparations

Making a confident diagnosis of haemangioblastoma on smear preparations is a challenge. It is important, by knowing the clinical and radiological features of the case, to have the diagnosis in mind. Haemangioblastomas often smear rather poorly into densely vascular thick clumps of cells. The cells tend to have medium-sized or rather large nuclei which are oval or elongated. The cytoplasm is indistinct. Mitotic figures are absent. There may be evidence of previous episodes of haemorrhage in the form of haemosiderin pigment. Mast cells, the granules of which stain metachromatically with toluidine blue, may be recognized. Although not entirely specific for haemangioblastoma these cells are rarely seen in other CNS tumours and their presence should raise a strong suspicion of this diagnosis.

Frozen sections

Frozen sections give the potential to view the characteristic features of haemangioblastoma which make it so readily recognizable on paraffin histology. These include 'stromal cells' with round nuclei and abundant vacuolated cytoplasm. The typical dense meshwork of capillaries may be surprisingly indistinct and recognition of the characteristic histological features depends on the quality of the frozen sections and on whether the area of tumour sampled is typical.

14.4.4. Differential diagnosis

If part of the cyst wall which does not contain haemangioblastoma is biopsied then the presence of astrocytic cells, often with Rosenthal fibres, may prompt the diagnosis of **pilocytic astrocytoma**. Haemangioblastomas frequently, although not invariably, have a meningeal attachment giving rise to confusion with **meningioma**. Confusion may arise with a **vascular glial tumour**. Even when paraffin histology is available it may be difficult to distinguish haemangioblastoma from a **metastatic renal carcinoma**, particularly as both of these tumours may occur in the context of von Hippel-Lindau disease.

14.5. OTHER NON-MENINGOTHELIAL MESENCHYMAL TUMOURS

Although they occur very rarely it is important to recognize that other mesenchymal tumours may arise in the meninges. Benign examples of such tumours include **osteocartilaginous tumours**, **lipoma** and **fibrous histiocytoma**. Malignant mesenchymal tumours which may arise from the meninges include **haemangioendothelioma**, **angiosarcoma**, **chondrosarcoma**, **malignant fibrous histiocytoma**, **rhabdomyosarcoma** and meningeal **sarcomatosis**.

14.6. PRIMARY MELANOCYTIC LESIONS

Exceptionally unusually primary melanocytic lesions may arise in the meninges. Benign proliferation of meningeal melanocytes may be diffuse (**diffuse melanosis**) or nodular (**melanocytoma**). **Primary malignant melanoma**, cytologically indistinguishable from metastatic malignant melanoma (*see* Chapter 17), has also been described.

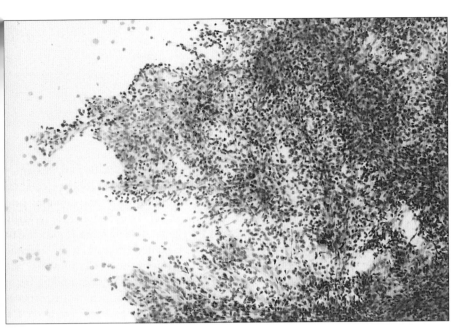

Figure 14.22
Haemangioblastoma. Male aged 63 years. Cerebellar lesion. Haemangioblastomas are generally tough tumours and smear poorly into thick clusters of cells giving the erroneous impression of a highly cellular tumour. The intense vascularity of the tumour is surprisingly inapparent. Smear preparation, toluidine blue, ×350.

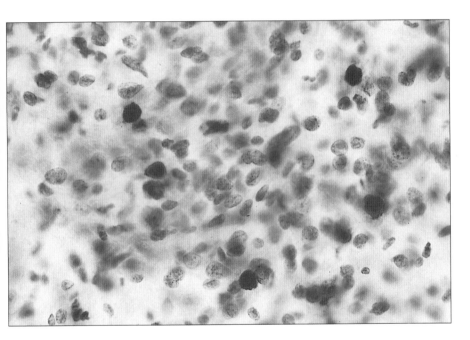

Figure 14.23
Haemangioblastoma. The same tumour as illustrated in Fig. 14.22. The cells have medium or large rounded nuclei and indistinct cytoplasm. The degree of pleomorphism may be pronounced raising a suspicion of malignancy but mitoses are not identified. Mast cells, which have metachromatic granules, may be identified and they may be numerous. Three are present in this field. If they are seen in smear preparations of a tumour serious thought should be given to the possibility of haemangioblastoma. Smear preparation, toluidine blue, ×1400.

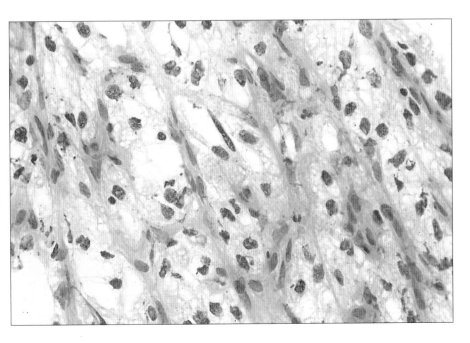

Figure 14.24
Haemangioblastoma. The same tumour as illustrated in the two previous figures. Good quality frozen sections show all the features of haemangioblastoma which are familiar from paraffin histology including the dense capillary meshwork and the intervening cells with round nuclei and abundant granular or vacuolated cytoplasm. Frozen section, haematoxylin eosin, ×1400.

FIFTEEN

LYMPHOID TUMOURS

15.1. PRIMARY CENTRAL NERVOUS SYSTEM LYMPHOMA

15.1.1. CLINICAL AND RADIOLOGICAL FEATURES

In the earlier decades of this century, primary CNS lymphoma was considered a rare neoplasm, accounting for around 1% of all CNS tumours. In the past two decades, there has been a considerable increase in the incidence of these tumours, which can only be partly accounted for by increased diagnostic recognition by neuropathologists as more antibodies for immunocyto-chemical diagnosis and typing of these tumours have become available. The increase in primary CNS lymphoma has occurred in both immunocompetent and immunocompromised patients; however, this group of tumours has a strikingly increased incidence in immunocompromised patients, particularly in the acquired immune deficiency syndrome (AIDS). In immunocompetent patients, the median age at diagnosis in most reported series is around 55 years with only a slight male predominance (as has been noted in systemic lymphomas). In immunocompromised patients, as a consequence of the AIDS epidemic the ratio of males to females is higher (17:1) with a median age of around 38 years. A wide range of disorders resulting in immune deficiency can predispose to primary CNS lymphoma, including genetic and acquired disorders. However, the most common predisposing factors are AIDS and immune suppression occurring in organ transplant patients, particularly with renal transplants. Most primary CNS lymphomas are supratentorial, with the cerebellum being the second commonest site involved. Within the cerebrum the frontal lobe and temporal lobes are most commonly involved and the tumour can spread from one hemisphere to another via the corpus callosum. The brain stem and spinal cord are rarely the sites of primary disease, but can be involved if the tumour spreads throughout the CSF pathway. The commonest clinical signs and symptoms in primary CNS lymphoma reflect the typical disease sites, with personality change, cerebellar signs and motor dysfunction being particularly common along with the non-specific manifestations of raised intracranial pressure.

Radiologically, primary CNS lymphomas show a high signal intensity on non-enhanced CT scans, with multifocal disease being observed in up to 45% of cases. Lesions are typically identified in the periventricular white matter involving the corpus callosum, thalamus and basal ganglia, in contrast with secondary cerebral lymphoma which tends to involve the subdural and subarachnoid spaces. CNS lymphomas are usually hypo-intense on T1-weighted imaging and iso-intense to hyper-intense on T2-weighted images with variable intense gadolinium enhancement. The tumours are usually sharply demarcated from the surrounding brain with a small rim of oedema. Treatment with corticosteroids can cause small tumours to 'melt away' on CT scans after a short period of time, but enhanced MRI scans will usually reveal a small residual abnormality.

15.1.2. SURGICAL FINDINGS

In past decades, the diagnostic approach to primary CNS lymphoma was craniotomy followed by a tumour excision or debulking. In gross excision specimens, these tumours appear as bulky and irregular masses merging into the surrounding oedematous brain. The tissue is usually soft with focal areas of necrosis and haemorrhage, although cystic change is uncommon. The recognition that extensive surgery has a limited role in the management of primary CNS lymphoma has prompted the widespread use of stereotactic biopsy as a means of obtaining tissue for diagnosis.

15.1.3. INTRA-OPERATIVE PATHOLOGY

Smear cytology

In view of the association between primary CNS lymphoma and AIDS, it is important to establish prior to surgery whether a patient with a suspected lymphoma is infected, or is in a recognized risk group for infection, with HIV. HIV infection is not a contraindication for neuropathological intra-operative diagnosis provided the appropriate facilities for tissue handling are available and the recommended procedures for dealing with unfixed HIV tissues are followed.

Most primary CNS lymphomas are soft enough to make good smear preparations, and since classification of these tumours depends extensively upon their cytological features, a diagnosis can often be made on smear preparations alone. Touch and imprint preparations, often used in the intra-operative investigations for systemic lymphoma, offer no significant advantages over smear preparations. Smear preparations of primary CNS lymphoma usually contain abnormal blood vessels, not of the type with hyperplastic endothelium

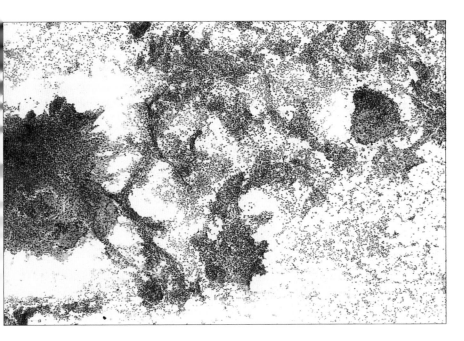

Figure 15.1
Cerebral lymphoma. Male aged 62 years, left parietal lobe. On low power examination, the vascular network of malignant CNS lymphomas is prominent, with tumour cells densely aggregated around the hyperplastic endothelium. Smear preparation, haematoxylin eosin, ×70.

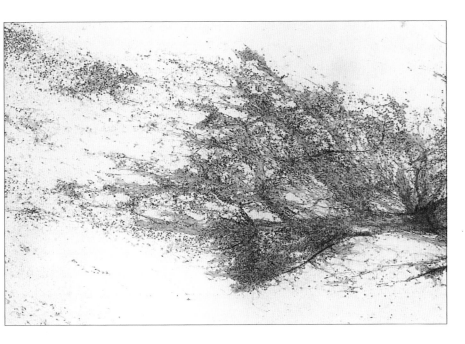

Figure 15.2
Cerebral lymphoma. Male aged 55 years, right parietal lobe. Smears of lymphomas show neoplastic cells spreading away from prominent blood vessels in a monolayer. The vascular endothelium is thickened and at low magnification resembles the hyperplastic endothelium found in malignant gliomas. However, a gliofibrillary matrix is not evident in this case. Smear preparation, haematoxylin eosin, ×70.

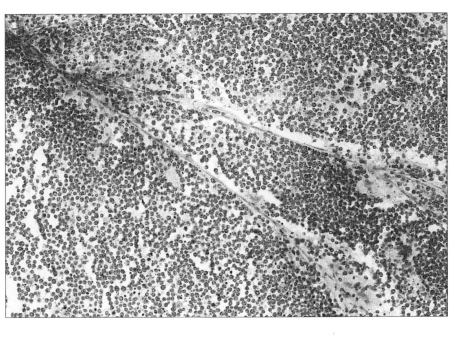

Figure 15.3
Cerebral lymphoma. Female aged 59 years, central white matter. Large pleomorphic tumour cells spread out from blood vessels in a monolayer, with occasional small non-neoplastic lymphocytes present adjacent to the capillary endothelium. Smear preparation, toluidine blue, ×140.

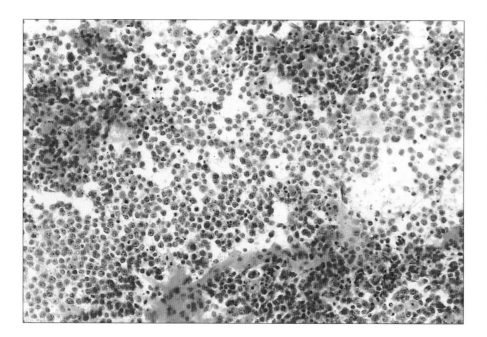

Figure 15.4
Cerebral lymphoma. Male aged 67 years, left cerebellar hemisphere tumour (see Fig. 15.8). The tumour cell population in the monolayer in malignant lymphoma shows no cellular cohesion, with well-defined cytoplasmic boundaries and a clear nuclear outline. Smear preparation, haematoxylin eosin, ×350.

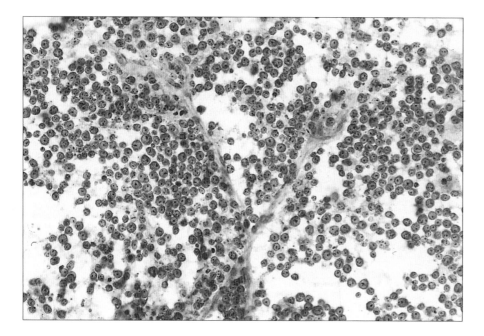

Figure 15.5
Cerebral lymphoma. Male aged 35 years with AIDS, left basal ganglia tumour. The neoplastic cells in malignant lymphoma are intimately associated with the prominent vascular endothelium and show widespread mitotic activity. Smear preparation, toluidine blue, ×350.

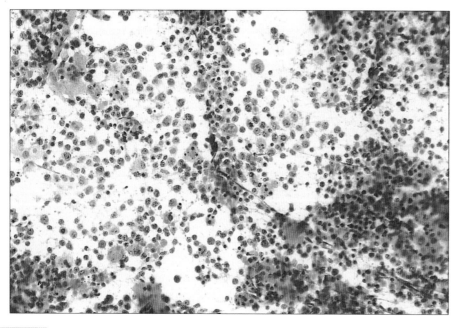

Figure 15.6
Cerebral lymphoma. Male aged 27 years with AIDS, right temporal tumour. Most malignant lymphomas exhibit a wide range of nuclear pleomorphism and include large immunoblastic cells which can be identified on low power examination, and stand out in contrast to the small non-neoplastic perivascular lymphocytes. Smear preparation, haematoxylin eosin, ×350.

present in gliomas, but with expansion of the vessel wall and perivascular connective tissue which are infiltrated by neoplastic cells. The tumour cells spread evenly away from the blood vessels in most cases, thus facilitating inspection of their cytological features.

Most primary CNS lymphomas are **high-grade B cell non-Hodgkin's lymphomas** and contain large immunoblasts and centroblasts, with a high nucleus/cytoplasm ratio and prominent nucleoli. Even in high grade tumours, plasmacytoid cells may be identified and lymphoplasmacytoid cells may predominate in low-grade neoplasms. There are a few reports of well-differentiated low-grade lymphocytic lymphomas occurring as primary CNS tumours, and Burkitt-type lymphomas have also been reported, although they are rare.

A population of small non-neoplastic lymphocytes (usually T-lymphocytes) can often be identified adjacent to the blood vessels within smear preparations. This population of reactive cells can be prominent in some cases and may lead to the erroneous diagnosis of an inflammatory process. However, inspection of the cellular monolayer away from the blood vessel will reveal characteristic cytological features of the tumour cells. Mitotic figures are often identifiable in high grade tumours and areas of necrosis and haemorrhage may also be seen in smear preparations. A toluidine blue stain is particularly suitable for studying the nuclear morphology of primary CNS lymphomas, and the Giemsa technique may also be used on smear preparations of CNS lymphomas to facilitate the study of nuclear morphology.

Frozen sections

Primary CNS lymphomas are often difficult to diagnose on frozen section since their nuclear morphology is not readily identifiable. However, frozen sections may reveal blood vessels in which the wall is infiltrated by tumour cells, an appearance characteristic of primary CNS lymphomas, which should not be mistaken for the perivascular cuffing seen in reactive inflammatory states and within occasional gliomas (*see* Chapter 5). Frozen sections in HIV patients with primary CNS lymphoma may reveal additional pathologies including toxoplasmosis and CMV infection, which are commonly associated with primary CNS lymphoma in this context. Poor nuclear morphology in cryostat sections may lead to the erroneous diagnosis of a reactive inflammatory condition in these cases if only one pathology is actively looked for.

15.1.4. GRADING AND MALIGNANCY

As in systemic lymphomas, a number of classification schemes have been proposed for cerebral lymphoma over the years, often leading to a confusing complexity of nomenclature, particularly for the non-specialist. A consensus classification (the REAL classification) has

recently been published and it is hoped that this will form the basis for future classification schemes. Most classification schemes depend upon the accurate identification of cellular and nuclear morphology, combined with demonstration of a B- or T-cell lineage within the tumour cell population. The latter can readily be performed using immunocytochemistry with commercially available antibodies on paraffin sections and no longer requires the use of frozen section material for this purpose. As indicated above, most primary CNS lymphomas are high grade B-cell neoplasms, although **primary cerebral T-cell lymphomas** are becoming increasingly recognized and in some series form up to 10% of all primary CNS lymphomas. T-cell lymphomas may be identified in smear preparations by their characteristic nuclear morphology, with cleaved and convoluted outlines, and a general lack of immunoblastic cells. A definite diagnosis of primary T-cell lymphoma will require appropriate immunophenotypic studies in paraffin sections.

Previous attempts to correlate patient survival with cellular morphology has been disappointing, as often no clear-cut correlation between tumour grade and survival has been obtained, particularly in immunosuppressed patients who may have co-existing disease processes. However, a number of reports have described patients with low and intermediate grade lymphomas as having a better prognosis than those with the predominant high-grade tumours, and so it is worthwhile to make an attempt to reach an accurate morphological and immunophenotypic diagnosis, while recognizing that prospective studies in larger individual cohorts of immunosuppressed and immunocompetent patients are required for accurate information on this problem.

15.1.5. DIFFERENTIAL DIAGNOSIS

On clinical and radiological grounds, the differential diagnosis of primary CNS lymphomas include other lesions which arise within the cerebral and cerebellar white matter, including **gliomas** (particularly **glioblastoma multiforme**, which can give rise to a 'butterfly' lesion across the corpus callosum, thus mimicking lymphoma), **metastatic carcinoma**, and **intracerebral infections** including **toxoplasmosis** in AIDS. However, these lesions are usually associated with hypodense areas with ring enhancement and calcification or haemorrhage and cyst formation. Superficially located lymphomas may be confused radiologically with **meningiomas** although angiography will help differentiate these lesions.

On morphological grounds, primary CNS lymphoma can be distinguished from glioblastoma multiforme and other gliomas by the lack of vascular endothelial proliferation, the wide dispersal of tumour cells away from blood vessels (which does not occur in gliomas) and the absence of a gliofibrillary matrix or perivascular orientation of tumour cells. Necrosis and haemorrhage however can occur in lymphomas as well as in glioblastomas, but the

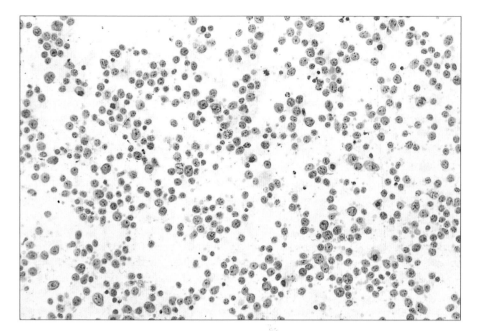

Figure 15.7

Cerebral lymphoma. Male aged 48 years, frontal lobe. Lymphoplasmacytoid differentiation is evident in some low-grade cerebral lymphomas, with a few binucleate plasmacytoid cells present (centre and bottom left). Nuclear pleomorphism is not pronounced in the population of smaller cells, but binucleate plasmacytoid cells are extremely uncommon in reactive conditions within the CNS. Smear preparation, toluidine blue, ×350.

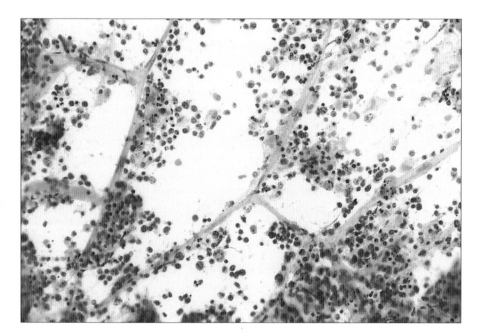

Figure 15.8

Cerebral lymphoma. Male aged 67 years, left cerebellar hemisphere tumour (see Fig. 15.4). The hyperplastic endothelium in malignant lymphomas can show a complex branching pattern resembling that seen in a malignant glioma. The resemblance may be reinforced by the presence of necrosis in the tumour cell population (right). Smear preparation, haematoxylin eosin, ×350.

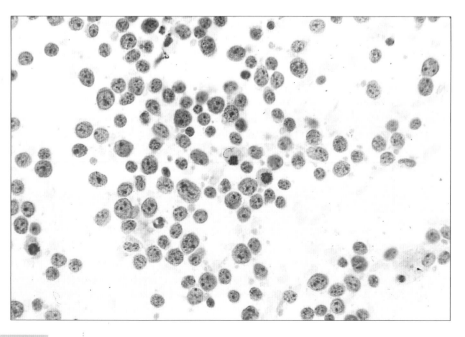

Figure 15.9

Cerebral lymphoma. Female aged 73, central white matter tumour. Malignant lymphomas are readily distinguishable from other primary CNS tumours by their nuclear chromatin pattern, often with multiple nucleoli and clear nuclear margin. Mitotic figures are often present in smear preparations. Smear preparation, toluidine blue, ×700.

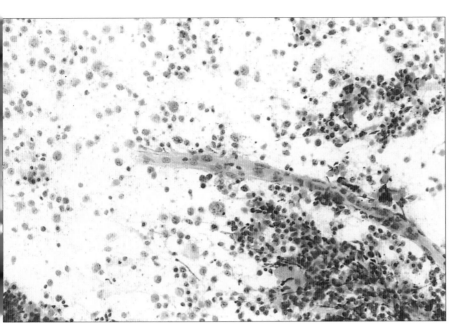

Figure 15.10
Cerebral lymphoma. Male aged 41 years with AIDS, corpus callosum tumour. Patchy necrosis and perivascular haemorrhage (right) are often present in high grade malignant lymphomas in immunocompromised patients, particularly in the context of AIDS. Smear preparation, haematoxylin eosin, ×350.

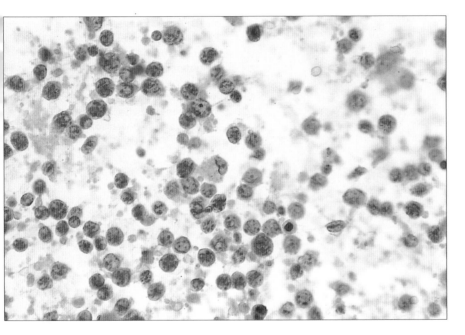

Figure 15.11
Cerebral lymphoma. Male aged 28 years with AIDS, thalamus. Deep-seated CNS lymphomas in AIDS patients are often necrotic, and the presence of abundant necrotic material at low magnification can raise the suspicion of co-existing toxoplasma infection. However, most cases of toxoplasma contain identifiable cysts on smear preparations, with intracellular parasites evident at higher magnification. Smear preparation, haematoxylin eosin, ×700.

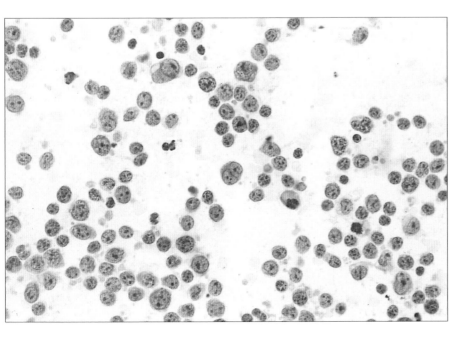

Figure 15.12
Cerebral lymphoma. Male aged 27 years, tumour in right basal ganglia. The malignant lymphomas occurring in AIDS patients are high grade tumours which usually contain large immunoblastic cells, with occasional multinucleate cells (centre) and mitotic figures. Smear preparation, toluidine blue, ×700.

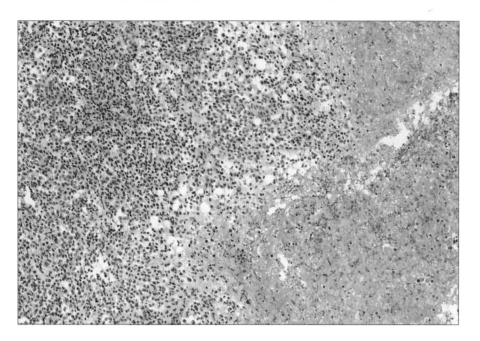

Figure 15.13

Male aged 41 years with AIDS, corpus callosum tumour (see Fig. 15.10). Extensive necrosis (right) occurs in some high grade malignant lymphomas, particularly in patients with AIDS. On low power examination the pattern of necrosis and vascular endothelial hyperplasia may resemble a malignant glioma; this difficulty will be resolved by study of the tumour cell cytology. Cryostat section, haematoxylin eosin, ×70.

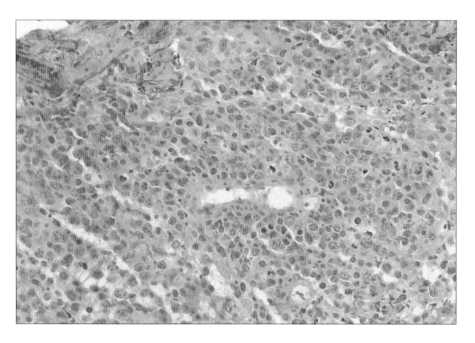

Figure 15.14

Female aged 66 years, right frontal tumour. Expansion of the blood vessel wall and infiltration by tumour cells (centre) is a characteristic feature of malignant CNS lymphomas. The neoplastic cells extensively infiltrate the oedematous parenchyma. Cryostat section, haematoxylin eosin, ×700.

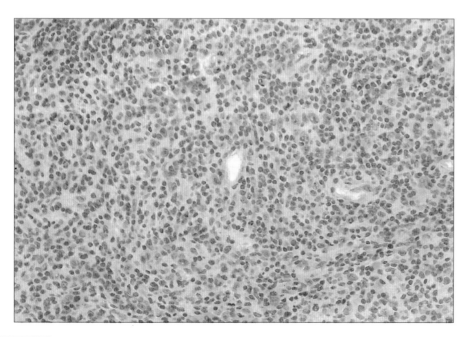

Figure 15.15

Cerebral lymphoma. Male aged 70 years, left temporal tumour. Occasional CNS lymphomas are low grade tumours, with relatively uniform tumour cells infiltrating the parenchyma in a more even distribution than in high grade tumours. Necrosis is absent, but the vascular endothelium is hyperplastic. Cryostat section, haematoxylin eosin, ×350.

characteristic multinucleate giant cells of glioblastomas are absent in lymphomas. The presence of small rounded tumour cells with prominent nuclei and a distinct cell margin in primary CNS lymphomas can be confused with **oligodendroglioma**. However, finely branching capillary blood vessels and calcification are usually absent in primary CNS lymphoma, although characteristic of oligodendroglioma. Furthermore, oligodendroglial tumours usually exhibit a perivascular orientation of tumour cells, which contain more abundant cytoplasm than in primary CNS lymphoma. The chromatin pattern in most oligodendroglioma does not include prominent single or multiple nucleoli, and the cleaved nucleus characteristic of the uncommon primary T-cell CNS lymphoma is clearly distinguishable from oligodendroglioma.

Similarly, a distinction from metastatic carcinoma can usually be made in smear preparations, particularly since lymphomas lack the characteristic clustered or cohesive groups of cells that are present in metastatic carcinomas and usually contain cells with a high nucleus/cytoplasm ratio. Diagnostic confusion may arise with **metastatic small cell anaplastic ('oat cell') carcinoma**, although the carrot-shaped nuclei which are usually present within these tumours on smear preparations are absent in lymphomas. Cryostat sections will usually facilitate this distinction and reveal the epithelial sheets of tumour cells present in the metastatic carcinoma. **Cerebellar medulloblastoma and cerebral PNET**, although uncommon in adults, may be confused with lymphomas on cryostat sections if nuclear morphology is poor. Smear preparations will usually allow a clear distinction between these groups of tumours, since medulloblastomas and PNET have more irregular cohesive cells with elongated or carrot-shaped nuclei without prominent nucleoli. Inexperienced pathologists may confuse normal **cerebellar granular neurones** for lymphoma cells, particularly in smear preparations, in view of their round shape, scanty cytoplasm and rounded nucleus. However, closer inspection will reveal a lack of nuclear pleomorphism, a uniform chromatin pattern which is unusual for lymphoma, and no associated abnormal blood vessels. Frozen sections will help clarify this difficulty and in particular will demonstrate the characteristic location of the granular neurones within the cerebellar cortex.

Primary CNS lymphoma is unlikely to be confused with **meningioma** on either smear or cryostat preparations, since the presence of arachnoidal cell whorls, or clusters of arachnoidal cells with ill-defined cell boundaries, psammoma bodies, and nuclear cytoplasmic 'inclusions' are never encountered in primary CNS lymphomas. This distinction will be particularly evident on cryostat section, where the architectural features of the meningioma will be more readily apparent.

Primary CNS lymphomas require to be distinguished from other lymphoid neoplasms which can occur in the CNS including **Hodgkin's disease**, although this is extremely rare both as a primary or a secondary tumour. The presence of binucleate Reed-Sternberg cells is characteristic of Hodgkin's disease, but their identification in both smear and cryostat sections is not always easy during the intra-operative procedure. Paraffin sections are usually required for a distinction between Hodgkin's disease and other forms of lymphoma. **Lymphomatoid granulomatosis** is a rare lymphoproliferative disorder which is now believed to relate to malignant T-cell lymphoma. In this rare disorder, multiple cerebral lesions may occur in association with pulmonary lesions. The cellular morphology of this disorder is complex and includes numerous macrophages and T-lymphoid cells with characteristic cleaved nuclei. Other lymphoreticular neoplasms including **plasma cell tumours** and **systemic non-Hodgkin's lymphomas** can occur as metastatic deposits within the brain, and their distinction from primary CNS lymphomas can be impossible on morphological grounds until additional clinical information and staging data is available. **Angiotropic lymphoma (intravascular B-cell lymphoma)** is an extremely uncommon disorder which is often not diagnosed until autopsy. However, reports exist of biopsy specimens in this condition, in which malignant lymphoma cells accumulate within intracerebral blood vessels and can variably infiltrate to the surrounding parenchyma.

Primary CNS lymphoma may be confused with **inflammatory disorders** in both smear and cryostat preparations, including **viral encephalitis** with perivascular lymphocytic cuffing, although the abnormal nuclear morphology in the smear preparations away from blood vessels should facilitate their differentiation. Other infective processes may co-exist in AIDS patients alongside primary CNS lymphoma, particularly **toxoplasmosis** and **CMV encephalitis** and their presence should always be looked for and suspected in patients with a relevant history.

15.2. PLASMA CELL TUMOURS

15.2.1. CLINICAL AND RADIOLOGICAL FEATURES

Plasma cell tumours involving the CNS usually arise in the coverings of the brain or in the adjacent bone. These may occur as solitary plasmacytomas or as multiple myeloma, which predominantly involve the thoracic spine. Intracranial involvement by solitary plasmacytoma is rare within the substance of the brain, although a few intrasellar examples have been reported which clinically mimicked a pituitary adenoma. Both solitary plasmacytoma and multiple myeloma tend to occur in middle-aged or elderly individuals, with no association with immunosuppression or AIDS. Patients tend to present with local signs and symptoms relating to bony involvement and compression of neural tissue, particularly with vertebral column lesions.

Radiologically, intracranial plasmacytomas are usually dural-based lesions which are hyper-intense on CT scans and enhance uniformly after intravenous contrast. The tumours are also hyper-intense on T2-weighted MRI scans and give variable enhancement after gadolinium. Spinal tumours are usually also located in the dura, but may extend along and out from the intervertebral foramen. These tumours should be distinguished from multiple myeloma deposits radiologically; myeloma deposits more often involve the vertebral bodies rather than the spinal dura although some lesions can involve both sites.

15.2.2. SURGICAL FINDINGS

Intracranial and intraspinal plasmacytomas are usually firm rubbery tissues firmly attached to the dura, and may appear encapsulated, with a pink/white appearance. Haemorrhage and necrosis are uncommon but the tumours may be adherent to adjacent vital structures including nerves and blood vessels.

15.2.3. INTRA-OPERATIVE PATHOLOGY

The rubbery consistency of many plasmacytomas make smear preparations difficult to make without crush artefact. However, successful preparations will clearly demonstrate the plasmacytoid nature of these lesions with little associated vasculature and a tendency to form a uniform monolayer spread. The degree of plasma cell differentiation can vary substantially both within tumours and from one lesion to another. The tumours may exhibit a spectrum of B-cell differentiation including occasional immunoblasts and smaller lymphoplasmacytoid cells. Mitotic activity, necrosis and haemorrhage are usually absent in cryostat sections, but the plasmacytoid morphology is usually evident, with solid sheets of cells and little intervening stroma or

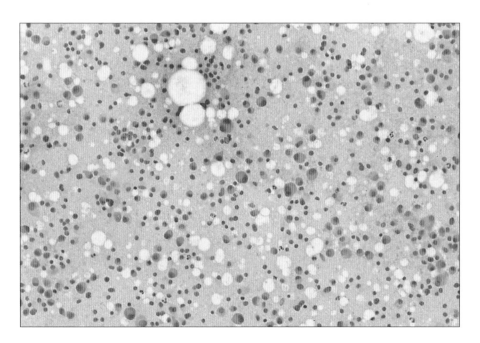

Figure 15.16
Spinal plasmacytoma. Male aged 58 years, T8 region. Most plasmacytomas are easily recognized in smear preparations by the appearance of a pleomorphic plasma cell population (including binucleate cells) with occasional cells containing Russell bodies (centre). The population of smaller lymphocytes in this smear preparation shows none of the nuclear features associated with malignant lymphoma. Smear preparation, haematoxylin eosin, ×350.

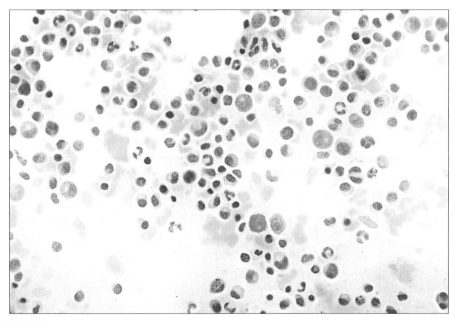

Figure 15.17
Spinal plasmacytoma. Male aged 58 years, T8 region (same case as Fig. 15.16). Plasmacytomas show variable staining of the cytoplasm in the malignant cells, with a characteristic dispersed chromatin pattern. A variety of plasma cell differentiation can be identified in these tumours, with many small well-differentiated plasma cells present in this case. Smear preparation, toluidine blue, ×700.

associated blood vessels. As in smears, a spectrum of B-cell differentiation may be evident, and small reactive lymphocytes can be identified both around blood vessels and within the tumour cell population.

15.2.4. GRADING AND MALIGNANCY

The presence of numerous immunoblastic cells with readily identifiable mitotic figures should raise the suspicion that a plasma cell tumour may represent a multiple myeloma although it must be emphasized that this is a clinical diagnosis which requires additional investigations including staging. It is therefore not possible to give an accurate prognosis on morphological grounds alone.

15.2.5. DIFFERENTIAL DIAGNOSIS

The clinical and radiological differential diagnosis of solitary plasmacytoma includes **meningioma**, **metastatic carcinoma** and, in the spinal cord, **Schwannoma** and **neurofibroma**. These tumours should be readily distinguishable both on smear and cryostat preparations, although a cryostat preparation of a plasma cell tumour may not always be readily distinguishable from a metastatic carcinoma. However the smear preparations, if available, will be helpful in this respect since plasma cell tumours show no tendency to form sheets or aggregates in smears.

Differentiation from a **primary or secondary lymphoma**, however, may be less clear-cut and additional investigations on paraffin sections including immunophenotypic studies to investigate light chain restriction and heavy chain expression are required. This is particularly true with **spinal epidural lymphoma**, which can occasionally extend through the dura to mimic a plasma cell tumour. In the case of skull lesions, a differentiation from **histocytosis X** may be required in younger patients. Most histocytosis X lesions contain a predominant population of large macrophages with prominent cleaved and irregular nuclei, and a variable admixture of other cells including lymphocytes, plasma cells and eosinophils. This polymorphous cellular population can usually be distinguished readily from a plasmacytoma, with its more uniform cellularity. Radiological distinction is also usually possible; the skull lesions of histocytosis X have a characteristic 'punched-out' appearance.

Plasmacytoma also requires differentiation from inflammatory conditions, including **tuberculosis, osteomyelitis** and **other chronic inflammatory conditions**. The relative monomorphic appearance of plasmacytoma, along with the spectrum of differentiation confined to the B-cell lineage, usually allows such distinctions to be made; absence of haemorrhage and necrosis are other helpful features. In reaching a final diagnosis of plasmacytoma it is important to have all the requisite clinical information available including the results of staging and bone scans, serum biochemistry and electrophoresis, and urinary protein studies. These are not often all available at the time of neurosurgery, but should be considered mandatory clinical information before a final report is issued.

15.3. SPINAL EPIDURAL LYMPHOMA

15.3.1. CLINICAL FEATURES

Lymphomas occur in the spinal epidural space most commonly as a manifestation of systemic tumour spread from other sites, or rarely as a primary lesion. Primary spinal epidural lymphomas occur most often in adults aged 50–60 years, but a wide age range has been reported from childhood to extreme old age. Most patients present with lumbar radicular pain, which is followed by signs and symptoms of spinal cord compression, often within a week or a few days. The clinical differential diagnosis includes intervertebral disc herniation and metastatic carcinoma.

The radiological investigation of choice in the past was a myelogram, but MRI studies can now demonstrate the site and size of the lesion and its relationship to adjacent structures. Primary spinal epidural lymphomas occur most frequently in the mid-thoracic region, but cervical and lumbar lesions have been reported. Most tumours extend over 2–3 vertebral bodies, but more widespread lesions have been described. The tumour mass is often dural-based, but may extend into the intervertebral canal, or occasionally involve the vertebral body. The tumour mass may be fusiform or lobulated, producing irregular compression of the spinal cord. Spinal epidural lymphomas are hyper-intense on CT scans, with uniform contrast enhancement. T1 MRI images usually show a hypodense mass, which is isodense or hyperdense on T2 images and gives variable enhancement after gadolinium.

15.3.2. SURGICAL FINDINGS

Most cases of spinal epidural lymphoma are treated by decompressive laminectomy, which reveals a pale rubbery lobulated lesion which is often attached to (and may occasionally penetrate) the spinal dura. Nerve root involvement is less common, but the neoplasm may invade the adjacent bone, or extend through the intervertebral canal to produce a dumb-bell-shaped mass.

15.3.3. INTRA-OPERATIVE PATHOLOGY

Spinal epidural lymphomas are often firm and rubbery, which makes it difficult to produce satisfactory smear preparations, in which case imprint preparations may be produced for cytological examination. Softer cases

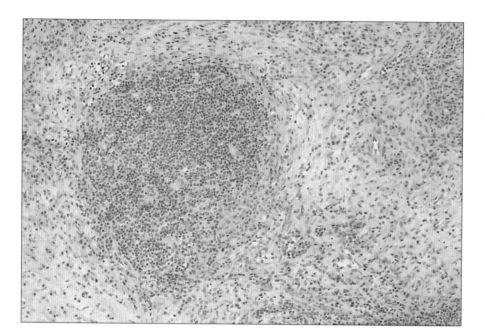

Figure 15.18
Spinal epidural lymphoma. Male aged 66 years, T10–11 region. Low grade spinal epidural lymphomas often have a follicular architecture, with a population of small and relatively uniform neoplastic cells which infiltrate the adjacent connective tissue. Cryostat section, haematoxylin eosin, ×140.

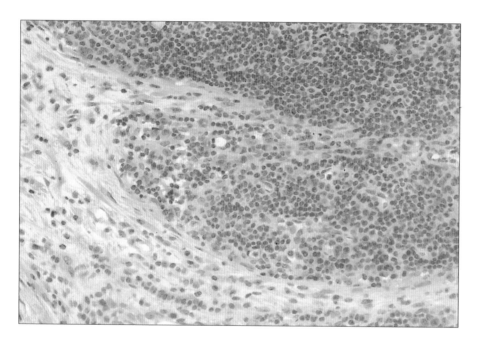

Figure 15.19
Spinal epidural lymphoma. Female aged 70 years, L 2–4 region. Sampling of tissue at the margin of the lesion allows inspection of the infiltrating tumour cell population, particularly around the edge of neoplastic follicular structures. This feature is helpful in distinguishing a low grade malignant tumour from a benign lesion. Cryostat section, haematoxylin eosin, ×350.

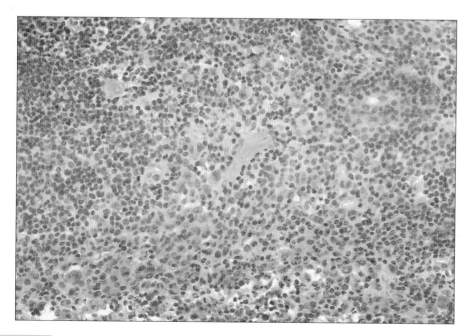

Figure 15.20
Spinal epidural lymphoma. Male aged 61 years, L1–4 region High grade malignant spinal epidural lymphomas usually comprise sheets of pleomorphic tumour cells with no follicular structure, containing prominent vascular endothelium. Cryostat section, haematoxylin eosin, ×350.

will smear more easily, to reveal a population of neoplastic lymphoid cells which is often markedly pleomorphic. Vascular endothelial structures are not as prominent as in cases of primary cerebral lymphoma, and necrosis is uncommon. The morphological spectrum of spinal epidural lymphomas encompasses a wide range, from low grade follicular centre cell lymphomas to diffuse large B-cell and occasional T-cell tumours.

Frozen section examination is helpful in this category of tumours and shows the architectural pattern of the tumour, which may be follicular or diffuse. Detailed cytological examination is not usually possible on frozen sections, although the major tumour subtypes may be identified. Frozen section examination also allows a preliminary study of the extent of tumour invasion, which may be required to confirm an intra-operative complete tumour resection.

15.3.4. GRADING AND MALIGNANCY

Accurate grading and classification of spinal epidural lymphomas is best performed on paraffin-embedded sections, using a standardized system (the REAL Classification). Although most primary tumours at this site are diffuse large B-cell lymphomas, occasional low grade B-cell tumours have been identified, as well as peripheral T-cell tumours. The spinal epidural space may occasionally be involved in Hodgkin's disease, but is an extremely rare site for the initial presentation and diagnosis of this form of lymphoma. It is important for treatment and prognosis to establish whether any other site in the body is involved, so staging investigations should be performed on each patient with an apparent primary lymphoma.

15.3.5. DIFFERENTIAL DIAGNOSIS

The differential diagnosis for spinal epidural lymphoma is similar to that for a solitary plasmacytoma in the epidural space. The clinical and radiological differential diagnosis includes **meningioma**, **Schwannoma**, **neurofibroma** and **solitary plasmacytoma** for discrete tumour masses, with **metastatic carcinoma** to be considered particularly when there is vertebral body involvement. These tumours should each be readily identified on smear and cryostat preparations; the lack of cellular cohesion in smear preparations of lymphomas and their characteristic nuclear morphology usually allow a clearcut distinction to be made. Differentiation between a solitary plasma cell tumour and a B-cell epidural lymphoma with plasmacytoid differentiation is more difficult and may require additional clinical information including the results of bone scans, serum biochemistry and electrophoresis, and urinary protein studies.

Spinal epidural lymphoma also requires differentiation from **tuberculosis**, **osteomyelitis** and **other chronic inflammatory conditions** involving the spine. Apart from the relevant clinical data, both the cytological and architectural features of lymphomas are helpful in this respect; none of the inflammatory conditions has either the range of nuclear pleomorphism present in a malignant lymphoma or the characteristic tumour architecture (even in diffuse tumours) of solid sheets of malignant cells which infiltrate adjacent structures.

15.4. SECONDARY LEUKAEMIC DEPOSITS INCLUDING 'GRANULOCYTIC SARCOMA'

These lesions are of importance primarily as a differential diagnosis in solitary plasmacytoma. Typically, they occur in patients with known leukaemia and in the case of 'granulocytic sarcoma' (a virtually obsolete term) this is usually of the acute myeloid type. The diagnosis on smear preparations is facilitated by the presence of variably differentiated neoplastic granulocytes which spread in a monolayer, although other cell types may occasionally be present, including macrophages, plasma cells and megakaryocytes. These are uncommon lesions and it is essential to obtain full clinical and haematological information before arriving at a final diagnosis.

SIXTEEN

PITUITARY ADENOMAS

16.1. CLINICAL AND RADIOLOGICAL FEATURES

Functioning pituitary adenomas of any size can present with clinical evidence of tumour hormone secretion. The commonest clinical syndromes are those caused by corticotroph adenomas (Cushing's disease), growth hormone cell adenomas (acromegally or gigantism) and prolactin cell adenomas (amenorrhoea and infertility). Of these, corticotroph tumours are the most likely to be microadenomas, too small to be associated with any other signs or symptoms. Larger adenomas will usually produce evidence of mass effect, which may be the sole means of presentation if they are endocrinologically silent lesions. Those with suprasellar extension typically cause visual disturbances due to pressure on the optic chiasm, particularly homonymous field defects. In addition, large suprasellar adenomas are frequently associated with headaches due to raised intracranial pressure. Adenomas encroaching on the cavernous sinuses commonly present with eye movement palsies involving the III, IV and VI cranial nerves, but headache can also be a feature here. Even quite small non-functioning tumours may also present with secondary endocrine disturbances, including hypopituitism due to pressure on the adjacent gland and clinical prolacti-naemia relating to stalk compression syndrome. In pituitary apoplexy, there is an acute presentation with headache, ophthalmoplegia and visual loss. It occurs when a pituitary adenoma rapidly swells due to haemorrhage or infarction within the tumour.

Plain skull X-rays have largely been superseded by MR and CT scans in the investigation of pituitary tumours, but they remain a sensitive way of picking up balloon-ing and erosion of the bony fossa caused by larger adenomas. Using scans, the results are dependant on the size of the tumour. Microadenomas are defined as being less than 10 mm in diameter and are very difficult to identify using CT scans. In T1-weighted MR images they are usually hypo-intense compared to the surrounding gland, but there is no gadolinium enhance-ment and the changes can be quite subtle. Larger tumours are more readily visible in CT scans, with heterogeneous signal, stalk shift and elevation of the diaphragma as common features. MR scans, however, are probably the most useful method of defining the limits of those adenomas which breach the bounds of the sella. The tumour tissue is iso-intense to grey matter using T1 weighting but diffusely hyper-intense in T2-weighted images. As with CT scans, there is moderate to strong enhancement of larger adenomas when contrast media are used.

16.2. SURGICAL FINDINGS

Microadenomas are usually approached trans-sphenoidally and occasionally may be difficult for the surgeon to locate, as for example with very small Cushing's tumours. They characteristically appear as very soft, whitish nodules embedded in the anterior gland tissue. Most examples are well circumscribed, but distinction from anterior gland tissue may cause problems if they are multiple or there is associated gland hyperplasia. Larger tumours fill the expanded fossa, flattening the gland to one side. They may push the diaphragma upwards in a dome-like fashion, extend laterally to fill one or other cavernous sinus, or invade down into the nasopharynx and air sinuses as lobulated masses. The tumour tissue is typically soft and brown in colour, and may be partly cystic. Calcification is not usually seen. There is a marked haemorrhagic tendency, and most adenomas bleed profusely when manipulated. Haemorrhage may occur distant from the part of the tumour being resected and this can lead to post-opera-tive haematoma if excision has been incomplete. The largest adenomas grow massively up through the diaphragma and are likely to require an intracranial approach. They can entirely envelope or displace the optic chiasm, pushing extensively up into the base of the brain and the third ventricle. When such behaviour is not associated with obvious expansion of the fossa, it may be difficult for the surgeon to decide whether the lesion is a pituitary adenoma or a primary suprasellar tumour such as a meningioma.

16.3. INTRA-OPERATIVE PATHOLOGY

Smear cytology

The majority of pituitary adenomas have a very soft texture and smear easily into a thin film. The pattern taken up by the smeared tissue varies both with the intrinsic architecture of the tumour and the way in which it has been smeared. Most characteristically there is a smooth monolayer of cells, which is spread across the slide in a similar fashion to a blood film. The cells in these areas do not mould against each other and show little or no cohesive tendency. Some tumours may not smear quite so easily as this, with the tissue clump-ing into loose aggregates. Even so, there remains a distinct tendency for individual cells to dissociate from the edges of the larger tissue masses, sometimes with a monolayer of discohesive cells in the background. In other cases, the smear can produce well-formed papil-lary structures, with cuffs of tumour cells clinging to branching blood vessels. Once again, however, individual cells usually smear out easily from the margins of these structures to form an intervening monolayer. Very occasionally, cell rosettes may be encountered, without relationship to blood vessels. These usually lack a true lumen and are mostly rather ill-defined structures, merging with the surrounding sheets of tumour cells. Blood vessels are not usually prominent in smear preparations, despite the intrinsic vascularity of most pituitary adenomas. They are mostly confined to the centre of papillary formations or larger clumps of tissue and may be hard to visualize. Most are thin-walled, capillary vessels with a delicately branched pattern. There is often abundant fresh blood mixed in with the smeared tissue, which produces a greenish background colour in toluidine blue stained preparations.

At higher magnification, the cytology usually suggests a single population of cells, even with adenomas of mixed hormonal cell type. In typical cases, the nuclei are centrally placed, very uniform and rounded in shape, and have finely speckled chromatin with no distinct nucleolus. In some adenomas there can be quite pronounced nuclear pleomorphism including multinucleated cells, but this is not common and does not necessarily indicate a malignant tendency (see below). It is sometimes stated that cytoplasmic detail in pituitary smears is more clearly seen using HE staining, but in our experience this is not always the case. Depending on the individual tumour being smeared, either toluidine blue or HE can be more informative cytologically, and this is perhaps one type of lesion where it is worth routinely performing two stains in parallel. The tumour cell bodies are rounded and discreet, without processes. They usually have clearly defined cytoplasmic margins, most easily appreciated where the cells are separated in thin sheets. When the tissue is poorly preserved or over-smeared, however, the cytoplasm of some cells can be very indistinct, with apparently denuded nuclei set in a granular or amorphous background. In some sparsely

granulated prolactin and growth hormone cell adenomas, a prominent Golgi body is visible in smear preparations, with an eccentric nucleus and a clearly defined pale zone in the adjacent cytoplasm. In general it is not possible to predict the tinctorial or hormonal subtypes of pituitary adenomas using smear preparations, nor is it usually necessary to attempt this intra-operatively. Chromaphobe and basophil (ACTH cell) adenomas are certainly not reliably identifiable on cytological grounds alone, regardless of the stain used. In some acidophil (densely granulated) growth hormone cell adenomas the tumour cell cytoplasm may be strikingly eosinophilic in HE preparations, or bright turquoise if toluidine blue is used, but the same is also true of null secretory adenomas which have undergone oncocytic change.

Following pituitary apoplexy, smear preparations usually show infarcted tissue admixed with fresh blood, often with a prominent polymorph infiltrate. Tumour tissue which is entirely necrotic is amorphous and greasy in appearance, but there are often areas where the ghost outlines of partly viable tumour cells are visible and an intra-operative diagnosis is usually possible if the clinical history is taken into account.

Frozen sections

The varied architecture of pituitary adenomas is readily apparent in cryostat sections, which are particularly useful in helping to distinguish tumour from normal anterior gland tissue. In addition, some adenomas will need frozen sectioning because they are simply too tough to make satisfactory smear preparations. This is usually due to an increased collagenous stroma, a feature sometimes associated with prolactin cell adenomas, especially after bromocriptine therapy. As in paraffin sections, pituitary adenomas may show a predominantly sinusoidal or papillary architecture, or simply a sheet-like growth pattern. The uniformly packeted arrangement of the anterior gland is absent,

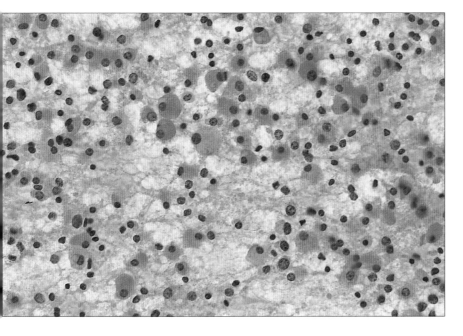

Figure 16.1

Normal anterior pituitary gland. In contrast to pituitary adenomas, smears of anterior gland tissue show cytological heterogeneity, with cells of differing size, tinctorial quality and nuclear pattern. These correspond to the various cell types present in the normal gland, although only the brightly staining acidophil cells are easily recognizable in smear preparations. In addition, the tissue is often tougher than that of adenomas and consequently less willing to smear into an even monolayer of cells. Smear preparation, haematoxylin eosin, ×350.

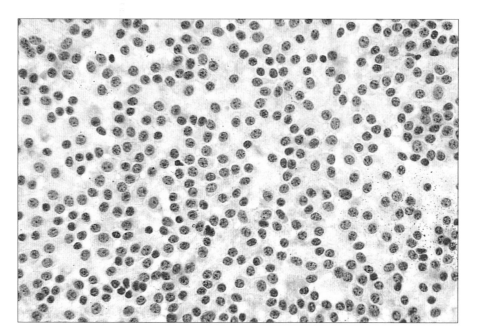

Figure 16.2
Pituitary adenoma. Male aged 58 years with Cushing's disease. Most pituitary adenomas are very soft and smear easily into a smooth, even monolayer of individual cells. The cells show little cohesive tendency and do not exhibit moulding. The impression is typically that of a single cell population, with uniform, rounded nuclei and monotonous cytological features. Smear preparation, ACTH cell microadenoma, haematoxylin eosin, ×350.

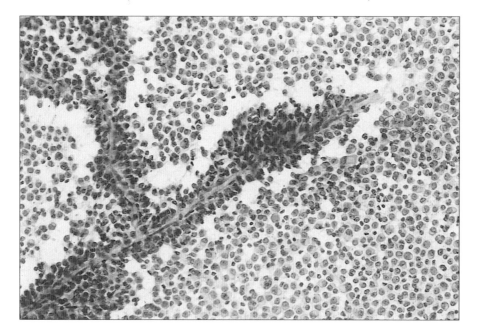

Figure 16.3
Pituitary adenoma. Male aged 33 years presenting with acromegally and visual impairment. In some cases, adenoma smears show papillary formations with central blood vessels and a surrounding cuff of tumour cells. Individual tumour cells smear out very easily from the edges of these structures and there is usually a background monolayer of discohesive cells. Smear preparation, growth hormone cell adenoma, toluidine blue, ×220.

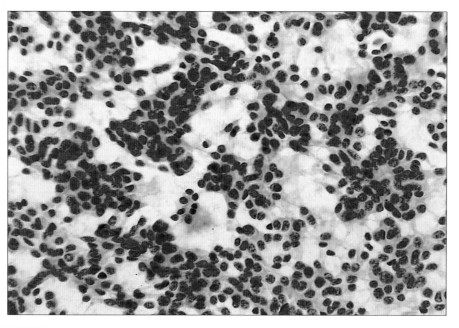

Figure 16.4
Pituitary adenoma. Female aged 41 years presenting with secondary amenorrhoea. In this tumour, the cells have smeared out less evenly than usual, producing a clumped effect. Individually smeared cells are also present, however, and the tissue still has quite a loose, discohesive appearance. Smear preparation, prolactin cell adenoma, haematoxylin eosin, ×350.

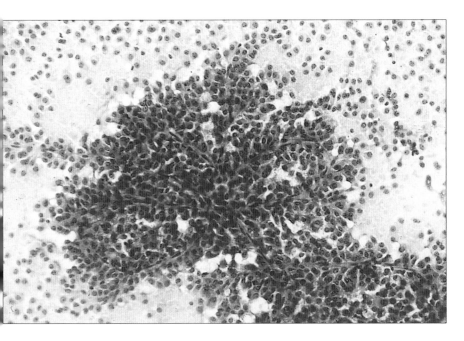

Figure 16.5
Pituitary adenoma. Female aged 65 years with Cushing's disease. Blood vessels are not a prominent feature in most pituitary adenoma smears and tend to be confined to papillary formations (*see* Fig. 16.3) or larger clumps of tissue, as here. They are mostly of thin-walled capillary type, and have a delicate branching or anastamosing pattern. Note the individual cells easily smearing away from the margins of the tissue into the background. Smear preparation, ACTH cell microadenoma, toluidine blue, ×175.

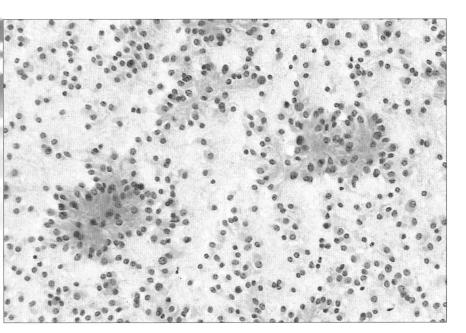

Figure 16.6
Pituitary adenoma. Male aged 60 years with acromegally. Rather uncommonly, some areas of a smear may show large rosettes, usually without a discernible lumen. They tend to have ill-defined margins, merging with the background of cells which surround them. This was an acidophil (densely granulated) adenoma and the tumour cell cytoplasm is quite eosinophilic, especially in the rosettes. Smear preparation, growth hormone cell microadenoma, haematoxylin eosin, ×220.

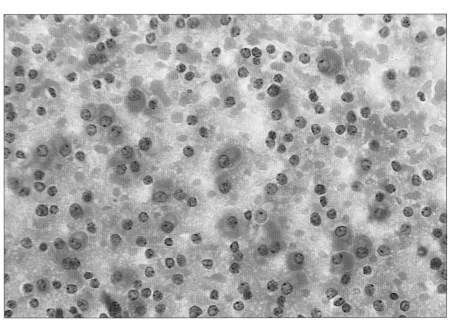

Figure 16.7
Pituitary adenoma. Same case as Fig. 16.6. In toluidine blue stained smears, acidophilia is sometimes apparent as a bright turquoise colour in the cell cytoplasm. Adenomas cannot be reliably classified in this way, however, and a similar appearance may be produced by null-secretory tumours which have undergone oncocytic change. Note the abundant, green-coloured fresh blood in the background. Smear preparation, growth hormone cell adenoma, toluidine blue, ×350.

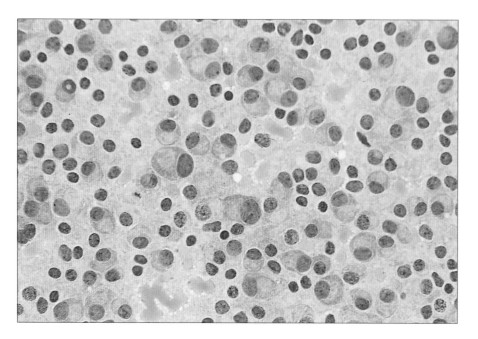

Figure 16.8
Pituitary adenoma. Male aged 45 years presenting with headache and chiasmatic compression. The prominent Golgi bodies of some sparsely granulated adenomas are visible in smear preparations as a pale zone which displaces the nucleus. This tumour also shows some variation in the size of the tumour cells and their nuclei, which is not in itself of clinical significance. Note again the fresh blood mixed in with smeared tissue. Smear preparation, prolactin cell adenoma, toluidine blue, ×440.

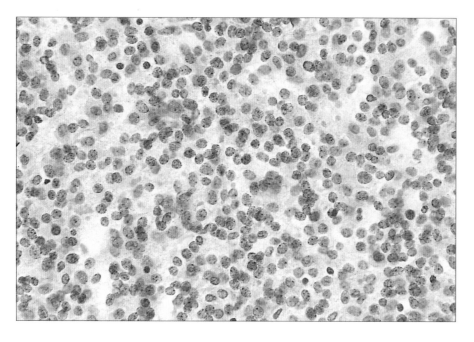

Figure 16.9
Pituitary adenoma. Male aged 68 years presenting with the mass effects of a large, predominantly suprasellar tumour. In smear preparations of most adenomas, the cell cytoplasm is discreet and well defined (see Figs 16.2,3,7,8), but it can be very indistinct if the tumour tissue is poorly preserved or over-smeared. As seen here, the result is a sheet of monotonous, round nuclei set in a faintly granular matrix, without discernible cytoplasmic margins. Smear preparation, null-secretory adenoma, toluidine blue, ×350.

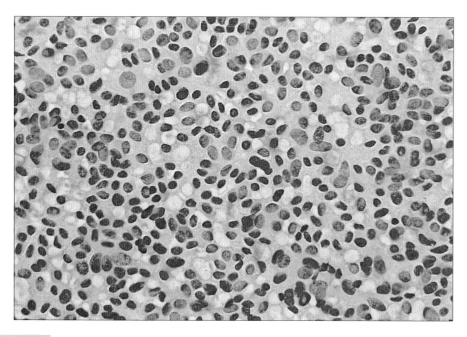

Figure 16.10
Pituitary adenoma. Male aged 58 years with visual field impairment. This case shows a moderate degree of nuclear and cytological pleomorphism which was not felt to have any prognostic implications. No mitoses were found, either in the intra-operative smears or the subsequent paraffin sections, and the tumour had not infiltrated parasellar tissues. The modest suprasellar extension was completely removed using a trans-sphenoidal approach. Smear preparation, null-secretory adenoma, haematoxylin eosin, ×350.

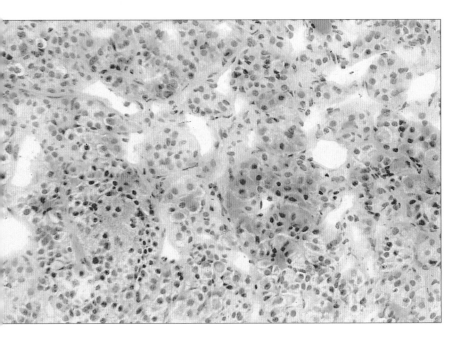

Figure 16.11
Normal anterior pituitary gland. Frozen sections clearly demonstrate the sinusoidal and packeted architecture of the anterior gland, which is particularly useful in the distinction of gland tissue from adenoma. There is a mixture of cell types of differing size and staining pattern, and these are randomly grouped together in compact clusters between the prominent network of vascular channels. Frozen section, haematoxylin eosin, ×220.

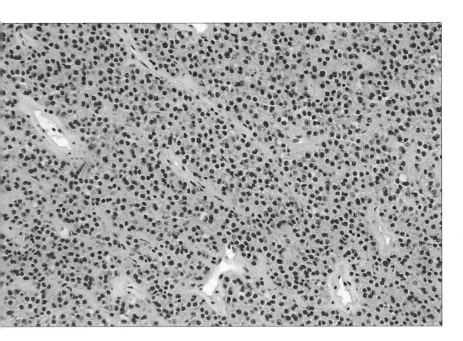

Figure 16.12
Pituitary adenoma. Female aged 43 years presenting with a mass in the sphenoid sinus region. A sheet-like growth pattern like this is most commonly encountered in frozen sections, but some adenomas may show papillary or sinusoidal architecture. The packeted arrangement of the anterior gland is always effaced. As in smear preparations, the tumour cells are usually monotonous in appearance, with uniform, rounded nuclei and homogeneous intensity of cytoplasmic staining. This example showed faint acidophilia on trichrome stains. Frozen section, non-functioning TSH and growth hormone cell adenoma, haematoxylin eosin, ×220.

but may be seen in distorted form if the tissue sampled is from an area of hyperplasia rather than true tumour. Symptomatic hyperplasia is very rare and is virtually restricted to cases of Cushing's disease, with or without a coexisting adenoma. The vascularity of adenomas is more easily seen in frozen sections than smear preparations, with abundant thin-walled capillaries or larger sinusoidal channels. As in smears, cytoplasmic eosinophilia may be due to genuine acidophilia (i.e. a densely granulated tumour type) or just oncocytic change. Once again, it is probably unwise to try and predict the subtype of a pituitary adenoma on the basis of intra-operative frozen sections.

16.4. GRADING AND MALIGNANCY

All pituitary adenomas have a natural capacity to infiltrate local structures, but predicting which tumours will behave badly on the basis of their intra-operative pathology is notoriously difficult. Cytological pleomorphism and atypia correlate rather poorly with invasive behaviour, which may occur in adenomas with very uniform and monotonous microscopic features. Moreover, significant pleomorphism and giant cell formation is quite uncommon, whereas macroscopic invasion of the fossa walls occurs in over a third of all cases. Tumour necrosis is more often encountered, but in most cases this reflects spontaneous infarction rather than a malignant growth pattern. Identifying mitoses is probably the only safe way to try and predict malignant behaviour, and rapid growth should be suspected if more than an occasional mitotic figure is seen in smears or frozen sections. In many cases, however, malignant adenomas will have already declared themselves by the time of surgery with obvious infiltration of parasellar tissues. It is therefore essential to examine the radiological scans before making an intra-operative diagnosis of

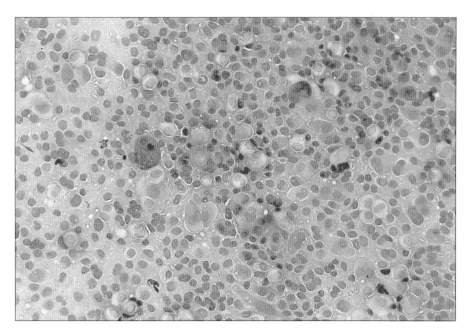

Figure 16.13
Malignant pituitary adenoma. Male aged 80 years. The tumour shows very marked pleomorphism, including giant cells and other cytological atypia. Mitoses were easily found in some areas of the smear. There is also quite pronounced eosinophilia due to oncocytic change. Clinically, there was extensive suprasellar growth, which had erupted through the diaphragma and invaded the base of the brain in the region of the third ventricle. Smear preparation, null-secretory adenoma, haematoxylin eosin, ×220.

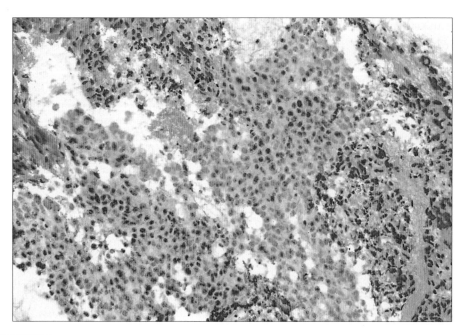

Figure 16.14
Malignant pituitary adenoma. Female aged 27 years presenting with clinical evidence of a large suprasellar mass. There is only mild cytological pleomorphism, but a high mitotic rate was apparent in the intra-operative smears. The tumour had extensively infiltrated suprasellar structures and the cavernous sinuses, and it recurred despite radical surgery and post-operative radiotherapy. Smear preparation, null-secretory adenoma, toluidine blue, ×350.

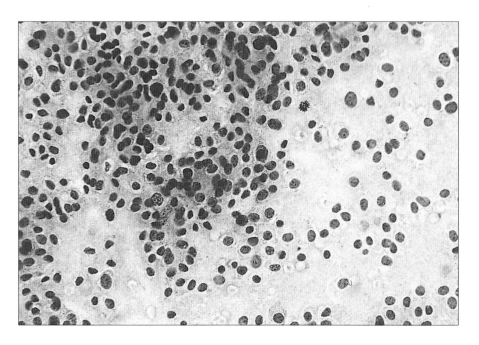

Figure 16.15
Malignant pituitary adenoma. Female aged 69 years presenting with headache and rapidly progressive visual loss. This tumour showed very extensive haemorrhagic necrosis and the original clinical diagnosis was that of pituitary apoplexy. Mitotic figures were present in the sections, however, and radiology showed that the lesion was widely infiltrating the cavernous sinuses and adjacent skull base. Frozen section, null-secretory adenoma, haematoxylin eosin, ×220.

malignancy. Indeed, there is an argument for avoiding the concept of malignant adenomas entirely and simply classifying them as invasive or non-invasive on the basis of their observed behaviour. In a similar fashion, we feel that the term 'pituitary carcinoma' is best defined by a demonstrated capacity to metastasize, rather than purely by cytological or histological criteria. It is nonetheless worth noting that the rare pituitary tumours which do metastasize also exhibit quite marked pleomorphism and a high mitotic rate.

16.5. DIFFERENTIAL DIAGNOSIS

Functioning adenomas

Functioning pituitary adenomas which are large do not usually present much of a problem for intra-operative diagnosis, provided the results of pre-operative serum hormone assays are known at the time. This is important because the endocrinological effects of many FSH, LH and TSH cell adenomas may not be apparent clinically, despite active hormone secretion and raised serum levels. The same is also true of prolactin cell adenomas in men and postmenopausal women, although care is needed not to misinterpret the modestly raised serum prolactin levels associated with stalk compression syndrome.

Functioning microadenomas can present more of an intra-operative challenge for surgeon and pathologist alike, even when there is a clinically obvious syndrome such as Cushing's disease or acromegally. A transsphenoidal or similar approach is often used, and sometimes it can be difficult for the surgeon to locate the smallest adenomas or distinguish them from the surrounding anterior gland tissue. Using smear preparations, adenomas differ from the anterior gland in being softer and more easily smeared into a thin monolayer. Unlike gland tissue, the cells are of uniform type with similar cytoplasmic staining characteristics. This can sometimes be easier to appreciate with an HE stained preparation. Frozen sections are also very useful in distinguishing tumour from normal gland, and will demonstrate both the cellular heterogeneity of anterior gland tissue and its uniformly packeted architecture. The latter is not found in adenomas, although it is present in distorted form in the rare cases of pathologically functioning hyperplasia of the anterior gland. Anterior gland tissue may also be encountered in **lymphocytic hypophysitis**, an equally rare chronic inflammation of the gland which almost exclusively affects women at or shortly after childbirth and can present clinically as a pituitary mass lesion.

Non-functioning adenomas

The differential diagnosis of large non-functioning adenomas includes most other types of tumour which occur in suprasellar or parasellar sites. The list of theoretical possibilities is quite extensive, but can be narrowed in practice by knowledge of the predominant location and extent of the lesion.

- For those tumours confined to an expanded fossa, a **metastasis** should be considered, especially if the smears or frozen sections show cytological evidence of malignancy. Acinar formation is also more suggestive of metastatic carcinoma than pituitary adenoma, but carcinomatous acini must not be confused with the ciliated Rathke's cleft remnants sometimes incorporated in adenoma tissue. **Pilocytic astrocytomas** of the posterior gland should be easily distinguished from adenomas by their prominent gliofibrillar stroma, and hypophyseal **granular cell tumours** because of the characteristically swollen cells with abundant, granular cytoplasm.
- Where the tumour is predominantly suprasellar, it may be difficult to ascertain radiologically or surgically whether the lesion has grown up out of the fossa, or whether it is a primarily suprasellar tumour which has invaded downwards. It is important to remember that pituitary adenomas with massive suprasellar extension can sometimes produce little expansion of the fossa itself. Third ventricular or optic chiasm **pilocytic astrocytomas** need to be considered in this context, as do **metastases**. **Meningiomas** are also an important differential diagnosis at this site, and show a similar radiological contrast enhancement to pituitary adenomas. They tend to smear much less thinly than adenomas, and typical fibroblastic or whorled features are usually apparent using either smears or frozen sections. Less commonly, **ectopic germinomas** may present in a suprasellar location. Regardless of the intra-operative preparation used, these should be identifiable by their characteristic mixture of lymphocytes and large malignant cells. It is worth noting that both meningiomas and germinomas can be occasionally confined entirely within the pituitary fossa. Most cystic suprasellar lesions are readily distinguished from pituitary adenomas radiologically and surgically, but some **craniopharyngiomas** may cause a problem, particularly if they are predominantly solid lesions. The presence of calcification virtually excludes a pituitary adenoma and craniopharyngiomas are almost inevitably too tough to permit smearing. Using frozen sections, they can usually be distinguished from adenomas by their adimantinous pattern and basaloid palisading, even if keratinization is not a prominent feature.
- Some pituitary adenomas invade almost exclusively in a parasellar or infrasellar direction, and may again show little expansion of fossa itself. Invasion of tough connective tissues means that smear preparations may not be possible in these circumstances and even frozen sections may be hazardous if bony fragments are incorporated. Parasellar lesions such as **chordomas**, **mucocoeles** and **primary bone or cartilaginous tumours** can usually be excluded on surgical and radiological grounds. **Nasopharyngeal carcinomas** will usually show clear evidence of malignancy, often combined with evidence of

squamous differentiation. **Olfactory neuroblastomas** tend to present in a younger age group than most non-functioning pituitary adenomas, and can be distinguished by their fibrillar stroma and characteristic rosette formation if frozen sections are used. **Paragangliomas** may be impossible to distinguish from pituitary adenomas using frozen sections and are almost always too tough to smear. However, they very rarely occur as primary lesions in the sellar region and will usually show radiological evidence of massive extension from an origin in the jugulotympanic region.

SEVENTEEN

METASTATIC TUMOURS

17.1. CLINICAL AND RADIOLOGICAL FEATURES

Central nervous system metastases which present a diagnostic problem are often the first evidence of neoplastic disease, occurring in patients without clinical evidence of a primary tumour or systemic dissemination. Intra-operative advice is more likely to be requested if the lesion is solitary, although by no means all multifocal tumours in the brain are metastases. The age of the patient is clearly very important when considering the diagnosis of unsuspected metastases, since these are most unlikely to be encountered in the first few decades of life but become increasingly common in older age groups. In addition to those lesions sited within the brain itself, the neurosurgeon may also be asked to operate on extradural tumour deposits in cranial or spinal bones, thus creating two distinct categories of specimen for the pathologist.

Tumour deposits of the cranial vault or base are not usually a presenting clinical feature of metastatic disease, and in practice the bony lesions which require intra-operative diagnosis are mostly those affecting the spinal column. Spinal metastases typically cause signs and symptoms of cord or root compression due to vertebral collapse. Back pain is also a frequent complaint and may be the only symptom if the tumour has an osteosclerotic tendency, like many prostatic carcinomas. Other common primary tumour types include breast and lung carcinomas, lymphomas and plasma cell tumours (myeloma). These last two are not always metastatic and are dealt with in Chapter 15. Radiologically, plain films generally show evidence of bony collapse if the tumour is not of sclerotic type. More than one adjacent vertebra may be affected, and when this is the case the disc spaces are usually preserved, in contrast to suppurative disease. Any part of the spine can be involved, but deposits are most commonly encountered in the thoracic region. Magnetic resonance scans are very useful to demonstrate disturbance of the spinal profile, with loss of high signal epidural fat and the normal delineation between cord and dura. Tumour tissue within the spinal canal is mostly iso-intense with cord using both T1- and T2-weighted sequences and nearly always enhances after administration of contrast media. Bony infiltration is less well shown, but tends to produce a loss of T1-weighted signal intensity due to replacement of marrow tissue.

Parenchymal tumour deposits encountered in neurosurgical practice are almost inevitably sited in the cerebrum or hindbrain, since dissemination to the spinal cord is usually a very late event, occurring in patients with widespread systemic disease. In cases with a solitary brain metastasis and no known primary tumour there is usually short history, with rapid progression of signs and symptoms relating to an expanding space occupying lesion. The clinical picture is often dominated by the effects of raised intracranial pressure, which can be largely due to widespread peritumoural oedema. Almost any type of primary malignant tumour may be involved, but perhaps the most commonly encountered are bronchial, breast and gastro-intestinal carcinomas and melanomas. Sarcomas are rare in this context because they tend to metastasize late, usually after the primary tumour has become clinically apparent. Most cerebral metastases are quite superficial in location and often correspond to the arterial watershed zones. The cerebral and cerebellar hemispheres are affected with equal frequency. Less common sites include the ventricular cavities, due to choroid plexus involvement, the cerebellopontine angles and the pineal region. The brainstem is only rarely involved. Radiologically, parenchymal metastases show very variable signal intensity in both CT and MR scans. Non-necrotic areas of tumour are often quite high density in T2-weighted MR scans, but they are likely to be iso- or hypo-dense compared to white matter with T1 weighting and in CT scans. Many examples show a central area of lower density due to necrosis, and as a result contrast enhancement is confined to a peripheral rim. Extensive surrounding oedema of the white matter and shift due to mass effect are also relatively constant radiological features.

17.2. SURGICAL FINDINGS

Bony involvement is usually extensive in symptomatic spinal metastatic disease, and thus very obvious at surgery. In some cases there may be no soft tumour within the spinal canal, forcing the surgeon to biopsy fragments of collapsed vertebra. This can obviously cause difficulties in the preparation of smears, and care is needed if frozen sections are not to harm the microtome blade. Often, however, the dura is enveloped by a carapace of tumour within the canal, which is free from bone fragments and can be easily biopsied. Rarely, the tumour can be confined to the epidural space within the spinal canal, without any evidence of bony involvement. We have seen this most often with lymphoma, but sometimes the surgeon turns out to have biopsied epidural fat rather than tumour in these circumstances. The dura itself is virtually never breached, although the surrounding tumour can be densely adherent and difficult to peel off.

Parenchymal metastases in the brain generally appear very well circumscribed to the naked eye. In some cases, they may seem to be entirely unattached to the surrounding white matter, which is usually softened and discoloured due to oedema. The tumours are typically spherical in shape with a firm, granular texture, although some mucin-secreting adenocarcinomas can be slimy. The central part of larger lesions is often necrotic and may appear as a softened, yellow area or a cystic cavity containing turbid fluid. Melanomas are more likely than most other types of metastasis to be haemorrhagic and the tumour tissue may also show obvious brown or black pigmentation at surgery. In quite a high proportion of cases, however, no discoloration is discernible to the naked eye, even when melanin pigment is easily found in smears or frozen sections.

17.3. INTRA-OPERATIVE PATHOLOGY

Smear cytology

Carcinoma metastases in the brain are usually soft enough to make good smear preparations, and in most cases an intra-operative diagnosis can be reached without too much difficulty. It needs to be emphasized, however, that the cytological features are very variable, and it is easy to overlook the possibility of metastatic disease entirely if there are no clinical clues. Most carcinomas exhibit at least some epithelial cohesiveness in smears, forming discreet clumps of tumour cells in addition to larger masses of thickly smeared tissue. Depending on the type of tumour, there will also be a variable dissociation of individual cells around the edges of the clumped tissue, and some softer tumours may even smear predominantly as a monolayer. Tumour cell nuclei are typically large and rounded with pale chromatin and prominent nucleoli, but this is by no means a constant feature. In some cases the nuclei may have a monotonous and bland chromatin pattern, whilst in poorly differentiated lesions they can be small and hyperchromatic. Mitotic figures are always present, but in some cases they can be very hard to identify, depending on the nuclear size and chromatin density. The degree of nuclear pleomorphism again varies considerably and care is needed not to be misled by lesions with very monotonous cytological features, as may occur with some renal metastases for example. Tumour cell cytoplasm is sometimes sparse and indistinct, especially in less well differentiated carcinomas, but it is useful if well-defined cell margins can be identified where the tissue is more thinly smeared. Moulding of adjacent cells where they form cohesive sheets is also a helpful feature. Reactive brain tissue may be present in some smears, particularly when the tumour is not being biopsied under direct vision, and contrasts sharply with the intermingled clumps of malignant epithelial cells.

Identification of the primary tumour type is usually neither possible nor necessary at the time of surgery, but when they are very well differentiated, **adenocarci-**

noma metastases may show glandular features in smear preparations. These include tubular acini, rosettes, papillary fronds and cell palisades with basally-orientated nuclei. Signet ring or ballooned cells with foamy cytoplasm may be identified in some cases, particularly those derived from the gastro-intestinal tract. Where extracellular mucous is present, it is usually visible as an amorphous or stringy background to the cells. This has a rather slimy look and is variably greyish or turquoise coloured in toluidine blue stained preparations but tends to be basophilic if an HE stain is used. Occasionally, smears of well differentiated **thyroid carcinoma** metastases contain recognizable follicular structures, although again this cannot be relied upon. Some **renal cell carcinomas** show pronounced clear-cell cytology, and the tumour cells can even be mistaken for foamy macrophages if they are of uniform, rounded shape. Metastases from **oat cell carcinomas** have a tendency to dissociate into a monolayer when smeared and lack the cohesive clumps of typical carcinomas. The cells have small, dark nuclei with very indistinct cytoplasm and may be difficult to distinguish from those of primitive neuroectodermal tumours. **Squamous carcinoma** metastases normally cannot be specifically identified in smears, and keratinized tumour cells or keratin nests are only to be expected in exceptionally well-differentiated examples.

Metastatic **melanomas** of the brain are typically very soft lesions which can be smeared easily into a thin film of tissue. The tumour cells are much less cohesive than those of most carcinomas and often show a marked tendency towards pleomorphism. Giant, multinucleated and bizarre cells are commonly encountered, often to an extent which is only matched by high grade glial tumours. Tumour cell nuclei are typically large, optically pale and have one or more prominent nucleoli. There is usually abundant, pale cytoplasm and a careful search will quite often disclose finely stippled cytoplasmic pigment in some of the tumour cells. This is greyish-green in toluidine blue stained preparations and golden brown if an HE stain is used. Old blood pigment has similar staining characteristics, but is more irregularly clumped and usually found in macrophages rather than tumour cells. Needless to say, the absence of demonstrable melanin pigment in a smear by no means excludes the diagnosis.

Frozen sections

Extradural spinal metastases are generally too tough for smearing and require frozen sections for intra-operative diagnosis, as will biopsies from skull base sites. In either case, care is needed to select areas of the tissue sample which are free from bony fragments if badly torn sections are to be avoided. Cryostat sectioning is also useful for unusually fibrous parenchymal metastases or those which cause diagnostic uncertainty in smear preparations. The malignant epithelial nature of most carcinomas is usually readily apparent in frozen sections, and in particular the glandular features of better differentiated adenocarcinomas may be easier to appreciate than

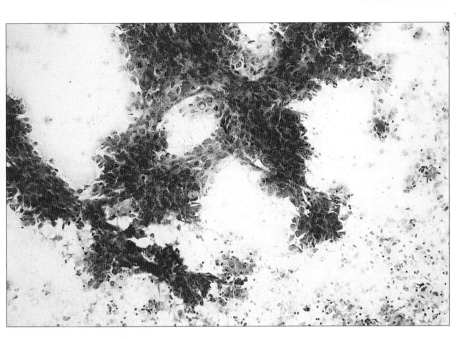

Figure 17.1
Metastatic carcinoma. Cerebral lesion in a male aged 65 years with no known primary tumour. The tissue shows typical epithelial cohesiveness and is forming well-demarcated masses. More thinly smeared, mostly necrotic tumour cells are visible in the background. Smear preparation, toluidine blue, ×110.

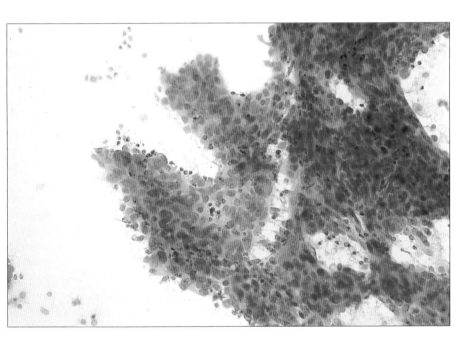

Figure 17.2
Poorly differentiated metastatic carcinoma. Cerebral lesion in a female aged 70 years with no known primary tumour. The smear has formed quite thick and cellular masses of tumour, with little tendency for individual cells to dissociate away from the margins. Considerable cytological pleomorphism is evident despite the thickness of the tissue. Smear preparation, haematoxylin eosin, ×175.

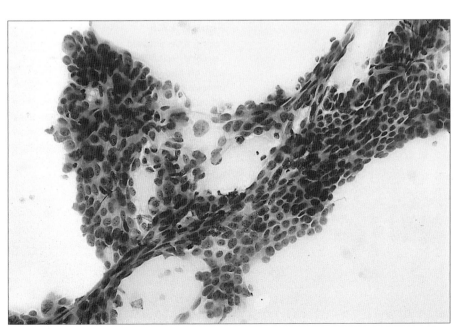

Figure 17.3
Metastatic duct carcinoma of breast. Cerebral lesion in a female aged 58. The tumour tissue has smeared quite thinly, although the cells are still very cohesive. There is nothing to suggest the glandular nature of the primary tumour in this smear, but the cells have a regular, sheet-like arrangement which clearly indicates their epithelial nature. Smear preparation, toluidine blue, ×175.

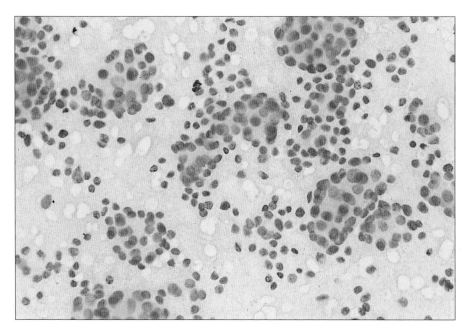

Figure 17.4
Metastatic adenocarcinoma. Thoracic spine lesion in a female aged 73 with no known primary tumour. The tumour tissue is smearing into small clumps but the cells are less cohesive than in many carcinomas. The cytoplasmic margins of individually smeared cells are indistinct and their nuclei show surprisingly little in the way of pleomorphism. Meningioma would need to be considered as a differential diagnosis if this lesion were intradural. Smear preparation, haematoxylin eosin, ×350.

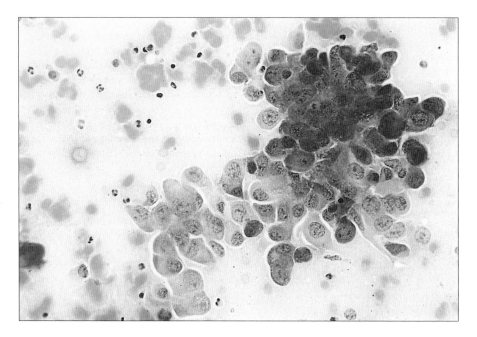

Figure 17.5
Metastatic adenocarcinoma. Cerebellar lesion in a female aged 52 years with no known primary tumour. This clump of cells shows typical cytological features of well-differentiated carcinoma tissue. The cells are cohesive, with circumscribed cytoplasmic margins which mould against each other in an epithelial fashion. The nuclei are large and rounded, with pale chromatin and variably prominent nucleoli. Smear preparation, toluidine blue, ×350.

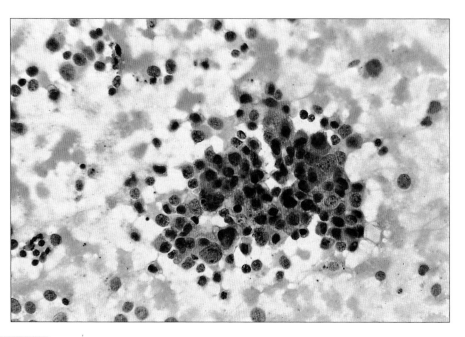

Figure 17.6
Poorly differentiated metastatic carcinoma. Cerebral lesion in a female aged 70 years with no known primary tumour. The tumour cells are mostly clumped together, although some have smeared out individually. Cytoplasmic margins are not as well-defined as in Fig. 18.5, and nuclei show a significant degree of hyperchromatism and pleomorphism. Smear preparation, haematoxylin eosin, ×350.

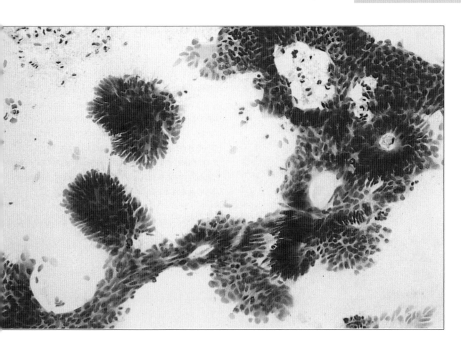

Figure 17.7
Metastatic adenocarcinoma. Cerebral lesion in a male aged 67 years with no known primary tumour. In addition to forming epithelial sheets, smears of this tumour show a distinct papillary pattern. A glandular origin is also suggested by the presence of well-defined tubular acini. Smear preparation, toluidine blue, ×175.

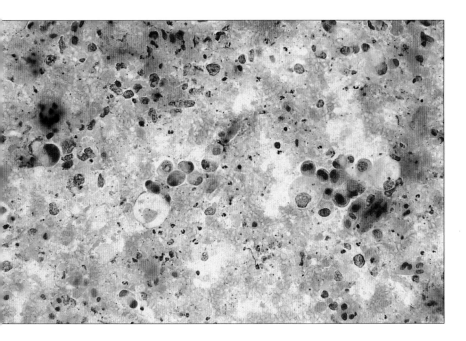

Figure 17.8
Mucinous metastatic adenocarcinoma. Cerebral lesion in a male aged 69 years with a colonic primary tumour. Many of the tumour cells contain clear mucin, and some examples show quite pronounced cytoplasmic ballooning. The background consists largely of red blood cells. Smear preparation, haematoxylin eosin, ×220.

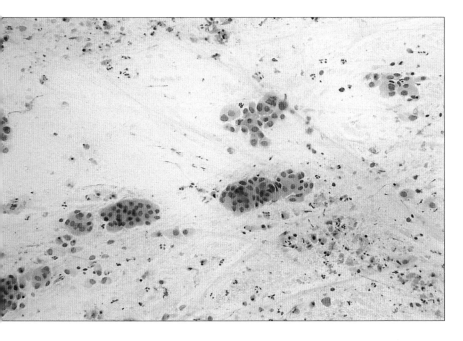

Figure 17.9
Mucinous metastatic adenocarcinoma. Biopsy from the thoracic spine of a male aged 70 years with a colonic primary tumour. Clumps of tumour cells are set in a background of abundant stromal mucin. This has a slimy, rather stringy appearance and is associated with scattered, brightly stained macrophages. Smear preparation, haematoxylin eosin, ×175.

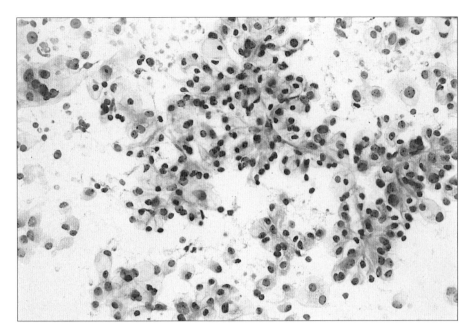

Figure 17.10
Metastatic clear-cell carcinoma. Cerebellar tumour from a male aged 59 years with a primary renal adenocarcinoma. The tumour cells have quite well-defined, foamy or granular cytoplasm. The nuclei can appear deceptively monotonous in this type of tumour and the cells may sometimes be confused with foamy macrophages. In this example, however, the papillary architecture clearly suggests an epithelial origin. Smear preparation, toluidine blue, ×220.

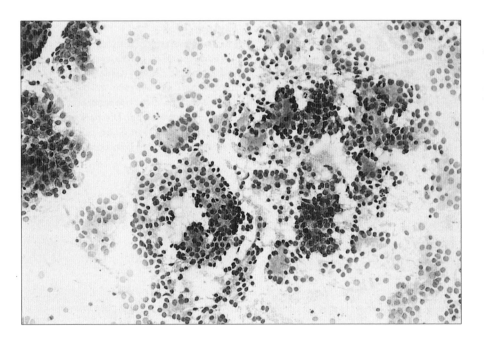

Figure 17.11
Metastatic follicular thyroid carcinoma. Thoracic spine tumour from a female aged 52. The cells are forming solid rosette-like structures which represent smeared tumour follicles. As in Fig. 17.10. the nuclei have deceptively monotonous appearance, and mitotic figures were extremely hard to find. Smear preparation, toluidine blue, ×220.

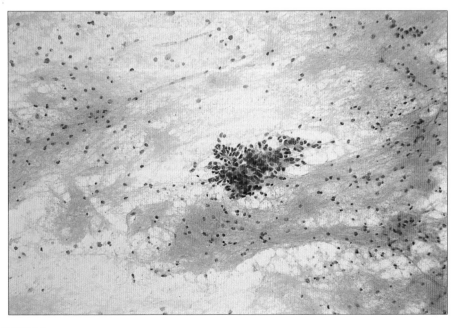

Figure 17.12
Metastatic adenocarcinoma. Cerebral lesion from a male aged 73 years with no known primary tumour. The majority of this biopsy consisted of reactive brain tissue, but careful examination of the smear revealed occasional small clumps of tumour cells with a papillary pattern. Smear preparation, haematoxylin eosin, ×110.

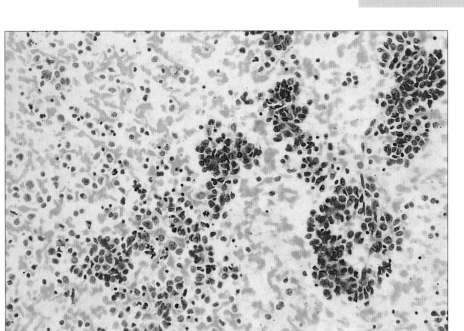

Figure 17.13
Metastatic small cell carcinoma (oat cell carcinoma). Cerebellar lesion from a male aged 61 years with a bronchial primary tumour. These tumours often show little cohesive tendency and may partly smear out in a monolayer. The cells have indistinct cytoplasm and small, hyperchromatic nuclei which exhibit moulding. The cytological appearances can be similar to those of some primitive neuroectodermal tumours, but the age of the patient usually makes this diagnosis unlikely. Smear preparation, toluidine blue, ×220.

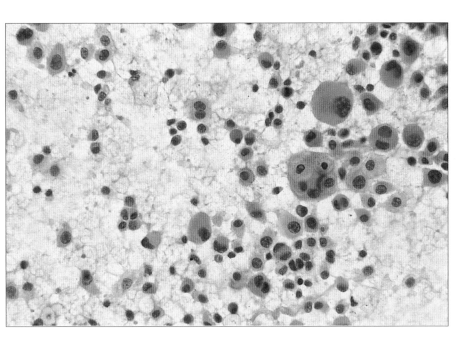

Figure 17.14
Metastatic melanoma. Cerebral lesion from a female aged 40 years with no known primary tumour. The tumour cells are entirely discohesive in this smear and show very marked cytological pleomorphism. Finely stippled brown pigment is just visible in the cytoplasm of one small tumour cell in the centre of this field. Smear preparation, haematoxylin eosin, ×350.

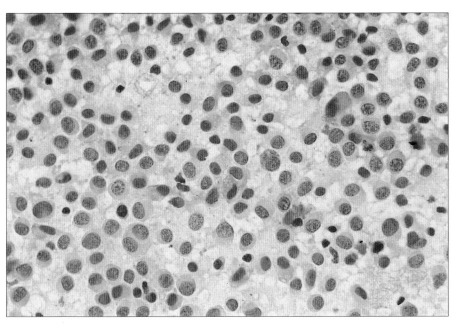

Figure 17.15
Metastatic melanoma. Cerebral lesion from a female aged 52 years with a history of a cutaneous primary melanoma removed several years previously. The tumour has smeared into a thin monolayer of cells which are less pleomorphic than those shown in Fig. 17.14. They have pale, quite well-circumscribed cytoplasm and large, rounded nuclei with dispersed chromatin. The tumour was macroscopically pigmented and fine brown pigment granules are present in one cell shown here. Smear preparation, haematoxylin eosin, ×440.

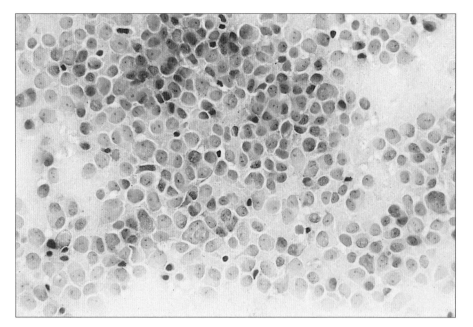

Figure 17.16
Metastatic melanoma. Same case as Fig. 17.15. Melanin pigment has a grey-green colour when toluidine blue staining is used, and is visible as a finely stippled cytoplasmic discoloration in several cells here. Iron pigment has similar staining characteristics but is more coarsely clumped and usually found in macrophages rather than tumour cells. Smear preparation, toluidine blue, ×350.

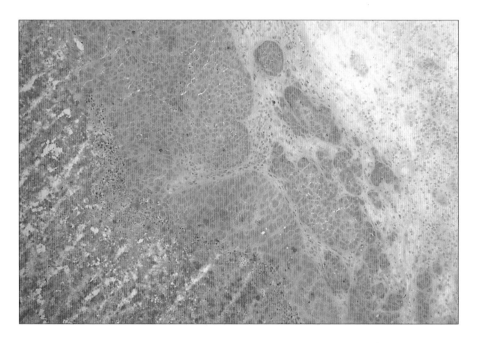

Figure 17.17
Metastatic carcinoma. Cerebellar lesion from a female aged 65 years with no known primary tumour. A mantle of epithelial tumour tissue surrounds a large area of central necrosis, visible bottom left. On the other side of the field, separate islands of tumour cells can be seen infiltrating adjacent reactive brain tissue in a characteristic fashion. Frozen section, haematoxylin eosin, ×90.

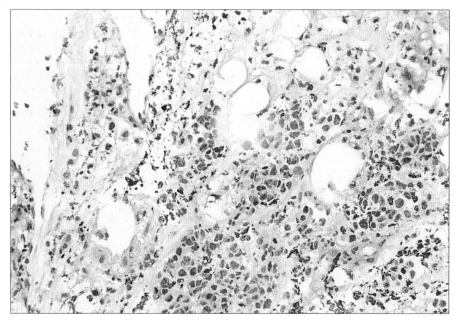

Figure 17.18
Poorly differentiated metastatic carcinoma. Thoracic spine lesion from a male aged 74 years with no known primary tumour. Tumour cells with poorly defined cytoplasm and angular, hyperchromatic nuclei are infiltrating extradural adipose tissue. Frozen section, haematoxylin eosin, ×220.

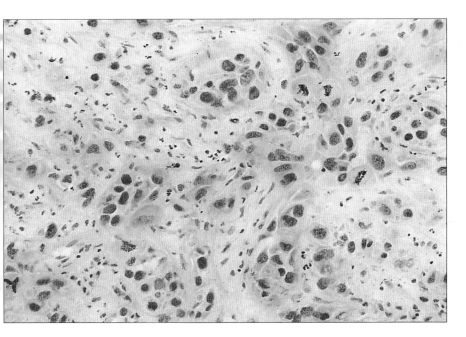

Figure 17.19
Metastatic large cell carcinoma. Thoracic spine lesion from a female aged 63 years with a primary bronchial tumour. Clumps of pleomorphic and clearly malignant tumour cells are set in a background of infiltrated collagenous tissue. There are frequent mitoses. This biopsy was taken from an area of collapsed vertebral body with no remaining bony fragments. Frozen section, haematoxylin eosin, ×220.

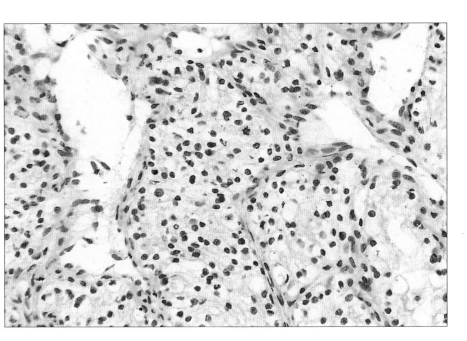

Figure 17.20
Metastatic clear cell carcinoma. Extradural lumbar spine lesion from a male aged 78 years with a primary renal carcinoma. Groups of tumour cells with clear cytoplasm and quite uniform, small nuclei are arranged in an alveolar pattern with some intervening vascular channels. Mitoses were easily found at higher magnification and the tumour showed extensive bony involvement with vertebral collapse. Frozen section, haematoxylin eosin, ×350.

in smears. Frozen sections can also be useful for demonstrating the patterns exhibited by the invading edge of metastatic tumours, whether into adjacent brain or extradural connective tissue. Where very dense collagenous tissue is infiltrated, however, even a gentle biopsy technique may sometimes result in severe squeeze artefact, such that histological detail of the tumour cells is entirely lost. Any metastasis may show widespread necrosis, and in some instances finding areas of viable tumour can be a problem. It is not unusual for extensively necrotic lesions to have an organoid growth pattern, with surviving tumour tissue cuffing blood vessels and forming thin mantles around the margins of confluent necrotic zones. For metastatic melanomas, the same comments regarding pigment apply as in smear preparations, and only finely stippled granules within tumour cell cytoplasm can be interpreted as conclusive. A prominent reactive lymphocytic infiltrate is sometimes a helpful feature, although by no means specific.

17.4. DIFFERENTIAL DIAGNOSIS

In the spine and the skull base, metastatic tumours need to be distinguished from **primary extradural malignancies,** including tumours of bone and cartilage and chordomas. Where the tumour is clearly epithelial in nature this is unlikely to cause much difficulty, but at the time of surgery it may not be possible to be sure whether a solitary tumour with sarcomatous features is primary or metastatic. It can only be repeated that soft tissue malignancies tend to metastasize late in the disease course, when the primary lesion has already become clinically apparent. Some carcinomas in the skull base may be direct extensions from a head or neck primary tumour, but again this is usually apparent surgically and radiologically.

In the brain, some rapidly growing **glioblastomas** can be clinically and radiologically indistinguishable from metastases, and on occasion may appear to be multi-centric. Cytological evidence of glial origin is usually apparent in smear preparations, although very poorly differentiated cases need care in interpretation even if frozen sections are used. **Primitive neuroectodermal tumours** are often very difficult to distinguish from small cell anaplastic carcinomas in either smears or frozen sections. Fortunately the two entities are usually confined to very different age groups and an intra-operative diagnosis of PNET should not be entertained lightly in middle aged or elderly patients. When the tumour is intraventricular the same comments apply to primary **choroid plexus carcinomas**, which cannot be reliably distinguished from metastatic papillary carcinomas using intra-operative techniques. **Primary cerebral lymphomas**, by contrast, tend to arise in later adult life and have very different immediate management implications from carcinoma metastases. Of the two, lymphomas tend to be deeper seated lesions and are less likely to show radiological evidence of central necrosis. Pathologically, they can usually be recognized by their distinctive smear cytology and angiocentric growth pattern in frozen sections (*see* Chapter 15). Metastatic clear cell carcinomas can easily be confused with **haemangioblastomas** in frozen sections, and in some cases a careful search may be needed to demonstrate histological evidence of malignancy. Identification of mitoses or tumour necrosis is essential, since haemangioblastomas may show quite pronounced pleomorphism. It is worth remembering that haemangioblastomas are generally much tougher lesions and unlikely to produce a satisfactory smear preparation. A clear cell metastasis is also more likely if the tumour is supratentorial and lacks a cyst.

Metastases arising at unusual intracranial locations perhaps require particular care in differential diagnosis.

Those in the **suprasellar region** need to be distinguished from pituitary tumours and craniopharyngiomas. Even large, endrocrinologically silent pituitary adenomas are most unlikely to show evidence of true malignancy and will often be associated with radiological evidence of long-standing bony changes in the pituitary fossa (*see* Chapter 16). Craniopharyngiomas are mostly recognized surgically and radiologically, but if there is clinical doubt frozen sections will normally demonstrate their typical, well differentiated squamous features. In the **cerebellopontine angle**, solitary carcinoma metastases need to be included in the differential diagnosis of meningioma and acoustic Schwannoma. The latter is unlikely to cause much confusion with carcinoma in frozen sections or smears, but it can be more difficult to be certain that a cellular meningioma without obvious whorls is not in fact a rather monotonous, well-differentiated carcinoma metastasis. In the **pineal region**, it should be remembered that primary germinomas are pathologically identical to metastatic seminomas, which must always remain a possibility in young adult males. The prominent lymphocytic component of either lesion is usually helpful in the distinction from metastatic large cell carcinoma. In contrast to lymphoma, the lymphocyte infiltrate has entirely benign cytology. Pineoblastomas can have a very similar cytological appearance to small cell anaplastic carcinomas, but as with other PNETs the age groups involved are too disparate to pose much of a dilemma in practical terms. Teratomas of the pineal region again occur mostly in infancy or childhood, but in younger adults the diagnosis still needs to be considered as an alternative to metastatic carcinoma. Definite distinction between the two can be impossible on the basis of intra-operative smears or frozen sections if the teratoma is predominantly epithelial or the metastasis very poorly differentiated.

EIGHTEEN

LESIONS THAT DO NOT SMEAR WELL

Most lesions of the central nervous system are soft in texture and therefore are readily amenable to examination using the smear technique. However, there are certain tumours and tumour-like lesions which because of their tough consistency may not produce satisfactory smear preparations and this chapter deals with the best approach to their intra-operative diagnosis. Lesions which more often than not, or which on occasion, pose such a problem are listed in Tables 18.1 and 18.2. Not surprisingly the list contains several dural-based and extradural lesions. Many lesions which simply prove difficult to smear on occasion are noted here in Table 18.1 and are dealt with more completely in the relevant chapters elsewhere. Some other lesions, which are not dealt with elsewhere, are listed in Table 18.2 and described in more detail below.

With tissue that is simply tough or rubbery it is usually worthwhile attempting to make smear preparations. It is often surprising how much information can be gained from a preparation even when the tissue has smeared poorly. In this situation the tissue forms thick clumps on the slide which may be largely impenetrable to the lens. When attempting to examine tissue which has smeared in this way it is important to remember that, being much thicker than a normal smear preparation, the tissue appears much more cellular than it would in a normal smear preparation or in a frozen section. By skirting around the margin of the tissue clumps, or by scanning the intervening spaces, there may well be clusters of cells which provide useful diagnostic information. Examples of tumours which may succumb to diagnosis in this situation include, for example, meningioma or carcinoma in which only a few cells, when seen clearly enough, are sufficient for a diagnosis.

If smear preparations have been made from pieces of tough tissue and proved unhelpful when examined under the microscope then it is usually appropriate to proceed to frozen sections. Little has been lost, only 3 or 4 minutes in time, in the attempt to make and examine smears. Indeed if, when the smear preparations are made and before they have been stained and examined under the microscope, the impression is that they will be unhelpful then it may be appropriate to proceed immediately to select a sample of the specimen for frozen section. The smears and frozen sections are then processed in parallel.

A further category which predictably poses problems for the smear technique is that of lesions arising in bone of the spine, skull base, or skull vault. Examples of such lesions include metastatic carcinoma, myeloma and primary bone tumours. With metastatic tumours and myeloma in particular it is often possible, by searching through the material available, to find a few small pieces which are soft enough to be smeared. It may be appropriate to liaise with the neurosurgeons in the operating theatre and to specifically request that they send the softest pieces of abnormal tissue which they can find. Even if all of the available material is hard and calcified it can be surprising that gently pressing a piece of abnormal-looking bone to form an imprint on the slide will not infrequently yield a few cells which are identifiable as myeloma or carcinoma. This is really the only option available with which to attempt an intra-operative diagnosis in this situation. Frozen sections cannot be cut from heavily calcified tissue. If all fails then it is simply necessary to report this fact to the neurosurgeons and to indicate that further information will only be available following fixation, decalcification and processing for paraffin histology.

18.1. INTRADURAL LESIONS: CRANIOPHARYNGIOMA

18.1.1. CLINICAL AND RADIOLOGICAL FEATURES

Craniopharyngiomas arise in the suprasellar region and present typically in childhood and young adult life with visual symptoms or hypopituitarism. Radiologically, craniopharyngioma appears as a well-circumscribed lobulated mass which may be cystic and show evidence of calcification. Craniopharyngiomas vary considerably in size and may be very large tumours which project into the third ventricle to cause hydrocephalus. They are slowly growing and essentially benign lesions. Frequently, however, they are not amenable to complete excision as a consequence of the location, which is problematic from a neurosurgical point of view, the tight adherence of the wall of the tumour to adjacent structures and the presence on occasions of fingers of tumour extending into the surrounding tissue. If not completely excised craniopharyngiomas tend to recur.

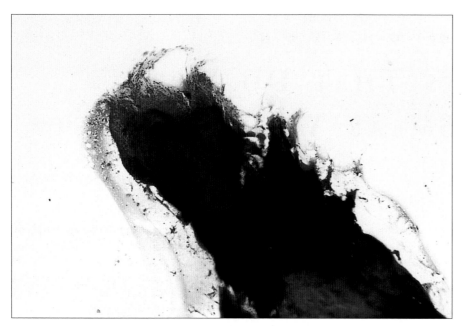

Figure 18.1
Desmoplastic carcinoma. Female aged 41 years, spinal extradural mass. This lesion was too tough to make satisfactory smear preparations and the tissue appears mostly in the form of thick, deeply stained impenetrable clumps. A few pleomorphic cells are visible at the upper margin of the clump illustrated and although tumour was suspected a diagnosis could not be made with confidence. Smear preparation, toluidine blue, ×175.

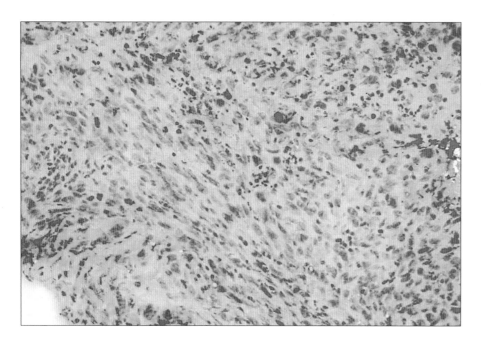

Figure 18.2
Desmoplastic carcinoma. Female aged 41 years, lumbar spinal extradural mass. This is a frozen section of the lesion illustrated in Fig. 18.1. In contrast to the smear preparation there is now little difficulty in identifying a pleomorphic malignant spindle-cell tumour suspected to be metastatic carcinoma and subsequently confirmed as such with the benefit of immunohistochemistry. Frozen section, haematoxylin eosin, ×700.

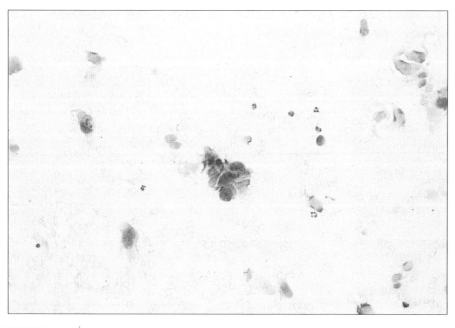

Figure 18.3
Metastatic carcinoma. Male aged 87 years, spinal extradural mass. This lesion macroscopically had the appearance of abnormal bone. Smear preparations or frozen sections could not be made from the specimen. Imprints were made by gently pressing the specimen several times onto a slide. These preparations revealed malignant cells, some of which were arranged in small clusters, allowing a diagnosis of tumour, probable carcinoma, to be made at the time of surgery. Imprint preparation, toluidine blue, ×700.

Table 18.1

Tumours which may not produce satisfactory smear preparations (these are dealt with elsewhere in the relevant chapters)

Astrocytic tumours
    glioblastoma (with desmoplasia)
    gliosarcoma
    pilocytic astrocytoma
    pleomorphic xanthoastrocytoma
    subependymal giant cell astrocytoma
Ependymal tumours
    subependymoma
Neuronal tumours
    ganglion cell tumours
Pineal region tumours
    teratoma
Primitive neuroectodermal tumours
    desmoplastic medulloblastoma
Nerve root tumours
    peripheral nerve sheath tumours
Meningeal tumours
    meningioma (especially fibrous and psammomatous
      variants, infiltrated bone, meningioma en plaque)
    haemangiopericytoma
    haemangioblastoma
    osteocartilaginous tumours
    meningeal sarcoma
Lymphomas and plasma cell tumours
    lymphoma (bone metastasis)
    myeloma
Metastatic tumours
    carcinoma (bone metastasis or desmoplastic carcinoma)
    melanoma (bone metastasis)

Table 18.2

Other lesions which may not produce satisfactory smear preparations

Intradural
    Craniopharyngioma
    Nervous system cysts
      Rathke's cleft cyst
      colloid cyst
      epidermoid cyst
      dermoid cyst
      enterogenous (endodermal) cyst
      neuroglial cyst
      arachnoid cyst
    Vascular lesions
    Lipoma
Extradural
    Chordoma
    Sequestrated prolapsed intervertebral disc
    Non-neoplastic bone lesions
      fibrous dysplasia
      Langerhan's cell histiocytosis
      aneurysmal bone cyst
    Tumours arising in bone
      osteoma
      chondroma
      osteochondroma
      giant cell tumour of bone
      osteosarcoma
      chondrosarcoma
    Tumours arising in soft tissue

18.1.2. SURGICAL FINDINGS

Craniopharyngiomas typically lie above the diaphragma sellae, below the third ventricle and behind the optic chiasm. The visible surfaces are smooth and lobulated although the surface is usually tightly adherent to structures with which the tumour has come into contact. Cysts within the tumour contain viscous brown fluid, classically described as 'machine oil', which glistens as a consequence of cholesterol crystals suspended within the fluid. The solid parts of the tumour are greyish-white in colour, tough and focally calcified.

18.1.3. INTRA-OPERATIVE PATHOLOGY

Smear cytology

Craniopharyngiomas are tough and generally smear reluctantly. However, smear preparations may reveal clumps or sheets of cohesive, uniform epithelial cells. The cysts in craniopharyngiomas frequently contain macrophages with abundant foamy cytoplasm and these may be present in smears. Smears of central nervous tissue immediately adjacent to a craniopharyngioma may show a florid reactive gliosis. As a result of the characteristic clinical and radiological features of this tumour there is usually little doubt as to its identity at the time of surgery. Observation of the microscopic features described above, although not entirely specific, is usually sufficient reassurance as to the correct identity of the mass.

Frozen sections

Provided the lesion is not intensely calcified, frozen sections will reveal the characteristic sheets or lobules of uniform epithelial cells. Cysts of varying size may be present appearing either empty or filled with amorphous eosinophilic material or macrophages. Cholesterol clefts may be identified. Areas of fibrosis are common and there may be a chronic inflammatory cell infiltrate. As mentioned above, if the specimen comes from central nervous tissue immediately adjacent to the tumour then a florid chronic reactive gliosis, often containing Rosenthal fibres, will be seen.

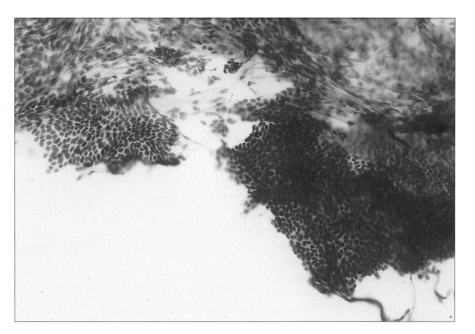

Figure 18.4
Craniopharyngioma. Female aged 31 years, suprasellar mass. Although craniopharyngiomas are usually tough they often can be made to reveal clumps or sheets of cohesive uniform epithelial cells in smear preparations. Although the cytological appearances are not entirely specific, given the characteristic location of the lesion, there is little doubt as to the correct diagnosis. Smear preparation, toluidine blue, ×700.

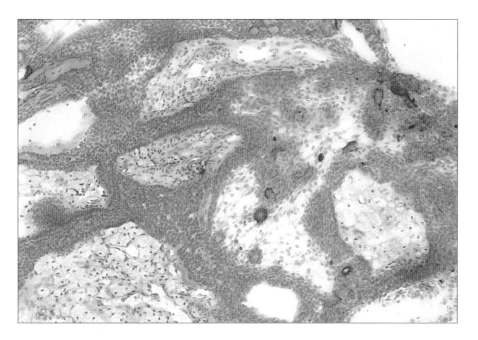

Figure 18.5
Craniopharyngioma. Male aged 61 years, suprasellar mass. Frozen sections show the instantly recognizable appearance of a craniopharyngioma with sheets of uniform epithelial cells enclosing cysts. Some of the cysts contain macrophages with abundant cytoplasm. Small areas of calcification are also included. Frozen section, haematoxylin eosin, ×350.

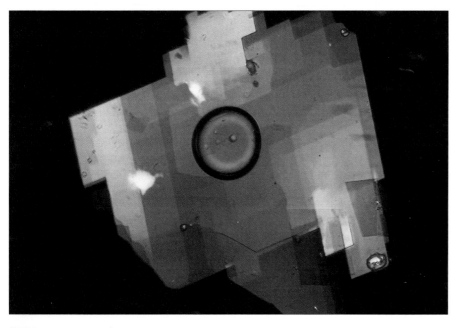

Figure 18.6
Craniopharyngioma. Male aged 23 years, suprasellar mass. Fluid was drained from a cyst which had re-accumulated several years after a de-bulking operation. A tissue diagnosis of craniopharyngioma had therefore been made previously. Wet preparations of the fluid, which had the characteristic 'machine oil' appearance, was found to contain cholesterol crystals when viewed with polarized light. Identification of cholesterol crystals may be diagnostically helpful when surgery is performed to drain a suprasellar cyst without tissue being obtained for histology. Unstained wet preparation, polarized light, ×1400.

Cyst fluid preparations

If smear preparations and/or frozen sections prove unhelpful or if tissue is not available then examination of wet preparations of cyst fluid is often rewarding. These are made simply by placing a few drops of fluid on a slide and overlaying this with a cover slip. Examination of the fluid under polarized light will show cholesterol crystals with the characteristic appearance illustrated. On occasions the only specimen obtained at a neurosurgical procedure on a craniopharyngioma is a sample of fluid drained from a cyst. In this situation the identification of cholesterol crystals in the fluid, in the appropriate clinical and radiological setting, is virtually diagnostic.

18.1.4. DIFFERENTIAL DIAGNOSIS

The clinical and pathological features of craniopharyngioma are so characteristic that there is usually little doubt as to the correct diagnosis. A craniopharyngioma with a large cyst lined by epithelial cells and with little in the way of a solid component may be difficult to distinguish from other forms of **epithelium-lined cyst**, such as a dermoid cyst. Indeed the existence of such lesions causes some blurring of the margins of these diagnostic entities. The epithelial nature of the cells in craniopharyngioma may give rise to confusion with a **metastatic carcinoma**. The distinction is made partly on the basis of the age of the patient as craniopharyngiomas infrequently present in middle life or old age and partly on the lack of malignant cytological features in a craniopharyngioma. If the surgical specimen provided is from the edge of the lesion it may be composed of central nervous tissue exhibiting a florid chronic reactive gliosis, including the presence of Rosenthal fibres, and may be misinterpreted as **pilocytic astrocytoma**. Pilocytic astrocytomas, which may occur in relation to the optic nerves, optic chiasm and hypothalamus, radiologically usually appear as expansions of these structures whereas they are typically indented by a craniopharyngioma.

18.2. INTRADURAL LESIONS: NERVOUS SYSTEM CYSTS

A single cyst or multiple cysts may form a prominent component of a wide range of tumours of the nervous system, mostly benign, and including the following: fibrillary astrocytoma, pilocytic astrocytoma, pleomorphic xanthoastrocytoma, ependymoma, ganglion cell tumour, dysembryoplastic neuroepithelial tumour, Schwannoma, haemangioblastoma, teratoma, choroid plexus tumour and craniopharyngioma. These lesions usually have an obvious solid component which if biopsied will lead to the correct diagnosis whether by smears or frozen sections. They are dealt with in the appropriate chapters covering specific tumour entities and cystic lesions are also mentioned in Chapter 5. In addition, benign cysts with thin walls lined by a variety of cell types may also occur and these are described in more detail below.

Benign thin-walled cysts are relatively uncommon. They tend to expand slowly and present clinically as a consequence of this expansion. On imaging all are well-circumscribed spherical or lobulated lesions, but the appearances vary somewhat mainly according to the material contained within the cyst. These lesions are amenable to cure if they can be completely excised, although this may not be feasible. Contamination of CSF with cyst contents may give rise to a chemical meningitis.

Rathke's cleft cyst is an intrasellar or, less commonly, suprasellar cyst which is lined by a single-layered cuboidal or columnar ciliated epithelium. The epithelium may undergo squamous metaplasia. The appearance on T1-weighted MR may be high or low signal depending on the cyst contents. Very small cysts of similar structure are commonly found lying between the anterior and posterior parts of the pituitary gland and are therefore sometimes encountered in smear preparations or frozen sections of pituitary adenoma.

Colloid cyst occurs specifically in the anterior part of the third ventricle and typically presents with features of acute hydrocephalus because of obstruction to flow of the cerebrospinal fluid. The appearances on imaging are those of a well-circumscribed smooth surfaced mass lying within the third ventricle often displaying a high signal on T1-weighted MR scans. Histologically the lesion is a thin-walled cyst, lined by a ciliated columnar epithelium, containing gelatinous material.

Epidermoid cyst may occur at any location although most frequently these lesions are found in the cerebellopontine angle or spinal canal. The appearance on T1-weighted MR is variable being either high or low signal depending on whether the cyst contents are high or low in lipid. They are well-circumscribed uniloculated cysts which have a smooth or lobulated external surface that has a characteristic pearly sheen. The cyst is lined by a multi-layered squamous epithelium and the cyst contains keratin. Keratin flakes have a characteristic appearance on both smear preparations and frozen sections and their recognition is very suggestive of epidermoid cyst, even in the absence of identifiable epithelial cells. However it should be borne in mind that the presence of a squamous epithelium does not necessarily identify the lesion as an epidermoid cyst as squamous metaplasia may occur in Rathke's cleft and enterogenous cysts.

Dermoid cyst has similarities with epidermoid cyst although the regional distribution differs. Most examples occur in the midline in the posterior fossa or lumbosacral spinal canal. They tend to present in childhood or young adult life which is in contrast to epidermoid cysts which often present later in life. Spinal examples may be associated with other features of spinal dysraphism. The cysts are well-circumscribed and contain cheesy yellow material in which hairs may be identified on macroscopic examination. Histologically, epidermoid cysts are lined by squamous epithelium lying beneath which are adnexal skin structures including sebaceous glands, sweat glands and hair follicles.

Enterogenous (endodermal) cyst lies within the spinal canal usually within the dural sheath and anterior to the spinal cord. The lining epithelium resembles that of the respiratory or intestinal tract complete with goblet cells producing mucin.

Neuroglial cyst is lined by ependymal cells or astrocytes. In the cranial cavity such cysts occur mostly in relation to a ventricle. A syrinx is a glial cyst of the spinal cord which may occur alone (syringomyelia) or in proximity to a focal lesion such as a tumour.

Arachnoid cyst lies superficially and is formed from a layer of leptomeninges enclosing CSF. The wall therefore is composed of collagen and meningothelial cells. Such cysts occur both within the cranial cavity and in the spinal canal.

18.2.1. SMEARS AND FROZEN SECTIONS

An intra-operative diagnosis may not be appropriate for the following reasons. First, the specimen may comprise minute fragments of the cyst wall and the most productive strategy may be to fix all of the available material for subsequent paraffin histology. In this case it is almost certainly inappropriate to prepare frozen sections because so little diagnostic material is available, although it may be helpful to use a very small part of the specimen to make smear preparations. Second, the neurosurgeon may excise the cyst in its entirety in which case, the surgeon having done so, little is to be gained from an intra-operative diagnosis. However if an intra-operative diagnosis is required abundant tissue is available and frozen sections are likely to be more informative.

If they are made smears may include cyst contents which, depending on the type of cyst, appears as amorphous, granular or wispy material, sometimes metachromatic, perhaps keratin and occasionally macrophages. With luck smears will contain cells representative of the cyst lining which tends to lie flat on the slide giving a plan or surface view of the epithelium rather than the cross section which is more familiar. In most of the cysts described above these are uniform epithelial cells which smear into sheets or clumps. It is generally not possible to distinguish between different types of epithelium in smears. Because the cyst walls are usually very thin, as well as cyst contents, smears will often include surrounding connective tissue or central nervous tissue. In frozen sections it will be possible to identify the lesion as a benign epithelium-lined cyst; the specific type of epithelium may or may not be discerned with confidence.

18.2.2. EXAMINATION OF CYST FLUID

In most neurosurgical procedures performed on cystic lesions sufficient tissue will be obtained to achieve a diagnosis and in this situation the different properties of the fluids contained within the cysts of each type of tumour is largely irrelevant. On occasions, however, drainage of fluid from a cystic lesion may be the only operative procedure to be performed and it then becomes important to gain as much information as possible from the fluid. It may be useful to know that the fluid of a cystic astrocytoma is clear and yellow or golden in colour, often clotting at room temperature as a consequence of its high protein content. In contrast the fluid from a craniopharyngioma cyst is dark brown and turbid, resembling machine oil. Cyst contents with the colour and consistency of soft cheese hints at a diagnosis of dermoid or epidermoid cyst and the presence of hairs in such material is virtually diagnostic of a dermoid cyst.

Fluid can be prepared for examination under the microscope in a variety of different ways. Wet preparations can be examined by placing a cover slip over a few drops of the fluid on a slide. Such preparations are particularly helpful for examining crystals. In particular cholesterol crystals are readily identifiable by their morphology and, in the appropriate clinical setting, strongly hint at a diagnosis of craniopharyngioma, as described above. It may be helpful to examine the cellular content of the cyst fluid by making cytospin preparations similar to those used for CSF examination. If additional preparations are spun onto slides these can be used subsequently to help identify the cells by immunocytochemistry. In our experience, with the possible exception of craniopharyngioma, examination of cyst fluid alone rarely provides helpful information intra-operatively. It is usually more productive to examine the tissue that is available.

18.3. INTRADURAL LESIONS: VASCULAR LESIONS

Vascular lesions may be categorized as arteriovenous malformation, cavernous angioma, venous malformation and capillary teleangiectasis. Of these, the cavernous angioma may be 'tumour-like' in that it takes the form of a dark red lobulated mass, resembling a mulberry, formed from closely opposed vascular channels. Cavernous angioma may occur at any site in the cranial cavity and presentation is usually with seizures. Vascular lesions are usually readily recognizable as such, both radiologically and surgically, and an intra-operative diagnosis is not required. In some cases, particularly if there has been haemorrhage or infarction with consequent space-occupying effect there may be uncertainty over whether tumour is present or not. If smears or frozen sections are prepared the vascular nature of the lesion is likely to be apparent. Frozen sections are preferable for examination of vascular features. Vascular malformation, haemorrhage and infarction are illustrated in Chapter 3.

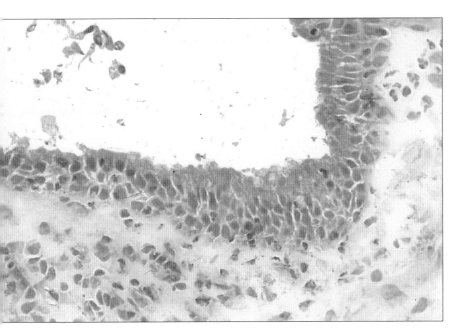

Figure 18.7
Rathke's cleft cyst. Male aged 40 years, intrasellar cystic lesion. Frozen sections reveal the lesion to be a benign epithelium-lined cyst. The cyst lining resembles respiratory epithelium being multi-layered, ciliated and columnar in architecture. In some examples the epithelium is composed of a single layer of cuboidal cells or there may be squamous metaplasia. Frozen section, haematoxylin eosin, ×1400.

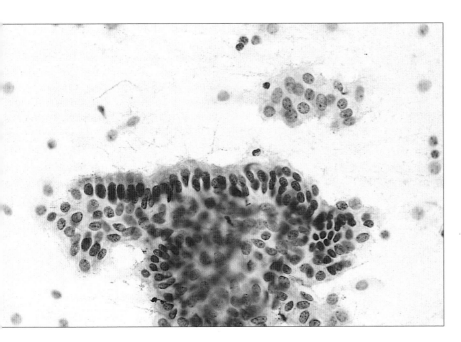

Figure 18.8
Rathke's cleft cyst. Male aged 40 years, intrasellar cystic lesion. In this smear clusters of uniform epithelial cells are readily identifiable. Although the cluster of cells illustrated here is mainly orientated *en face*, fortuitously the orientation of the cells at the edge of the clump reveals the columnar nature of the cells. Smear preparation, toluidine blue, ×1400.

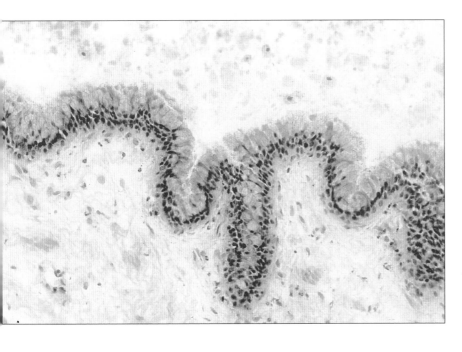

Figure 18.9
Colloid cyst. Male aged 28 years, third ventricular cyst. This example is lined by a multi-layered columnar epithelium with prominent goblet cells. The epithelium rests on a collagenous matrix. The cyst contents are eosinophilic, though pale-staining. Frozen section, haematoxylin eosin, ×700.

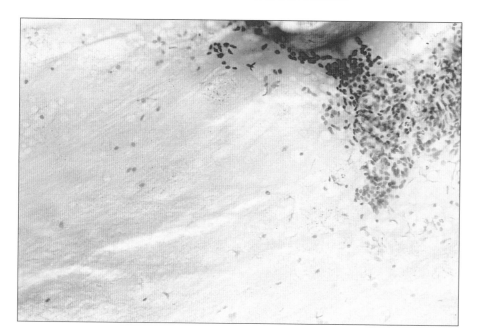

Figure 18.10
Colloid cyst. Male aged 34 years, third ventricular cyst. This smear shows mainly cyst contents which are amorphous and faintly metachromatic with toluidine blue. A few uniform round cells, probably derived from the lining epithelium, are included. Smear preparation, toluidine blue, ×350.

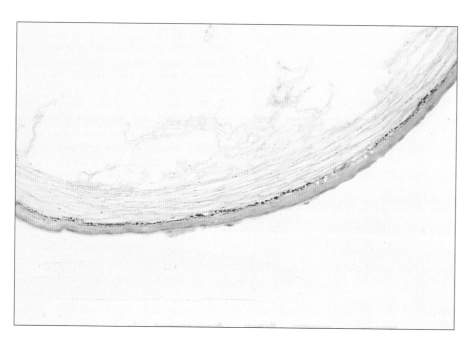

Figure 18.11
Epidermoid cyst. Male aged 56 years, cerebellopontine angle cyst. This frozen section shows the very thin cyst wall to be composed of a keratinizing stratified squamous epithelium. The absence of skin adnexal structures distinguishes the lesion from a dermoid cyst. Frozen section, haematoxylin eosin, ×700.

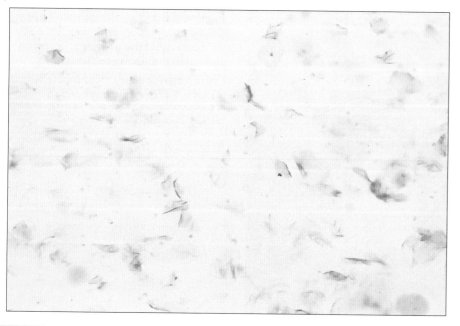

Figure 18.12
Epidermoid cyst. Female aged 38 years, lumbar spinal intradural lesion. Smears of the contents of this cystic lesion show the characteristic appearance of squames derived from the lining epithelium. They are polygonal in outline, often folded, have no discernible nuclei and take up little stain. Their recognition is highly suggestive of an epidermoid or dermoid cyst if no epithelium is available for examination. Smear preparation, toluidine blue, ×700.

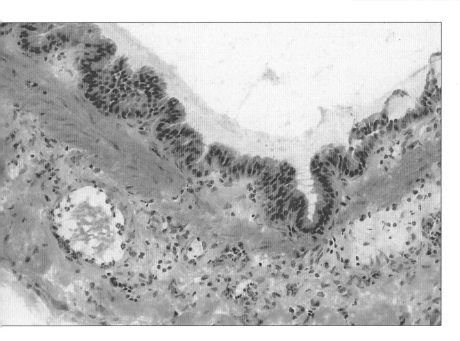

Figure 18.13
Enterogenous cyst. Female aged 26 years, spinal intradural, extramedullary cyst. The lining epithelium is multi-layered and columnar, somewhat resembling a respiratory or gastrointestinal epithelium. The epithelium rests on a collagenous membrane and pale-staining amorphous secretion is visible within the cyst. Frozen section, haematoxylin eosin, ×700.

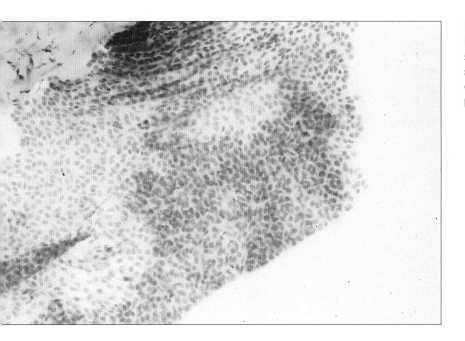

Figure 18.14
Enterogenous cyst. Female aged 48 years, spinal intradural, extramedullary cyst. This smear shows sheets of cohesive uniform epithelial cells viewed *en face*. Smear preparation, toluidine blue, ×700.

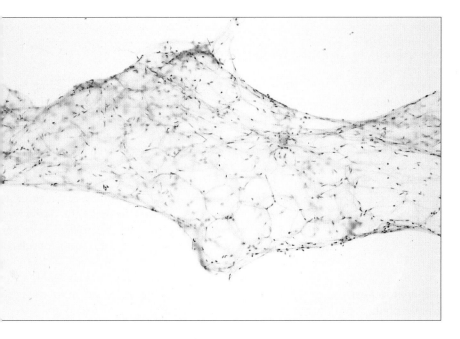

Figure 18.15
Lipoma. Male aged 21 years, corpus callosum lesion. Mature adipose tissue may be surprisingly difficult to smear. However, if smeared satisfactorily there is no mistaking the appearance of mature adipose tissue which is clearly of pathological significance if found at an intradural location. Smear preparation, toluidine blue, ×175.

18.4. INTRADURAL LESIONS: LIPOMA

Lipomas are composed of mature adipose tissue. In the central nervous system the tendency is for them to occur at midline sites. The commonest intracranial location is the corpus callosum. In the spine they occur in the lumbosacral region often in association with dysraphic abnormalities. Extradural spinal examples also occur rarely. Because of the high fat content lipomas characteristically have a very high signal on T1-weighted MRI. Macroscopically lipomas do not always have the bright yellow colour of adipose tissue, but may appear grey or brown. Smearing may rupture the cells leaving amorphous debris in the stained preparations or may show cells readily identifiable as mature adipocytes. Frozen sections may be difficult to prepare but will reveal the lipomatous nature of the lesion.

18.5. EXTRADURAL LESIONS: CHORDOMA

18.5.1. CLINICAL AND RADIOLOGICAL FEATURES

Chordoma is a slowly growing tumour which presents most commonly in adult life. The tumour arises in the midline originating from notochordal elements. In the cranial cavity the commonest site is the skull base where the mass is centred on the clivus. The tumour grows anteriorly to involve the pituitary fossa and cavernous sinuses and posteriorly to protrude into the posterior fossa where the brainstem may suffer compression. Presentation is typically with headaches, cranial nerve palsies and long tract signs. Although nearly all chordomas are extradural very occasional examples arise intradurally, most notably overlying the ventral surface of the pons. Chordomas also occur in the vertebral column where they lie anterior to the spinal canal. The majority of spinal chordomas arise in the sacral region and manifest themselves by compressing spinal roots. Radiologically chordoma appears as a lobulated osteolytic mass causing local tissue destruction. Chordoma is a tumour of relatively low grade malignancy which grows slowly and is very unlikely to metastasize. However, as a consequence of the location complete excision is often impossible and the typical clinical course is of repeated local recurrences over a period of many years or decades.

18.5.2. SURGICAL FINDINGS

The characteristic radiological and surgical appearances of chordoma mean that there is usually little doubt as to the correct diagnosis at the time of operation. The tumour appears as a lobulated mass of soft or firm translucent grey tissue causing local tissue destruction at the sites described above.

18.5.3. INTRA-OPERATIVE PATHOLOGY

Smear cytology

Although chordomas are often composed of tough or rubbery tissue they may be also at least partly soft and gelatinous in texture. Our experience is that smear preparations can usually be made fairly readily. A usually prominent, and diagnostically very helpful feature, is the presence of extracellular mucinous material which shows strong metachromasia with toluidine blue and is eosinophilic with H&E. The mucinous material often dominates the smear and the tumour cells, which may be relatively sparse, are arranged in small clusters or lie singly. The cells have rather uniform round nuclei and moderately abundant but indistinct cytoplasm which is often seen as being relatively unstained in contrast to the extracellular mucin. Occasionally vacuolation of the cytoplasm can be seen but it is generally not as apparent as in paraffin sections. Mitotic figures are rarely encountered.

Frozen sections

The characteristic architecture of chordoma, with the cells arranged in interconnecting strands, is often readily seen in frozen sections. Less commonly the cells may be arranged in compact sheets or lying individually within an abundant eosinophilic mucinous matrix. At low power the tumour often has a lobulated appearance. As in smear preparations the cells are seen to have rather small, uniform round nuclei and moderately abundant well demarcated cytoplasm. Cytoplasmic vacuolation may be seen but is not likely to be as striking a feature as it is in paraffin sections.

Differential diagnosis

Most chordomas arise in the classical setting of a tumour in the clivus or sacrum, with the typical macroscopic appearances, and the differential diagnosis is therefore a narrow one. In smear preparations and frozen sections distinction from a **chondroma** or **low grade chondrosarcoma** may be impossible. Even with the benefit of paraffin histology, if the typical architecture of chordoma is not present, it may be necessary to rely on immunohistochemistry to make the distinction. The presence of a tumour with vacuolated cells and mucin production may suggest the diagnosis of **adenocarcinoma**. However an adenocarcinoma is likely to have clearly malignant cytology and is unlikely to present as a slowly growing lobulated mass emerging from bone.

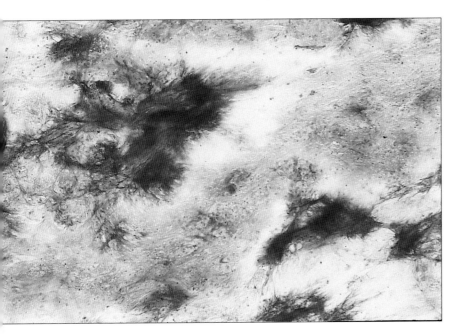

Figure 18.16

Chordoma. Female aged 52 years, mass arising from clivus. In smear preparations at low power the predominant feature is strongly staining mucin-like material which is metachromatic with toluidine blue. The material is smeared across most of the slide with more deeply staining focal aggregates. Smear preparation, toluidine blue, ×175.

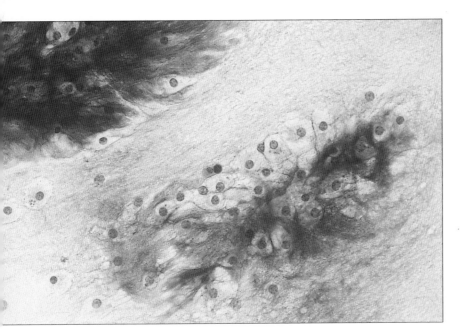

Figure 18.17

Chordoma. Female aged 61 years, mass arising from clivus. Higher power views of smear preparations of a chordoma show the amorphous nature of the metachromatic extracellular material. The cells, which are sparse, have uniform round nuclei and the pale-staining cytoplasm is seen set against the more deeply staining background. Smear preparation, toluidine blue, ×700.

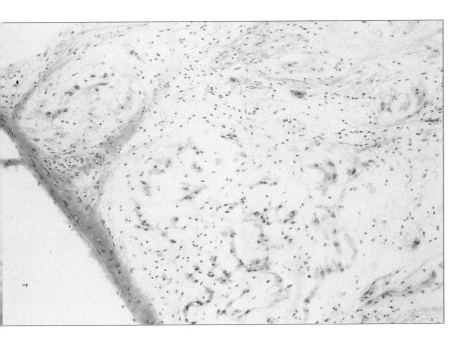

Figure 18.18

Chordoma. Female aged 52 years, mass arising from clivus. The same case as illustrated in Fig. 18.16. In frozen sections at low power the tumour often has a lobulated architecture as seen in this field. The tumour is sparsely cellular in keeping with the relatively low grade behaviour of the lesion. Frozen section, haematoxylin eosin, ×350.

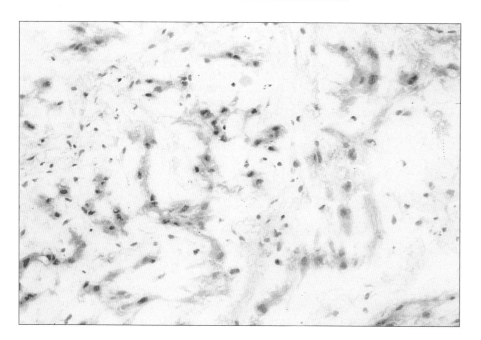

Figure 18.19
Chordoma. Female aged 52 years, mass arising from clivus. A higher power view of the field illustrated in Fig. 18.18 showing the strand-like arrangement of the tumour cells. The cells have uniform round nuclei and moderately abundant eosinophilic cytoplasm. Cytoplasmic vacuolation which is often a prominent feature in paraffin sections is not so readily seen in frozen sections. The extracellular matrix is pale-staining with H&E. Frozen section, haematoxylin eosin, ×700.

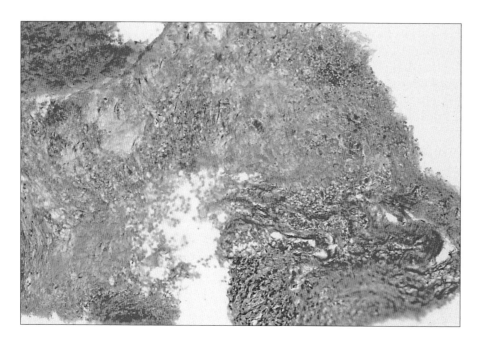

Figure 18.20
Sequestrated prolapsed intervertebral disc. Female aged 40 years, extradural mass within lumbar spinal canal. Frozen sections of degenerate or 'fossilized' intervertebral disc material could be interpreted as necrotic tumour. The material is eosinophilic and granular in texture, with few or no viable cells. Frozen section, haematoxylin eosin, ×350.

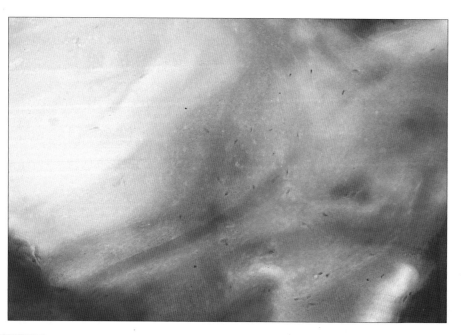

Figure 18.21
Sequestrated prolapsed intervertebral disc. Female aged 40 years, extradural mass within lumbar spinal canal. The same material as illustrated in Fig. 18.20 is shown here when smeared. The extracellular matrix of the disc material is amorphous and strongly metachromatic with toluidine blue. It resembles the extracellular matrix of a chordoma which is perhaps not surprising in view of their supposed common origin from notochordal tissue. Smear preparation, toluidine blue, ×175.

18.6. EXTRADURAL LESIONS: PROLAPSED INTERVERTEBRAL DISC

On occasions a prolapsed intervertebral disc may be misinterpreted at the time of surgery as a possible extradural spinal tumour. This is particularly so of a sequestrated prolapse, separated from its disc of origin. Frozen sections of degenerate intervertebral disc show granular eosinophilic material which is almost acellular and could be misinterpreted as necrotic tumour. In contrast smear preparations show material which is strongly metachromatic with toluidine blue.

18.7. EXTRADURAL LESIONS: NON-NEOPLASTIC BONE LESIONS

The calcified nature of the tissue poses problems for the intra-operative diagnosis of lesions arising in bone. Neither smear preparations nor frozen sections are ideal methods. However, smear preparations in particular may prove fruitful on occasions and an attempt at an intra-operative diagnosis may be worthwhile.

Fibrous dysplasia

In fibrous dysplasia there is focal or relatively widespread abnormal proliferation of fibro-osseous tissues which may involve the skull base or vault. Radiologically the appearances vary depending largely on the degree of calcification of the abnormal tissue. This condition usually presents in early adult life. Smear preparations, if they can be made, show calcified spicules with spindle-shaped cells lying in the intervening spaces. Frozen sections, again if they can be prepared, show the features familiar from paraffin histology with irregular trabeculae or islands of bone set in a matrix of fibrous tissue containing spindle-shaped cells.

Langerhan's cell histiocytosis

This disorder encompasses a spectrum which ranges from a solitary osteolytic lesion, most commonly in the skull vault of an adolescent, to multifocal skeletal lesions and extra-osseous involvement. If smear preparations are made they may show histiocytes with the characteristic large clefted nuclei and a variety of other inflammatory cells including eosinophils with bi-lobed nuclei. Frozen sections also show large histiocytic cells, which may be arranged in sheets or in groups resembling granulomas, and other inflammatory cells among which eosinophils may be prominent.

Aneurysmal bone cyst

This takes the form of an expansile tender lesion at any site in the skull or spine and occurs most commonly in early life. Histologically the lesion comprises abundant vascular channels with intervening spicules of bone. Smear preparations may show multinucleated cells amongst spindle-shaped cells.

18.8. EXTRADURAL LESIONS: TUMOURS ARISING IN BONE

Benign neoplasms which arise in bone include **osteoma, chondroma** and **osteochondroma**. The scope for intra-operative diagnosis with these lesions is severely limited because of their calcified nature. **Giant cell tumour of bone** may produce very striking appearances in smear preparations with abundant multinucleated giant cells. However a definite diagnosis, and

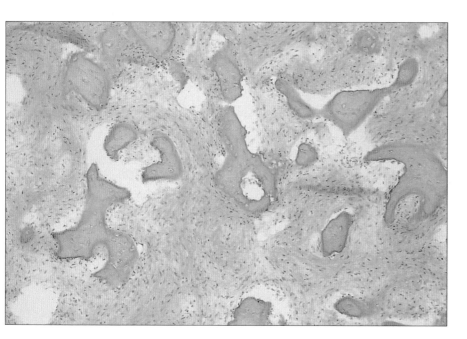

Figure 18.22
Fibrous dysplasia. Male aged 50 years, lesion in skull. If frozen sections can be prepared from the undecalcified tissue they reveal the characteristic appearance of bone spicules with irregular profiles embedded in a collagenous matrix containing spindle-shaped cells. Frozen section, haematoxylin eosin, ×700.

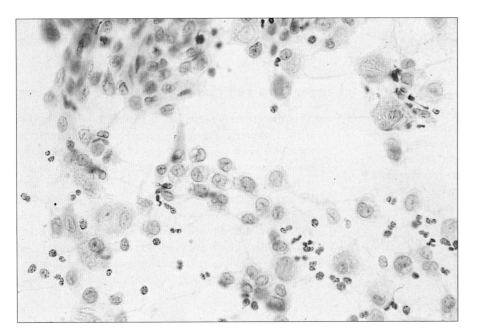

Figure 18.23
Langerhan's cell histioctyosis. Female aged 32 years, lesion in skull. If smears are made successfully the characteristic nuclear clefts of the large histiocyte-like cells can be seen more clearly than in sections. Also included is a mixture of smaller inflammatory cells including eosinophils recognizable by their bi-lobed nuclei. Smear preparation, toluidine blue, ×1400.

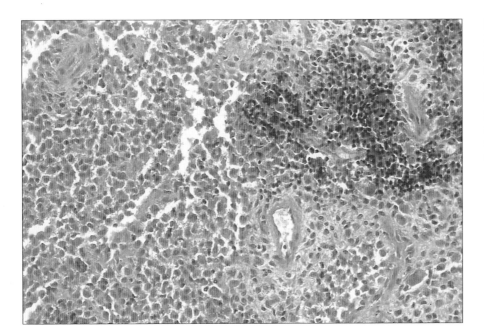

Figure 18.24
Langerhan's cell histiocytosis. Male aged 22 years, lesion in skull. Assuming a representative portion of the lesion is sampled, frozen sections show large histiocyte-like cells forming sheets or granuloma-like arrangements. Also visible is an aggregate of eosinophils in the top right of the field. Frozen section, haematoxylin eosin, ×700.

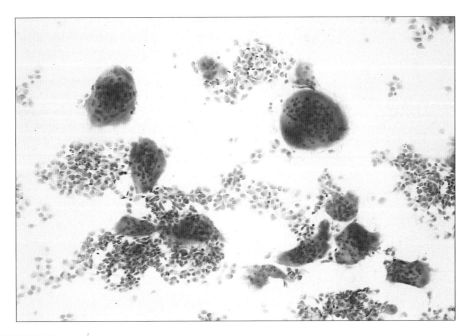

Figure 18.25
Giant cell tumour of bone. Male aged 30 years, lesion in spine. Multinucleated giant cells are readily recognizable in smear preparations. However their presence should be interpreted with caution as they may be a feature of several different lesions of bone including neoplasms, infections (e.g. tuberculosis) and non-specific reactive changes (osteoclasts). Smear preparation, toluidine blue, ×350.

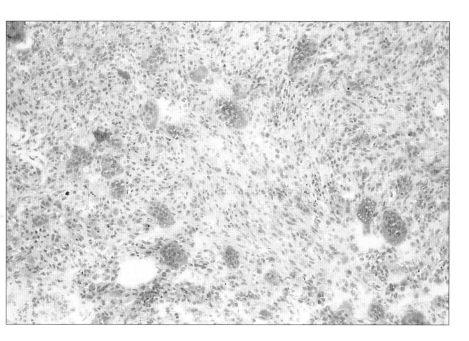

Figure 18.26
Central granuloma of facial bones. Male aged 52 years. Provided frozen sections can be made from lesions in bone multinucleated giant cells, if present, are readily apparent. An awareness of the spectrum of pathological processes with which they may be associated is essential. One of the most useful suggestions to be made intra-operatively may be to recommend tissue is obtained for microbiological investigations. It may well be wise to postpone a definitive diagnosis until paraffin histology is available. Frozen section, haematoxylin eosin, ×350.

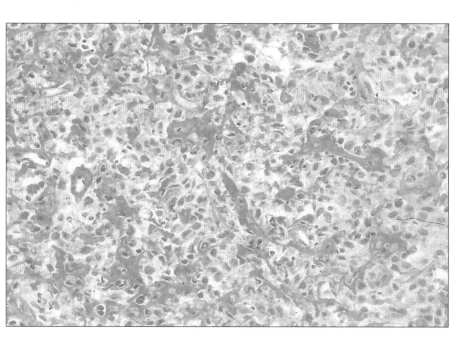

Figure 18.27
Osteosarcoma. Male aged 47 years, cervical spine. It may well not be possible to make preparations suitable for intra-operative diagnosis from tumours arising in bone because of the calcified nature of the tissue. If smears or frozen sections can be prepared then the diagnostic information provided to the surgeons at the time of the operation will depend on the adequacy of the sample, the quality of the preparation and the familiarity of the pathologist with lesions of bone. Frozen section, haematoxylin eosin, ×700.

in particular distinction from other lesions containing giant cells (e.g. other osteolytic lesions and tuberculosis) should await paraffin histology.

Malignant tumours arising in the bone of the skull and vertebral column include **osteosarcoma** and **chondrosarcoma**. If samples of the tissue provided at operation is sufficiently uncalcified then smear preparations or frozen sections may give evidence of the cytologically malignant nature of the lesion.

18.9. EXTRADURAL LESIONS: SOFT TISSUE TUMOURS

Soft tissue tumours may involve the nervous system when arising in extracranial or paraspinal tissues. Distinction between benign and malignant tumours can be made in smears and frozen sections on the basic cytological features. Further discussion of such lesions lies outside the scope of this book.

INDEX

Note: page references in *italics* refer to figures and tables; those in **bold** give the main discussion. The prefix 'cf.' to sub-entries indicates relevance to differential diagnosis.